Electrical Impedance Tomography for Tactile Imaging

A primer for experimentalists

Online at: https://doi.org/10.1088/978-0-7503-5402-8

IOP Series in Sensors and Sensor Systems

The IOP Series in Sensors and Sensor Systems includes books on all aspects of the science and technology of sensors and sensor systems. Spanning fundamentals, fabrication, applications and processing, the series aims to provide a library for instrument and measurement scientists, engineers and technologists in universities and industry.

The series seeks (but is not restricted to) publications in the following topics:

- Advanced materials for sensing
- Biosensors
- Chemical sensors
- Industrial applications
- Internet of Things (IoT)
- Lab-on-a-chip
- Localization and object tracking
- Manufacturing and packaging
- Mechanisms, modelling and simulations
- Microelectromechanical systems/nanoelectromechanical systems
- Micro and nanosensors
- Non-destructive testing
- Optoelectronic and photonic sensors
- Optomechanical sensors
- Physical sensors
- Remote sensors
- Sensing for health, safety and security
- Sensing principles
- Sensing systems
- Sensor arrays
- Sensor devices
- Sensor networks
- Sensor technology and applications
- Signal processing and data analysis
- Smart sensors and monitoring
- Telemetry

Authors are encouraged to take advantage of electronic publication through the use of colour, animations, video and interactive elements to enhance the reader experience.

A full list of titles published in this series can be found here: https://iopscience.iop.org/bookListInfo/iop-series-in-sensors-and-sensor-systems.

Electrical Impedance Tomography for Tactile Imaging

A primer for experimentalists

Elisabeth Smela
Department of Mechanical Engineering, University of Maryland, College Park, MD 20742, USA

With contributions from:

Ayush Nankani
Department of Mechanical Engineering, University of Maryland, College Park, MD 20742, USA

Carlos Cuellar
Department of Mechanical Engineering, University of Maryland, College Park, MD 20742, USA

IOP Publishing, Bristol, UK

ISBN 978-0-7503-5402-8 (ebook)
ISBN 978-0-7503-5400-4 (print)
ISBN 978-0-7503-5403-5 (myPrint)
ISBN 978-0-7503-5401-1 (mobi)

DOI 10.1088/978-0-7503-5402-8

Version: 20240201

IOP ebooks

British Library Cataloguing-in-Publication Data: A catalogue record for this book is available from the British Library.

Published by IOP Publishing, wholly owned by The Institute of Physics, London

IOP Publishing, No.2 The Distillery, Glassfields, Avon Street, Bristol, BS2 0GR, UK

US Office: IOP Publishing, Inc., 190 North Independence Mall West, Suite 601, Philadelphia, PA 19106, USA

Contents

Preface

The literature on electrical impedance tomography (EIT) has been, by its nature, highly mathematical. This book aims to bridge the gap between device-oriented experimentalists and the prior art. It aims to introduce the key concepts behind EIT starting at the level of undergraduate engineering mathematics. While it is possible to produce images from tactile imaging devices without understanding what is inside the 'black box', the process will remain largely mysterious without the concept of signal and image *modes*. Without these concepts one cannot properly appreciate the signal-to-noise considerations or understand the workings of the main 'dial', the hyperparameter λ, that controls the resulting images.

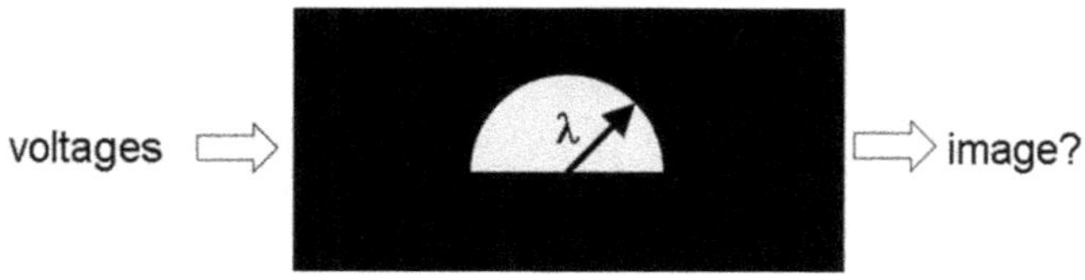

This book is focused on tactile imaging applications. The demands of this field are somewhat different than those of other application areas, including the medical imaging field that developed many of the EIT techniques and approaches.

There are seven chapters. In chapter 1 the field of electronic skins (e-skins) is overviewed to provide context for the use of EIT for tactile imaging. After a brief introduction to EIT, chapter 2 surveys the literature on the use of EIT for tactile imaging. Chapter 3 provides the details of the simulation methods and metrics used for image evaluation. The basic operation of EIT is examined in chapter 4. With that background, chapter 5 examines the effect of the hyperparameter in detail, and the closely related topic of noise is examined in chapter 6. Lastly, chapter 7 takes up practical approaches to choosing the hyperparameter and electrode patterns.

Acknowledgements

I would like to acknowledge the students and collaborators who have contributed to the work leading up to this book. Thank you to my colleagues Dr Miao Yu and Dr Hugh A Bruck for collaborating on the development of smart skins and to former PhD student Dr Ying Chen for starting our use of EIT, performing both experimental and simulation studies. Thanks also go to former postdoc Dr Ephraim Zegeye and to students Akshay Bajaj, Rahul Subramonian Bama, Faissal Hariri, Meghana Madarkal, Likhita Madiraju, Kevin McCright, Yonatan Saadon, Elizabeth Sauerbrunn, Shirley Shi, Ajeet Wankhede, and Hudson (Zepeng) Ye for their experimental work on devices employing EIT. Acknowledgements must also go to PhD, masters, undergraduate, and high school student alumni of the group who contributed to compliant strain sensors over the years: Kyle Archer, Eli M Barnett, Kimberly Berlic, Lee Dodds, Alex Edgerton, Dr Nehemiah Emaikwu, Danielle Fallon, Iver Jenstrom, Elisabeth Kuespert, Zeynep Karakas, Neelanjan Lahiri, Steven Lee, Ryan Lentz, Benjy M Levi, M Vidhiaza Leviandhika, Grace Lin, Julian J Lofton, Matthew McGraw, Kaitlin J Miller, Nick Papavizas, A Perez-Rosado, James A Tigue, Raymond Wang, Kaitlyn Watson, James Wissman, Vincent Wu, and Daniel Yoo; and those who, prior to that, worked on stretchable electrodes, which lead to the strain sensors: Dr Mark Kujawski, Dr Deepa Sritharan, Dr Mario Urdaneta, Remi Delille, Justin Di Palo, Kwuangwen (Wen) Hsieh, Z N Karakas, Justin D Pearse, and Brent Snyder.

Author biographies

Elisabeth Smela

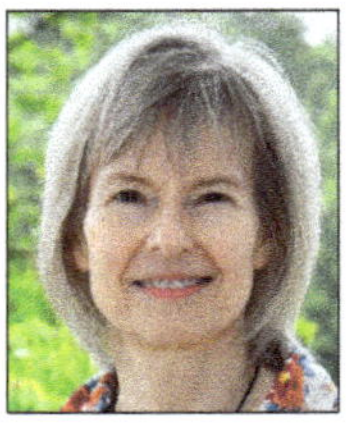

Elisabeth Smela is a Professor of Mechanical Engineering at the University of Maryland. She received a BS in physics from MIT and a PhD in electrical engineering from the University of Pennsylvania. Dr Smela then worked as a research scientist in Linköping, Sweden and in Risø, Denmark before becoming Vice President of Research and Development at Santa Fe Science and Technology, NM. Dr Smela's research interests have focused on polymeric and cell-based sensors and actuators. She spent a year as a Jefferson Science Fellow at the Department of State to stand up the US-ASEAN Smart Cities Network. She has recently been working with a group of engineering faculty to better integrate sustainability concepts throughout the undergraduate curriculum. Her interest in EIT stemmed from her work on strain sensors and tactile e-skins for various applications in robotics and healthcare, following earlier development of stretchable conductors.

Ayush Nankani

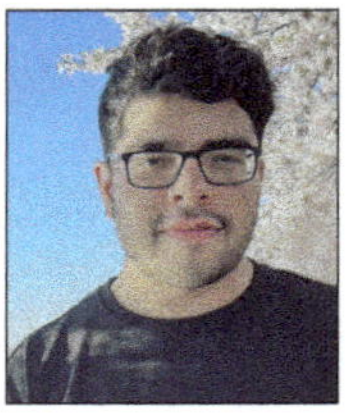

Ayush Nankani is an R&D engineer with a focus on medical robotics and pediatric innovation technologies at Children's National Hospital. He holds a Bachelor of Engineering degree in Mechanical Engineering from SVITS in Indore, Madhya Pradesh, India, and a Master of Science degree from the University of Maryland, College Park with Dr Smela. Ayush is currently working with a team at Children's National Hospital to improve healthcare outcomes for children.

Carlos Cuellar

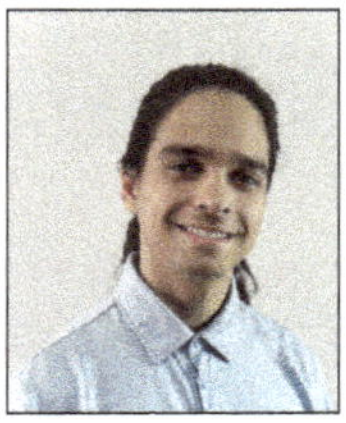

Carlos Edgardo Cuellar received a BS in Mechanical Engineering at the University of Maryland. As an undergraduate he conducted research on electronic skins for use in robotics and on nanocarbon-loaded paint-based sensors for structural health monitoring under the guidance of Dr Smela. He is currently working as an Automotive Test Engineer at Honda Development & Manufacturing of America.

Symbols

Measurement conditions	
I	current
I–M	injection–measurement pattern
$L; \Delta L$	length; change in length
r_T	target or touch radius, as a fraction of the sensor radius
$r_S; d_S$	sensor radius; sensor diameter
$R; \Delta R$	resistance, depends on sensor dimensions; change in resistance
ρ	resistivity, material property
ρ_0	reference state sensor resistivity
σ_0	reference state sensor conductivity, $1/\rho_0$
$\Delta\sigma$	difference in conductivity due to touch or, in simulations, of the target
t	thickness
x, y	target position coordinates
V	voltage
Data collection	
i	from 1 to m, measurement number, corresponding to a specific drive-measure combination
m	number of voltage measurements = frame size
$\mathbf{V}_{ref}$	$= [V_{ref}]$, frame (baseline set) of voltages
$\mathbf{V}_{touch}$	$= [V_{touch}]$, later frame of voltages
V_i	one measurement of a frame
$\boldsymbol{\Delta}$	$= \mathbf{V}_{touch} - \mathbf{V}_{ref}$, vector of m voltage differences Δ_i
$\mathbf{n}$	noise on each measurement, length m
$\mathbf{N}$	noise level (V)
Forward and inverse problems	
k	from 1 to n, specific mesh element
n	number of mesh elements
$\mathbf{J}$	sensitivity matrix, Jacobian, size m n, $\mathbf{J} = \mathbf{USV}^T = s_1\mathbf{u_1v_1}^T + s_2\mathbf{u_2v_2}^T + \ldots + s_r\mathbf{u_rv_r}^T$
$J_{i,k} = \partial V_i / \partial\sigma_k\|_{\sigma_{ref}}$	sensitivity matrix elements; i and k are indices
$\mathbf{J}_{reg}$	regularized matrix that is inverted
r	rank of $\mathbf{J}$, number of linearly independent columns
λ	hyperparameter
Ω	sensor area
Ω_k	sensor area elements or regions
$\Delta\sigma_k$	change in conductivity of region Ω_k
$\boldsymbol{\sigma}$	vector of conductivity changes $\Delta\sigma_k$
σ_T	conductivity of the target
$\mathbf{S}$	diagonal matrix of singular values s_i
s_i	singular values, $s_i = \mathbf{S}_{ii}$
i	singular value index
$\mathbf{U}$	left singular matrix of $\mathbf{J}$
$\mathbf{u}_i$	columns of $\mathbf{U}$, basis vectors for the voltage measurements
$\mathbf{V}$	right singular matrix of $\mathbf{J}$
$\mathbf{v}_i$	columns of $\mathbf{V}$, basis vectors for the conductivity changes

$\lvert \mathbf{U}^T \boldsymbol{\Delta} \rvert$	a spectrum that is a measure of the signal strength; T indicates the transpose of the **U**
$P_i = \lvert \mathbf{u}_i{}^T \boldsymbol{\Delta} \rvert$	Picard coefficients, units of volts, can be directly compared to the noise
$\lvert \mathbf{V}^T \boldsymbol{\sigma} \rvert$	a spectrum that reflects the effects of regularization on the image

Frequently used acronyms

Algorithms	
ANN	artificial neural network
EIDORS	electrical impedance and diffuse optical tomography reconstruction software
ML	machine learning
ROI	region of interest
Materials	
CB	carbon black
CNT	carbon nanotube
PDMS	poly(dimethyl siloxane)
PU	polyurethane
Other	
2D	2-dimensional
3D	3-dimensional
AC	alternating current
DC	direct current
DOF	degrees of freedom
HRI	human–robot interaction
PCB	printed circuit board
SHM	structural health monitoring

Chapter 1

Tactile imaging with electronic skins

Elisabeth Smela, with contributions by Carlos Cuellar

Tactile imaging is expected to find applications in human worn devices, such as prosthetics and personal health monitoring, as well as in robotics, such as for robot environmental awareness and for interactions with humans. Electrical impedance tomography (EIT) is a technique that can be used to interrogate a large-area sensor at its perimeter, producing an image of resistance changes resulting from tactile interactions on its surface. The sensors can be entirely soft and have arbitrary size and shape, while data collection can be controlled by simple hardware, and analysis by open-source, physics-based codes. While the use of EIT for tactile imaging is the focus of this book it is helpful to have a more complete context in which to understand that work, which is provided in this chapter.

It has been argued that electronic skin (e-skin) is critical for robots to function in real-world environments, particularly alongside people. As an example, socially-assistive robots, such as artificial pets with tactile sensors that respond to touch, have left the lab and are in use in care facilities. A strong motivation for the e-skin field is the realization of even more capable human-interactive robots able to safely perform tasks such as physically moving medical patients. EIT is well suited for e-skin applied to a robot's limbs or body (as opposed to end effectors for manipulation, which have different requirements).

Over the last two decades diverse tactile imaging prototypes have been demonstrated. Some are based on discrete rigid sensors that are assembled into arrays, others are fabricated on sheets, and still others are made from continuous stretchable materials. Stretchability has been achieved in numerous ways, including with elastomeric composites, fabrics, and encapsulated liquid metals. Many sensing modalities have been employed for e-skin, but tactile imaging has primarily made use of resistive and capacitive measurements. The requirement for e-skin to be applied over large, complex surfaces has thus largely been met.

doi:10.1088/978-0-7503-5402-8ch1

A challenge for tactile imagers is that there are many, often conflicting, requirements on their performance and on their integratability. For example, an e-skin should be able to accurately locate and quantify a wide range of tactile forces, while also being able to withstand impacts and changing environmental conditions; in addition, manufacturing must be cost-effective. Challenges to integration can be found at the sensor, application, and system levels and include forming robust electrical connections, minimizing noise and cross-talk, and meeting power requirements.

1.1 Applications and requirements for e-skin

As described in section 2.2.1, EIT is well suited for tactile monitoring of continuous large areas, particularly if stretchability or fitting over curved surfaces is needed—in other words, for e-skin technology. The envisioned applications of tactile e-skin are many: prosthetics, robotics, personal health monitoring, communication devices, automated surgery, and others. Thus, to provide context for understanding the requirements for tactile imaging, this section overviews the e-skin field.

1.1.1 Reviews of e-skin

There has been a surge in the number of reviews and literature surveys on the topic of tactile e-skin since 2010, a guide to which is given in table 1.1. E-skin generally refers to large-area devices that can sense multiple stimuli, from tactile to temperature and chemical. Some definitions of e-skin further require that they be self-healing and biocompatible, or that they include power, data storage, and processing. However, those requirements are not the focus of this work—here we concentrate only on large-area tactile e-skins and on applications involving tactile imaging, which is their most fundamental function. By tactile e-skin we refer to devices that can determine the spatial locations of contacts as well as the intensity, or strengths, of each contact, as opposed to strain or pressure sensors generally. Moreover, we emphasize large-area stretchable or fully ‘soft’ devices that can undergo strains of tens of percent, rather than flexible or rigid ones. Small-size sensors for artificial fingers, hands [1], or other end effectors used for grip or manipulation are not considered here, nor are topics on signal conditioning or transmission, information encoding, tactile perception, or control [2], even though those capabilities are essential. As has been pointed out in the literature previously, the challenge of creating e-skins is multi-disciplinary and multi-faceted, involving systems integration, signal processing and communication, materials development, patterning and processing, device characterization, power supply, and manufacturing.

Tellingly, most reviews have concentrated on the device level rather than the systems level. Research has focused on sensor characterization and demonstrations of function, with less attention paid to realizing the suggested applications or to issues related to implementing working systems.

Table 1.1. Review articles and literature surveys on tactile e-skin topics since 2010, presented chronologically. The final column indicates whether the work mentions EIT.

Ref.	Year	Subject	Topics	EIT
[2]	2010	Tactile sensing in robotics	Tactile perception, biological sense of touch, types and modalities of sensors, distributed sensing, system considerations	✓
[3]	2010	Stretchable electronic structures	Stretchable interconnections	×
[4]	2012	Stretchable and self-healing electronics	Overview of materials, architectures, encapsulation, interconnects, fabrication	×
[5]	2013	Stretchable and self-healing polymers and devices for e-skin	Stretchable semiconductors, substrates, sensors, solar cells, batteries, OLEDs, device examples; self-healing electronics	×
[6]	2013	Tactile sensor systems in robotics	History, system considerations and challenges: mechanical, electrical, sensor placement and survivability, feature extraction, data management and representation	✓
[7]	2013	Robotic tactile sensing technologies	In depth overview of transduction methods, materials, device structures	✓
[8]	2013	Evolution of e-skin	History, materials, sensing modalities, approaches to stretchability, healing and self-powering, integrated device examples	×
[9]	2013	Tactile sensing	Biological sensing, bio-hybrid tactile sensing, synthetic sensor modalities	×
[10]	2014	E-textiles	Materials, connections, fabrication, sensors, examples, strain and force sensors	
[11]	2014	E-skin	Stretchability, sensing mechanisms, device examples	×
[12]	2015	EIT for robotic skin	Tactile e-skin for robotics, operation of EIT, materials, data collection, metrics	✓
[13]	2015	Tactile skin for human–robot interaction (HRI)	Biological sensing, tactile communication, social HRI, touch interpretation	✓
[14]	2015	Flexible, stretchable electronics for health monitoring	Approaches to flexibility and stretchability, application examples	×
[15]	2015	E-skin	Transduction mechanisms, designs, fabrication, power, device examples	×
[16]	2015	Materials for e-skins for robotics	Approaches to achieve stretchability	×
[17]	2016	E-skin for prosthetics	Biological sensing, approaches to achieve stretchability, data encoding and signal readout	×
[18]	2016	Stretchable piezoelectric sensors	Piezoelectric effect, optimal materials and configurations, use in biomedicine	×

(Continued)

Table 1.1. (*Continued*)

Ref.	Year	Subject	Topics	EIT
[19]	2017	Tactile sensing for humanoid robotics	Sensing mechanisms, whole-body tactile systems, calibration, data representation, control	✓
[20]	2017	E-skin for wearable health monitoring	Approaches to stretchability, sensing mechanisms, health monitoring applications	×
[21]	2018	Textile-based wearable electronics (e-textiles)	Textile electronic devices, power, sensors	×
[22]	2018	Tactile sensing systems	Sensor requirements, iCub example, information processing, computation (including EIT)	✓
[23]	2018	Stretchable strain sensors	Electrically conductive polymer composite strain sensor mechanism, performance, filler types, morphology, other requirements	×
[24]	2018	3D printing of soft robots	Materials, printing technologies, sensor types, soft robot examples	×
[25]	2018	Polymer-based electronics	Stretchable semiconductors, sensors, displays, self-healing, biodegradation	×
[26]	2018	Flexible pressure sensors	Sensing mechanisms, materials	×
[27]	2019	Nano-material-based e-skin	Tactile sensor types, multifunctional sensing, organic thin-film transistors	×
[28]	2019	Polymer nanocomposite stretchable strain sensors	Thorough review; filled, sandwich, and coated types, sensing mechanisms, factors affecting performance	×
[29]	2019	E-skin	Components, power, data processing, applications, challenges	×
[33]	2019	Printable stretchable tactile sensors	Thorough review of printing methods and requirements, printed sensor examples	×
[34]	2019	Components and applications of e-skin	Existing capabilities, possible applications	×
[35]	2019	Graphene, graphite nano-platelet based tactile sensors	Devices based on capacitive, piezoresistive sensing	×
[36]	2019	Thermoelectric energy harvesting for e-skin	Existing capability	×
[37]	2019	Flexible, stretchable transistors and sensors	Tactile e-skin, printing	×
[38]	2019	Stretchable conductors for e-skin, e-textiles using nano-materials	Deep review of materials and properties, devices, sensors	×
[39]	2019	Flexible sensors	Multifunctional sensors, sensing modalities and materials	×

[40]	2019	E-skin overview	In-depth overview: approaches to stretchability, self-healing, tactile sensors, requirements, materials and designs, spatial sensing (including EIT), fabrication, integration	✓
[42]	2020	Pressure sensors	Sensing mechanisms, fabrication	×
[43]	2020	Flexible (not necessarily stretchable) pressure sensors	Sensing mechanisms, micro-structuring, applications, metrics	×
[44]	2020	Triboelectric nano-generators for e-skin	TENG mechanisms, examples, biodegradability	×
[45]	2020	Bioinspired e-skins	Bioinspired designs, wearable applications, challenges	×
[46]	2020	EIT for e-skin	Recent reconstruction algorithms, EIT tactile applications	✓
[47]	2020	Embodied tactile perception for robotics	Sensor placements, learning, perception	✓
[48]	2020	Tactile e-skin for soft robots	Applications for soft robots, use of machine learning (ML)	×
[49]	2020	EIT for structural health monitoring (SHM)	History, math, applications, recent advances, challenges	✓
[50]	2020	E-skin for human health	Brief overview of electrode materials, sensor device examples, integration	×
[51]	2021	Flexible (not necessarily stretchable) e-skin for human monitoring	History, materials and fabrication, sensors and application examples, power	×
[52]	2021	Soft multifunctional e-skin	Approaches to stretchability, sensor types, materials, structures, fabrication, self-healing	×
[53]	2021	Stretchable carbon material based multifunctional sensors	Multi-mode sensors, self-healing, biodegradable, power, system examples	×
[55]	2021	Skin-integrated devices	Sensing of physiological signals and motion, sensing optical, auditory, and tactile inputs, haptic interfaces for virtual reality	
[56]	2021	E-skin for health and biomonitoring	Sensing mechanisms, materials, approaches to stretchability, power	×
[57]	2021	Flexible pressure sensors	Requirements, sensing mechanisms, materials and structures, power	×
[58]	2021	Ionic tactile sensors	Materials, sensor types	×
[59]	2021	Sensor data processing for 'perception'	Biological sensing and perception, chip integration, memristors, synaptic transistors	×
[60]	2021	Electronic skin for medical devices	Requirements, wearable and implantable devices	×

(*Continued*)

Table 1.1. *(Continued)*

Ref.	Year	Subject	Topics	EIT
[61]	2022	Self-powered e-skin	Energy sources, integration, self-power, applications	×
[62]	2022	Overview of touch (focusing on hands) and vision perception	Sensing mechanisms, applications, vision-touch fusion	✓
[63]	2022	Multi-responsive e-skin	Sensing mechanisms, materials, sensor types, flexible circuits, applications, challenges	×
[64]	2022	Stretchable tactile sensors	Different types	✓
[65]	2022	Flexible electronics	Short review of sensing mechanisms, materials, sensor types, implantable	×
[66]	2022	Biodegradable e-skin	Sensing mechanisms, materials, applications, challenges	×
[67]	2022	Wearable tactile sensors	Bio-inspiration, biomimicry, requirements, biopolymer sensors	×
[68]	2023	Flexible sensors	Sensor-biology interfaces, power, sensor networks, environmental concerns, business, regulatory, and ethical considerations, intelligent flexible sensors	×

1.1.2 Envisioned applications of tactile e-skin other than robotics

In this section we address envisioned applications of e-skin other than robotics; the latter is addressed in section 1.1.3.

The rapid adoption of touch-screen technology attests to the usefulness of tactile interfaces. One might ask, what is the difference between a tactile e-skin and a touch screen? After all, touch screens register the position of contacts and can recognize gestures. Part of the answer is that a tactile e-skin should be conformal on 3D surfaces. Another part of the answer is that it should detect the intensity of contacts, not just their locations. A third is that in many cases, although not all, the skin should be compliant, or soft, or should give the impression of being soft even if the components are rigid.

1.1.2.1 Human-worn devices

The measurement of human motion represents a broad category of envisioned applications for e-skin, including gait measurement [69], sports training (e.g. knee joint monitoring [70]), health monitoring [71], physical rehabilitation, and recording the movement of a dancer. Smart textiles for wearable biomedicine [72], computing, and healthcare [73] have been under development for quite some time. Gloves have been made for reading human manual gesture [74, 75], skill training [75], and studying grasp mechanics [75, 76], with machine learning (ML) employed for gesture recognition and control [77].

Ultra-thin devices designed to attach directly to human skin ('second skins' [29]), or epidermal electronics, debuted in 2011 [78] as reviewed in [17, 20, 21, 51, 55, 56, 60]. Areas of potential application are health monitoring of vital signs such as heart rate, blood pressure, and respiration, or conditions such as epilepsy and sleep disorders (see e.g. [40, 51, 63]). For example, sensors for monitoring arterial pulse waves have been demonstrated [79]. Also of interest are monitoring of posture, gait, and tremors, as well as limb bending during activities, including exercise. There are, as of yet, no commercial second skins widely available on the market.

Soft skins have been proposed to overcome motion artefacts, inconsistent electrical contact, and stiffness mismatches between hard devices and soft tissue, which lead to errors in sensor measurements [60]. For health monitoring, devices should be flexible and stretchable to follow the bending of the body and associated skin deformation. Measuring muscle movements during speaking, breathing, or swallowing is of interest, as is measuring blinking and smiling [39]. Implantable sensors for disease diagnosis and post-surgery monitoring have also been contemplated [60, 65]. For example, it is of interest to monitor tendon strain without hindering the motion of the tendon [60]. Two important considerations for e-skin for health monitoring are cost and manufacturability, particularly for disposable devices [60]. In addition, device safety, longevity, and reliability are critical, as are means to power the devices [60].

Another group of applications comprise wearable tactile interfaces to machines [21], such as a wearable keypad [80] or data-glove [81]. A 'tactile internet' has been suggested with a human in the loop (TaHiL) [82]. Such an integration of sensor hardware with software on a network would need to have high speed to achieve the necessary low latency [82]. Virtual reality applications have also been suggested [83].

1.1.2.2 Human–machine interfaces

The area of human–machine interfaces (HMI) has attracted considerable interest [84]. One example of HMI that has received ongoing attention is tactile feedback from prosthetics [17, 85]. In this case, the tactile skin is not placed directly on the person but on the artificial limb worn by the person, for instance to detect grip and slip and for object and texture identification [31]. There is also interest in providing haptic feedback from robotic manipulators during surgery [86]. Soft devices for endoscopic surgery have been prototyped that are able to not only traverse tortuous paths to reach organs, but also provide surgeons with tactical feedback, and e-skins on balloon catheters are able to make measurements on the surface of tissue [60].

1.1.3 Applications in robotics

> *With robots starting to enter our lives in a number of ways (e.g., social, assistive, and surgery), the electronic skin (e-skin) is becoming increasingly important.* [29]

It has long been assumed that tactile e-skins will be essential for robots to collaborate with humans [87]. An e-skin would allow a robot to interact with the world and with people in intuitive ways, including collision detection, handling of objects, and human–robot communication by touch. In popular culture, a robot with a whole-body e-skin was epitomized in the 2014 film *Big Hero 6* [88]. An e-skin could confer awareness by a robot of its body surface, which is anticipated to help with navigating unpredictable situations and environments, as well as to complement vision and proprioception [89]. It would allow detection of contacts that occur elsewhere than on end effectors and allow interpretation of such contacts. However, e-skins are still far from mainstream for robots: the main sensors in use today are linear and rotational encoders (based on various principles, from optical to inductive), cameras, proximity sensors, and sensors for force, torque, and texture. Tactile sensors for robots have been the topic of reviews since the 1980s [90]. More recently, progress in e-skins for robotics was reviewed in [16, 91], and tactile systems for robots, including whole-body systems, were well reviewed in [19]. Systems considerations were highlighted in [2, 6]. Below we outline the main envisioned applications in robotics.

1.1.3.1 Safety: collision avoidance and mitigation

For robots to be able to work alongside humans (as 'cobots' [92]) or in complex, cluttered, uncontrolled environments, collisions must be avoided and potential damage from a collision mitigated. However, it should be noted that because there are non-contact methods of sensing object proximity, collision avoidance does not actually require an e-skin. Cameras have primarily been used for safety, with some use of point force or tactile sensors and laser scanners [93]. The Moxi robot (Diligent Robotics, Inc.), employed for delivery of small items in hospitals, uses sensor fusion, cameras, and artificial intelligence (AI) to avoid unsafe contact [94]. (Not to be confused with Moxie, Embodied, Inc., the social robot for children [95].) Although most industrial robots, which are heavy and high speed, have no environmental awareness, in some of them contact forces can be computed from torque sensors in the actuators at joints, and robots have been programmed with withdrawal reflexes. Nevertheless, they are kept physically separate from humans. Tactile sensors, which directly measure contact forces, have also been used for collision mitigation [19]. Soft robotic systems are thought to be intrinsically safer in case of human–robot contact due to their mechanical compliance.

An example of a robot with an e-skin for collision avoidance is the iCub, an open-source humanoid platform. It has been trained to build a representation of the extent of its body and the space around it (its 'peripersonal' space), allowing anticipation of contacts, by combining information from capacitance-sensing 'taxels', or tactile elements, with visual and joint-angle data [89].

Safety issues around human–robot coexistence (defined as humans and robots working in a shared space but with no shared goals), cooperation (working on a shared goal in a shared space), and collaboration (working simultaneously on a shared object) were reviewed in [93], along with relevant safety standards. Safety management for the Pepper healthcare robot (SoftBank Robotics Corp) were considered in [96]. Safety measures typically involve stopping motion entirely on detecting a human, or slowing speed or limiting force; it is also important for the human to be made aware of the robot's intentions and potential trajectories. Cushioning of rigid components has also been considered (e.g. [97]).

1.1.3.2 Environmental and self-awareness for task performance

Unlike for collision mitigation, there is a clearer need for e-skin for robots to interact with less-structured environments to better carry out complicated and dynamic tasks [8, 98]. For instance a stretchable sleeve with 25 discrete tactile sensors covering the forearm, wrist, and end effector of a humanoid robot and straddling the articulated joints enabled it to reach a target with reduced contact forces when maneuvering the arm through an array of columns [99]. Tactile feedback from multiple contacts were also used for force control during physical interactions with a user [100].

Tactile imaging can also supplement the visual systems of machines; examples are reviewed in [62], such as stacking objects into a tower, picking up books, and drawing. This is of particular interest in environments that are visually obstructed, for example by barriers such as walls or objects, or under conditions of poor visibility such as in darkness, smoke, or fog. Tactile feedback can also provide information on object characteristics such as compliance or weight [19]. Thus, tasks such as lifting have been shown to benefit from tactile imaging.

In one example of using an e-skin to help carry out a complicated task, a humanoid robot with a body-covering e-skin used information about surface deformations to stand up from sitting on a chair, pull a dummy on a bed toward itself, or pick up a box from a table [101]. The robot detected the initial shape and position of the objects, such as the table and box then planned motions that would transition the objects to a new state of contact. These jobs required a number of different body contacts and a complex sequence of maneuvers, illustrating the advantages of an e-skin.

Macra [102] and Macket [103] were two other, smaller humanoid robots with e-skin for whole-body interaction with objects. They were able to learn to perform behaviors such as, starting from a position of lying down on the back, rolling to the front side. Integrated behaviors, such as reaching something on a shelf by using an object as a support for leaning, which involved using environmental interaction to assist in the performance of target tasks, were also enabled by a smart skin [102]. An artificial skin was used to detect forces on a robot arm originating from perturbing human contacts, and the information was employed to compensate in controlling the arm's motion [104].

E-skins also offer robots proprioception, which is of particular value in soft robots [40, 105–108]. Bioinspired robots [109] using soft actuators [110–112] have been proposed for use in agriculture for such tasks as berry picking to avoid damaging delicate fruit. They have also been suggested for cluttered environments or tight spaces, since they offer highly dexterous manipulation [113], and for surgery, since their softness should make them safer in interactions with soft tissue [106]. Soft actuators, which are often pneumatic [114–116], have had limited or no sensing ability since they do not have the built-in position sensing capability of motors [117]. A stretchable e-skin could be used for detecting actuation-induced bending or length changes as well as externally-applied deformations [24]. The skin needs to be soft relative to the robot and able to achieve strains that can accommodate the robot's full range of motion. In one study, a stretchable tactile skin was retrofitted to the outside of a pneumatic bidirectional robot 'finger' actuator that detected its state of inflation. Delays, nonlinearities, and hysteresis in that all-polymeric system were well handled by employing ML in the controls [118].

1.1.3.3 Human–robot and human–machine interactions and collaboration

E-skins are considered to be indispensable for physical interactions between humans and machines [32]. Tactile human–robot interactions (HRI) were reviewed in [62, 119].

A driving vision for tactile e-skins is the eventual realization of service robots for healthcare settings or home elder care, as exemplified by RI-MAN [120]. Sensors in five locations on RI-MAN allow it to lift a human-size dummy (16 kg) in its arms by determining load and roll angle.

Socially-assistive robotics [121, 122] has been the primary commercially-viable application of e-skins. It has been claimed that tactile interaction with robot surrogate pets such as Paro has a calming effect [123, 124]. Paro had commercial success, with over 1700 sold, more than 100 of which were being used in institutions such as elder care homes in Denmark as of 2011 [125]. As of 2018, Paro continued to be sold at $6000 each [126]. The Huggable robot, also designed for hospitals and nursing homes, had a full-body touch-sensitive skin retrofitted inside a commercial teddy bear, together with compliant actuators and other sensors, and it could respond to touch by moving its head and limbs [127]. The system was able to distinguish nine touch modalities, including poking, patting, petting, and squeezing, including both direction of motion and intensity. A large humanoid robot that remains in the laboratory, HuggieBot, had soft stretchable tactile sensors to detect initiation and conclusion of a hug [128, 129]. The hugging was found to result in greater trust in the robot by the humans and to improved their moods. With the aim of realizing social robots, a soft, repairable, multi-modal tactile skin was demonstrated that used ML to classify touch modalities [130]. EIT-based sensors have also been used to identify types of touch [131–133].

Another class of applications for e-skins on robots involves communication by touch. The Institute of Electrical and Electronics Engineers (IEEE) has been holding the International Symposia on Robot and Human Interactive Communication (RO-MAN), since 1992, with contributions concerning touch. Communication robots with distributed soft skin were reviewed in [91]. The main aims are either to train or directly control the movement of a robot or, alternatively, to infer human intent based on human motions to improve human–machine collaboration on tasks, such as jointly carrying a large object [62] or dancing [134]. For an example of the former, a human holding a robot's hands could apply an upward force to command the robot to stand up [102]. However, a soft sensing skin is not always required: the Baxter robot interacted physically with humans by high-fives, fist bumps, and hand-clapping games using accelerometers in the wrist [135]. Human–robot collaboration (HRC) is hoped to increase the capability and productivity of industry [93]; HRC was reviewed in [136].

1.2 Approaches to e-skin design

Literature surveys (table 1.1) show wide diversity in the types of tactile imaging prototypes that have been demonstrated. E-skin has been defined to consist of a protective layer, a sensor layer, a signal processing layer, and a substrate [27], although not every skin integrates all of these as part of the skin itself, and the substrate may be a system onto which a skin is retrofitted. A feedback control layer [137] can also be included; although it may not be considered part of the skin, it may be needed to actually utilize the skin.

All e-skins must be able to conform to variously shaped, large-area surfaces. This section begins with two approaches to e-skin that are competitors to EIT—arrays of discrete sensors and row–column arrays—before we turn to continuous sensors that can employ EIT. As mentioned previously, here we focus exclusively on e-skins that sense pressure or strain, rather than other stimuli such as temperature. The descriptions below are mute concerning the sensing modality, which is taken up in section 1.3.2.

1.2.1 Rigid sensors: macro-scale discrete sensor arrays

There were early attempts to realize stretchable continuous sensor 'suits' for robots [91], but arrays of discrete tactile sensing elements, or taxels, became the preferred approach [19]. The latter were made using standard printed circuit board approaches rather than unconventional materials and processes. The use of either rigid or bendable substrates avoided the interconnection challenges encountered with stretchable skins. Their modularity allowed adjustment of sensor density based on the need for information from different parts of the body, and it granted sufficient conformability over the robot.

Arraying taxels over the surface requires connecting each of them with power and communication [138]. Ports at the periphery can connect neighboring taxels, simplifying the fitting process. A taxel, or small group of taxels, may have an associated microcontroller. At the system level it is necessary to recognize and deal with damaged taxels, for example by routing around or replacing them. To create an artificial 'flesh' that can be fitted to the surface, taxels have been covered with a protective layer of foam, or they have been embedded into a conformal material. To create smart textiles, taxels have typically been individually wired, integrating the leads into the weave of the fabric.

A wide range of sensor types has been deployed, including force-sensitive rubbers, optical technologies, semiconductor pressure sensors, piezoelectric sensors, graphite-loaded elastomers, 6-axis force-torque sensors, conductive gels, proximity sensors, capacitive pressure sensors, and multilayered fabrics [19]. A large variety of discrete sensors [6], as well as strip and small-area sensors, have been commercially available for some time.

The rigid modular approach to interconnections was applied in the iCub skin [89, 139]. The location of a taxel in a triangular skin module, and the location of the module within a skin patch, provided the location of the stimulus. By combining information from neighboring taxels, the speed of response could be dynamically increased and bandwidth requirements reduced. For the above-mentioned box-handling humanoid robot [140], sensors were mounted on flexible printed circuit (FPC) film that could not only be placed where desired, but also wrapped or folded, and even cut into smaller pieces. Each sheet included a microcontroller and serial bus terminators, reducing the number of wires. To add compliance, the sheets were covered with urethane foam and an outer package. For the humanoid RI-MAN, discrete rigid sensors were also mounted on FPC and embedded in an elastic layer [120]. Sensor data went to a single controller that shared it across a data network with a host PC and other controllers. Likewise, the Huggable robot [127] employed groups of sensors mounted on circuit boards, with multiplexers to reduce wiring and a silicone rubber 'flesh' for softness and protection of the electronics. Flexible commercial sensors were assembled into a bendable sheet in [141].

A different approach to softness was taken in the Macra and Macket robots, which embedded individual discrete sensor units inside a urethane foam [142]. The units had rigid components such as accelerometers and printed circuit boards. For the Marshmal robot, an artificial flesh was formed from an inner layer of shock-absorbing gel and an outer wrapping of cloth for wear protection [142]; this robot could fall off a table without damage. Soft sensors were developed for joint regions using knitted cloths of conductive yarn in combination with insulating yarn and metal electrodes [143]. A soft silicone flesh was proposed in an early paper with embedded sensing chips having integrated pressure sensing coils employing radio frequency inductive coupling for power and communication [138].

Regarding the number of sensors that have been used, the Macra and Macket robots had as few as 48 sensor units [142], while the RI-MAN prototype had 320 pressure sensors [120], the Huggable robot had 45 sensors for proximity and light touch on top of 1000 force sensors [127], and the box-manipulating robot had 1864 sensors [140].

1.2.2 Flexible and hybrid sensors

1.2.2.1 Row–column arrays

Due to their simplicity, row and column electrode formats are often used in laboratory prototypes. In resistive sensors the relative resistance changes of the rows and columns are monitored. For example, a stretchable system was developed from conductive fabric electrodes sandwiching patches of carbon black-filled piezoresistive silicone rubber [144]. Another piezoresistive stretchable array was created using Ag-filled silicone and carbon-filled polyurethane (PU) rubber; it was formed into a finger shape and used to distinguish among faces, edges, and corners of small objects [145]. Not all row–column arrays are rectangular—the electrodes may follow other paths, such as along the finger of a glove [76]. With row–column arrays, resolution is determined by the number of elements. One drawback of row–column systems is that damaging one area of the e-skin may render an entire row and column non-operational, potentially requiring complete replacement of the e-skin.

An example of a partially stretchable row–column sensing sheet was a 3×4 button keypad realized in PDMS containing channels filled with the conductive liquid eGaIn: pressing on the fluid caused dimensional changes of the fluid channel, leading to changes in resistance. A capacitive row–column array touch sensor worn on an arm has been demonstrated [146], but few row–column designs have yet been mounted on a robot.

1.2.2.2 Microfabricated and printed arrays

Also frequently employed have been arrays of sensors printed on sheets. Typically such sheets are bendable but not stretchable. For example, a Ge/Si nanowire active matrix field effect transistor (FET) array was created, comprising 342 pressure-sensitive rubber (PSR, carbon-filled silicone) taxels [147]. For this technology, the device had a relatively large area of 7 cm on each side; more typical sizes are 1 cm or smaller. The fabrication of these arrays can be complex. For [147], it involved electron beam and thermal evaporation, vapor–liquid–solid growth of nanowires, lithographic patterning, contact printing, atomic layer deposition, and oxygen plasma etching, among other steps. To realize stretchability, a similar transistor array on a bendable sheet with a sensing area of 4.4 cm on a side was perforated, allowing it to be stretched 50% and spread over curved surfaces and even folded [97]. The fabrication of this sensor was likewise complex.

Island-bridge designs have also been realized, in which the islands are not stretchable but the bridges are. Although it has been postulated that hybrid electronics comprising conventional chips with stretchable interconnects are most likely to be commercialized in the near future [40], the challenges associated with that approach remain significant.

Stretchable integrated e-skin systems are difficult to fabricate given the need for uniform layer-to-layer registration [40] and the fact that conventional lithography has difficulty handling stretchable materials [40], not to mention the large sizes required for applications like whole-body coverings. Furthermore, a high density of narrow interconnect lines, which have large parasitic capacitance and resistance, results in cross-talk and noise [40].

1.2.3 Soft sensors: continuous, stretchable sensors

Continuous sensors are the most straightforward to fabricate, involving no patterning, registration, or placement steps. For resistive sensors, only a single layer of sensing material is required. This layer can take a variety of forms: it can be a conductive fabric, a slab of piezoresistive rubber, or a coating applied to a substrate, all of which can be stretchable. For example, a thin film of carbon-loaded elastomer can be spray coated onto an elastomeric sheet. Capacitive sensors are normally slightly more complex, consisting of two conductors separated by an insulator, although the second conductor may be a human and the insulator may be the surrounding air. Continuous sensors can employ EIT, as described in section 2.2.2, with electrodes placed only at the periphery.

1.3 Designs, structures, and fabrication of soft tactile sensors

In this section, stretchable sensors are briefly reviewed, from the means used to confer stretchability to sensing modalities and fabrication. Since these topics have been extensively reviewed in depth in [5, 16, 24, 27, 51, 67] and other references in table 1.1, only the main points are touched upon here for completeness. We restrict attention to approaches that lend themselves to EIT, neglecting stretchable concepts such as embedded microphones [148] or optical pressure-mapping [149].

1.3.1 Sensor stretchability

Stretchability differs from flexibility or bendability and allows e-skins to be employed over soft materials and joints. Required strains are typically on the order of tens of percent, although that varies depending on the application, from several percent to over 100%. Approaches to stretchability fall broadly into two categories: (1) use of inherently stretchable materials such as elastomers and (2) patterning or structuring non-stretchable materials. The latter is often used to connect rigid or flexible 'islands', such as sensors or circuit elements, that have been manufactured using established fabrication processes. Routes to stretchability have been reviewed in [4, 5, 16, 38, 67, 150, 151].

1.3.1.1 Inherently stretchable materials

Among the most commonly used elastomeric materials are PU rubbers and silicones, such as PDMS (sold as e.g. Sylgard or Ecoflex). These materials can serve as substrates, flesh-like padding, or parts of the sensor. To form stretchable electrodes, for example, conductive carbon or metal nanoparticles (NPs) are mixed into the elastomer. The NPs provide a low percolation threshold so that the composite becomes electrically conductive while its stiffness remains close to that of the unfilled host elastomer. Sensors are produced the same way [5], but the amount of conductive filler (the 'loading') is lower because a higher resistance is needed. Encapsulation of liquid metals within channels in an elastomer is another route to stretchability [152].

As opposed to electronic conductors, there are also ionic conductors such as hydrogels. They are of interest for implantable and skin-wearable sensors because of their water content and biocompatibility [58]. An important class of salts for device applications are ionic liquids (ILs): these are room-temperature liquids containing no water, so the devices do not dry out. ILs have been employed in both resistive and capacitive sensors for strain and pressure [58].

One-dimensional materials, such as carbon nanotubes or silver nanowires, have been used not only in composites, but also alone as stretchable electrodes [153], as reviewed in [151]. They are typically deposited onto an elastomeric substrate. These highly conductive NTs maintain a percolating network under strain. Deposition of inherently rigid thin metal films on elastomeric substrates also allows some stretchability, the failure behavior being different from that of free-standing films [154, 155].

It must be observed that elastomeric materials are viscoelastic and therefore show hysteresis and other memory effects [8], such as large 'first-cycle' baseline resistivity shifts. Such memory effects have been challenging for sensor applications. ML is beginning to be applied to mitigate this complicating behavior.

1.3.1.2 Wrinkled or microstructured materials

Rigid materials such as metals can be made stretchable by creating out-of-plane topography, such as wrinkles or buckles [156, 157], or by allowing out-of-plane motion, such as by cutting (e.g. by laser ablation or etching); the latter was derived from the paper-cutting craft of kirigami. This approach has been called 'structure-derived elasticity' or 'geometric engineering' and the surfaces called 2.5-dimensional surfaces. Structures such as hemispheres, arch bridges, or spirals flatten under strain [158, 159]. In-plane serpentine patterns (zigzags, horseshoes, and other meanders) permit out-of-plane deformation during stretching [160]. Folding can also permit rigid materials to stretch [40]. Another form of micro- or milli-scale structuring is introducing pores into a material to increase its compliance [76, 161].

Micro-structuring can increase the sensitivity of tactile sensors [152, 162, 163]. A sensor design that had high sensitivity while also being able to withstand large impact forces was realized by geometrically defining voids in the sensing layer [164], using 'functional partitioning' to realize both performance metrics. A pressure-insensitive strain sensor was formed from a porous nano-carbon-loaded elastomer based on temporary separation of adjacent conductive pore walls [165].

A different approach to enabling rigid materials to stretch is depositing a film onto an elastomer in such a way that it forms a network of cracks; this allows rigid islands to separate and rejoin while staying in a 2D plane; more weakly adhered films or multilayers may result in the formation of overlaps with adjacent islands. Similarly, rigid materials can be rendered compliant by forming them into hollow spheres that connect to form a film, which can be deposited and patterned by printing or spray coating [166].

Patterning techniques used for these approaches include printing (e.g. screen printing, 3D printing), microfabrication (e.g. photolithographic definition, etching, electroplating), patterned deposition (e.g. spray coating through a stencil), material removal (e.g. laser ablation), and molding [151]. Many types of substrates can be used as molds for microstructured surfaces, from photo-lithographically defined etched silicon wafers to plastic microspheres or silk, as reviewed in [42]. An approach that does not require patterning is to pre-stretch the substrate prior to metal deposition; the elastic modulus mismatch results in a wrinkled surface upon subsequent relaxation.

Robustness has been raised as a problem with micro-structuring approaches. An even more significant problem is that these substrates are often small, on the order of a few cm on a side. As always, the challenges of making strong electro-mechanical connections to these materials cannot be overlooked. The most highly integrated systems have thus been flexible, but not stretchable.

1.3.1.3 Roles of the substrate and other layers

Soft padding has been used for mechanical protection, both to render a robot soft for human interaction and to shield sensors from damage. In addition, compliant padding allows strain sensors to be employed for force detection, with the range of forces determined by the stiffness of the underlying padding. Padding and other means of altering substrate compliance can moreover be used to enhance performance. Multiple layers of padding with different stiffness can, for example, extend the range of forces that can be detected [167]. Likewise, the compliance of the substrate can be altered by mini-structuring it: a rigid substrate with recesses of specific size underlying the sensor allows the sensor to respond solely to features of that size and smaller; larger features do not deform the sensor [168]. A sawtooth surface profile was also found to increase pressure sensitivity and range [166].

Stacking of layers has been used not only to combine different types of sensor, but also to add various electrode layers and encapsulation [15, 63]. On the other hand, stacking of elements can worsen hysteresis [169]. Considerations must also be given to how stress can be released after deformation [169].

1.3.2 Types of soft sensors

An enormous number of tactile sensor types based on various transduction mechanisms have been developed, including magnetic, optical, and others. The two most common types are resistive and capacitive. There has long been spirited discussion about the merits and disadvantages of these two, with some systems employing both for their different strengths. Both can in principle be used with EIT, but resistive sensors have dominated to date (table 2.3 in chapter 2). For completeness, the sensor types are briefly touched upon here; for in-depth discussions, the reader is referred to the reviews in table 1.1 and the historical literature. Most attention is here reserved for resistive sensors since they have been used for the large majority of tactile EIT systems.

1.3.2.1 Resistive sensors

Resistive sensors are attractive because they can have the simplest structure: a single layer of resistive material connected to wire leads. Their main disadvantage is high power consumption, since it is necessary to draw current to measure the resistance. The relationship between resistance R, an extrinsic (dimension-dependent) property, and resistivity ρ, an intrinsic (material) property, is:

$$R = \rho L/wt \tag{1.1}$$

where L is the resistor's length, w its width, and t its thickness. Some resistive sensors are based on dimensional changes alone, such as the fluidic sensors described in section 1.3.2.1.3. More typically, piezoresistive sensors are employed because of their higher sensitivity. In piezoresistives, the resistivity itself changes with strain. This is brought about by changing the ease of charge transport over an energy barrier, such as by changing the hopping or tunneling probability. In other cases, such as in sensors based on contact resistance, a combination of mechanisms contributes.

For resistive strain sensors, sensitivity is given by the gauge factor, GF:

$$GF = \frac{\Delta R/R}{\Delta L/L} = \frac{\Delta R/R}{\varepsilon} \quad (1.2)$$

where ε is the strain. A positive gauge factor is most typical and indicates that resistance increases with strain. For conventional metal foil strain gauges, GF = 2 due only to dimensional changes of the resistor, while for piezoresistives GF can be much larger.

Resistive sensors have been realized in numerous ways, as described below. While the discussion is divided into composites, fabrics, fluids, contact resistance, and other methods, in fact many devices mix these elements. For example, conductive fabric might be used as an electrical connection to a hydrogel, or a carbon-loaded composite may be mounted to a fabric.

1.3.2.1.1 Composites

As mentioned previously, piezoresistivity can be conferred by adding a conducting phase, in the form of nano-scale particles, as a filler into an insulating host. Electrons hop or tunnel between the particles. The amount of filler is critical: too little, and the particles do not form a conductive network through the material, too much and the material is always highly conducting. For sensors, the filler concentration, or *loading*, should be near the percolation threshold, which is the point at which the conductivity–concentration curve is steepest and has an inflection in the transition from insulating to conductive. At that point, small changes in loading lead to large changes in conductivity. Importantly, straining the material also leads to a change in inter-particle separation, and thus changes in conductivity. It must be noted that these materials are, as a result, also inherently sensitive to temperature and humidity, which also alter electron transport between particles.

In addition to loading, for stretchable sensors the size of the filler particles is also critical: they must be small, preferably nano-scale in at least one dimension, so that the host material remains elastomeric at the percolation threshold and is not stiffened by the filler. Furthermore, the shape of the particles and their adhesion to the host play important roles in sensor behavior, as does their alignment and distribution within the host. Sensors made from such composites were reviewed in [28]. Nano-carbons are the most frequently used particles in piezoresistive sensors, including nano-scale carbon black [76, 144, 170], carbon nanotubes (CNTs) [171], and graphite or 'graphene' nano-platelets (GnPs) [71, 172]. Occasionally, nano-scale Ag has been employed [73, 173].

Elastomeric composites are most useful for large-strain sensing applications, although with a sufficiently high GF they can also detect smaller strains. Punctures can, however, lead to tears and failure under strain. Therefore, elastic fabrics have been embedded into rubber composites to increase their durability [174], and carbon-loaded elastomers have been attached onto textiles, for example as was done to form a sensing glove [76]. Commercial sheets of pressure-sensitive and conductive rubber (e.g. CS57–7RSC, PCR Technical, Japan) are available that are conductive when compressed but otherwise insulating.

1.3.2.1.2 Fabrics

Fabric has numerous advantages for use in tactile imaging: it is stretchable and lightweight; it can be folded, twisted, and bent; it can be cut and sewn for facile integration into smart textiles; it can be washed; eyelets and other hardware can be added by piercing; and it can be embroidered, for example with a more conductive yarn. A whole-body sensing suit for a humanoid robot was made from a conductive knit [91] (and it was suggested that EIT be used in the future). To form sensors, conventional fabrics or yarns can be coated with conductive or sensing layers, including metals and conjugated polymers (also known as inherently conductive polymers, ICPs). Alternatively, conductive fibers can be used: fibers with a conductive core and insulating shell have been 3D-printed [175] and formed into sensing meshes. In addition to strain sensors, fiber-based transistors and memory devices have been demonstrated, as well as energy-harvesting and energy-storing fibers.

Woven fabrics are stretchable, but they are anisotropic and nonlinear [91]. (For EIT, compensating the effects of anisotropy on imaging should be further studied.) Non-woven fabrics (e.g. felts) have also been used for sensing, but they are not stretchable. Stretchable thread, for example nylon-spandex blends, is advantageous for stitching the fabric sensors. Conductive yarns can be used to make a stretchable electrical connection to the sensing area.

Fabric strain sensors generally have negative gauge factors, unlike most other piezoresistive sensors, meaning that resistance decreases with strain. This is because the contact resistance between fibers is reduced as the fabric stretches and the yarns come into more intimate contact. Like composites, fabrics are often used to detect large strains. Sensors based on multiple layers of fabric have been demonstrated [81]. Carbon-coated textiles have been coated with an elastomer to improve durability [176]. EIT has been used with several fabric-based sensors (table 2.3), including [169, 176–179].

Piezoresistive and conductive fabrics (such as Eeontex from Eeonyx Corp) can be obtained commercially [180]. The fabrics are coated with a conjugated polymer such as polypyrrole or poly(3,4-ethylenedioxythiophene) (PEDOT) [181]. They were developed for antistatic, electromagnetic shielding, and resistive heating applications, but have become popular as stretchable sensors. Fabric-based pressure sensors are also available [182].

The general field of textile-based electronics, or 'textronics' has also been extensively reviewed, including [10, 21, 54, 183–186]. Two approaches have been taken: mounting of electronic components onto textiles and weave-based approaches that use conductive and functionalized yarns. Challenges with the former include difficulty with interconnections and with the rigidity of the devices in a wearable, and with the latter challenges include poor mechanical and chemical stability of the fibers.

1.3.2.1.3 Liquids and fluidics

As discussed above, ionic resistive sensors have been developed, particularly for wearable applications. In these sensor materials, such as hydrogels and conjugated polymers, the signal is due to ion transport rather than electron transport. In one example, a strip of hydrogel changed its impedance with strain [187]. With the aqueous hydrogels, the loss of hydration due to evaporation, or conversely swelling due to water uptake, is the main challenge. Damage due to freezing may also need to be considered, depending on the application. Thus, researchers have explored the use of ionic liquids (ILs), which are room-temperature liquid salts. Ionic materials have primarily been explored for chemical sensing, but ionic gels, consisting of ILs within a polymer, undergo large capacitance changes with pressure, making them attractive for pressure sensing [40].

Another approach to resistive sensors is based on liquid metal-filled micro-channels in an elastomer sheet [75, 80, 188–190]; the metal is typically eutectic gallium–indium (eGaIn or gallinstan). Pressure or strain on the sheet leads to changes in the cross-sectional area and length of the sealed channel, changing its resistance (equation 1.1). Multi-level orthogonal channel structures have been achieved to form taxels at the intersections. A 'discrete' impedance tomography sensor based on a network of fluid channels was demonstrated [191]. Higher sensitivity can be achieved by combining IL-filled channels for sensing with eGaIn channels for electrical connections [74]. Because eGaIn oxidizes when it comes into contact with air, it can be patterned by direct ink writing onto a lower elastomer sheet, followed by electrical connection and encapsulation [192].

Typical methods of manufacturing these sensors involve molding silicone rubber (PDMS, Ecoflex, etc), lamination to seal the channels, and filling the channels with a syringe. Wires are inserted through the elastomer to contact the liquid metal or, to improve the robustness of the wire connections, conductive Ag thread can be sewn into the elastomer with multiple serpentine turns. Device sizes have been small, on the order of a few cm up to hand-sized. An attractive alternative to molding is filling an elastomeric foam with liquid metal [193].

1.3.2.1.4 Contact resistance

A number of EIT devices have employed changes in contact resistance with pressure in the form of stacked contact resistance sensors (SCRSs). Broadly, pressure increases the number of contact points and their cross-sectional areas, lowering the resistance between two conducting layers. In one example, the first conductive layer was a stretchable yarn net [177] or a carbon-loaded fabric [194, 195], and the second was an array of squares of silver-coated fabric mounted to a non-stretchable but flexible substrate. The disconnected pieces in the second layer allow detection of multiple contact points. In another example, a conductive fabric and a conductive paint-coated object were separated by small rubber insulators [196]. More recently, a stack of two piezoresistive composite sheets was used [197]. In one SCRS, the mesh of an insulating woven fabric between two conducting layers was altered to adjust the sensitivity [198].

1.3.2.1.5 Other methods

Percolation in 3D composites has a 2D analog: micro-cracked films that undergo a change in conductivity as the contacts between conductive islands are made or broken with strain, as reviewed in [23]. These films are typically metals. Micro-cracking was previously introduced in the context of stretchability in section 1.3.1.2.

Foams, sponges, and other porous materials have been coated, loaded, or filled with conductive materials to create resistive pressure sensors, as reviewed in [161]. In addition, conductive composites, as in section 1.3.2.1.1, can be rendered porous to yield lightweight, highly compliant sensors. Changes in percolation and contact resistance may both occur in these materials.

1.3.2.2 Capacitive sensors

Capacitive pressure sensors have the advantages of low power consumption and high sensitivity to small deformations. However, they have more constituents than resistive sensors, an insulating material (dielectric) located between two conductors, and they require more complex electronics. Given that the capacitance $C = \varepsilon A/d$, where ε is the dielectric constant, A the sensor area, and d the electrode spacing, there are many ways to effect a change in capacitance. Analogously to equation (1.2), the sensitivity of a capacitive pressure sensor is given by $S = (\Delta C/C)/\Delta P$, where P is the pressure. Similar definitions characterize sensors based on varying the dielectric constant or the area. Capacitive sensors benefit from a high dielectric constant [65], which may be difficult to achieve in soft devices. A large variety of placements of the dielectric with respect to the conductors has been demonstrated, but the configurations are primarily either sandwich (parallel plate) or planar.

A dual-mode touch sensor was created by printing electrodes on both sides of a fabric, which served as a compressible dielectric layer [146]. The proximity of a human finger changed the capacitive coupling between electrodes on the same side of the fabric; at the same time, a pressure sensor resulted from electrodes on opposite sides of the fabric. Other examples of capacitive pressure sensors include: thin metal electrodes on either side of an elastomeric foam dielectric [199], conductive fabrics sandwiching insulating layers of either foam [143] or a microstructured elastomer [200], and nanowire-loaded elastomers sandwiching a porous tape [201].

1.3.2.3 Self-powered sensing

Self-powered sensors could be based on triboelectric, piezoelectric, electrostatic, thermoelectric, magnetoelectric, or pyroelectric mechanisms [63]. These sensors detect *changes* in deformation, making them most appropriate for dynamic signals, such as experienced in tactile interactions.

Triboelectric nano-generators (TENGs) have been successfully implemented in e-skin applications [44, 51] and offer an intriguing possibility for use with EIT. (TENGs should not be confused with thermoelectric generators, or TEGs.) Triboelectric charge (static electricity) is generated by friction, and polymer pairs (e.g. Kapton+PET or PVC+gel) that occupy different levels in the triboelectric series producing an output voltage when stacked, although the effect is still often unpredictable. This voltage output can directly be the signal, or they can produce electrical energy to power a different sensing device. For example, an array of TENG sensing taxels was able to image poking [201, 203]. Alternatively, the energy from tapping a stretchable TENG was able to light an LED [202]. Elastic fibers were 3D printed and made into a row–column array that could sense touch at the connection points based on the triboelectric effect [175].

Piezoelectrics have long been used for sensing: they respond to changes in dimension with changes in surface charge. Work on piezoelectric sensors was reviewed in [18]. While piezoelectric polymers exist, a barrier to their use is conferring the required alignment by 'poling' at high voltage. These materials are rarely employed in tactile skins, although a capacitive tactile imaging array was made by weaving piezoelectric strips comprising polyvinylidene fluoride (PVDF) sandwiched between metal electrode films through a mesh of compressible tubes; this structure could alternatively be used to generate power [204]. Recently, a piezoelectric material was combined with a TENG and integrated into a glove to recognize gesture with the aid of ML [77].

1.3.3 Fabrication

A key advantage of continuous piezoresistive EIT sensors is that, unlike stretchable arrays, they require no patterning or multiple layers. Fabrication comprises only material preparation, in some cases film coating, and electrode attachment steps.

Molding is often used to create more elaborate piezoresistive and capacitive elastomeric sensors. For small features and areas, photolithography has been used to create the mold [159], whereas milling can be used to create molds with larger features for skins of up to tens of cm in size [205]. For UV-curable materials, direct photopatterning is an option.

Additive manufacturing has been envisioned to be a central technology for fabricating e-skins for wearable health monitoring or soft robots [60], which includes methods such as fused filament fabrication, aerosol jet printing, inkjet printing, direct ink writing, and electrohydrodynamic printing, as reviewed in [33]. Thus, 3D printing has been used to co-fabricate resistive sensors and the body of a soft robot [206]. While elastomers such as Ecoflex and PDMS are normally molded, they can be printed under special conditions, such as pre-mixing the two components and using a heated printing bed [207]; a special formulation of 'very fast' Dragon Skin (Smooth On) can also be printed. Miniature 3D stretchable tactile sensors to detect human movement have been printed, varying the Ag content of the host silicone to create insulating, resistive, and conductive layers and a spring-shaped sensor [208]. Likewise, compliant resistive soft sensors were realized using a Connex3 Objet350 multi-material printer with commercial photopolymers of various conductivities [206]. Multi-material printing was explored in the creation of sophisticated fingertips with capacitive pressure sensors for a robot hand [209]. Screen printing has also been employed, for example to create a piezoresistive pressure sensing array [145]. Nanoparticles can be incorporated in the print, respecting the requirements for 'ink' formulation, to make sensing layers and metal-containing composite electrodes [33].

In some cases, such as with soft robots, it is advantageous and feasible to create the sensor as part of the robot structure itself. By using compatible elastomers, sequential printing or molding can create sensors on or in the walls of the robot. In other cases, such as with rigid robots, it is desirable or necessary to retrofit soft sensors onto an existing system. For retrofitting, the issues are fitting, mechanical clearance and compliance, connecting, and other concerns that arise when joining two separate systems.

1.3.4 Sustainability

Increasing concern has been expressed in the recent literature about the environmental impact of electronic waste (e-waste) and the need to manage its rapid growth [66]. There are now consistent calls for the use of greener materials that are non-toxic and biodegradable, particularly for disposable wearables. Examples of biodegradable e-skins were reviewed in [66]. The use of biopolymer-based substrates, such as cellulose [66], has been explored, and materials other than precious metals can be considered for the conducting leads. Compromises in performance may be required, because, for example, organic materials have lower charge mobility than inorganic materials. Of course, the carbon footprint for producing the devices should be minimized. Furthermore, the number of different elements used in the devices should be limited, and their sources and abundance considered.

1.4 Tactile e-skin requirements

From the foregoing discussion of e-skin applications, the requirements and desirable features become apparent, as elucidated in [101, 210], and the other reviews in table 1.1. As discussed in [2, 57, 164], tactile imagers are tasked with fulfilling a large number of requirements. Table 1.2 lists the main ones, from the sensor to the application to commercial realization.

As noted by [211], the specific requirements for tactile e-skin depend on the application. For example, a medical robot to carry patients requires a high upper limit for force measurement compared to a keypad, and it has different needs for cleanability. It has been estimated that if a medical robot must also be able to detect a hand resting gently on its arm, a force range of 0.1–90 kPa is required [120, 212]. Such a robot will need to be covered with thick, soft padding, including over joints, so the tactile sensors will need to be stretchable and to have customizable shapes [213]. The resolution requirements may, however, be coarse: on the order of several cm on the forearm and even larger on the torso. Since the robot may experience

Table 1.2. Requirements for tactile e-skins. Although virtually all the requirements depend on the particular application, those that are more application-dependent are indicated by a '*'.

Sensing requirements	*Application requirements*
• accurate amplitude • appropriate, possibly large, dynamic range for the task • appropriate sensitivity for the task • appropriate resolution for the task • appropriate lifetime and repeatability for the application • reproducible output • real-time detection of multiple simultaneous contacts • low latency (fast response time) • linear response • minimal memory effects or compensatable for memory effects (drift, first-cycle effects, hysteresis, viscoelasticity and relaxation) • isotropic and uniform • large area *	• low power consumption • small number of required connecting wires • low noise • lightweight • real-time operation • stretchable ('soft') to conform to curved and complex surfaces, use over bending joints • compensatable for changes in ambient conditions (temperature, humidity) • durable to long-term use • robust to high strain, mechanical impacts, wear and tear, fluids • can be made in various shapes • straightforward installation; mountable or retrofittable onto existing systems * • work in harsh environments * • impervious to fluids, UV light * • able to handle heat from machine or robot * • safe (has mechanical damping) * • full-body coverage (for robotics) • comfortable for interaction (for human–machine interactions)
System commercialization and integration	*System integration nice-to-haves*
• low cost • manufacturable at high yield • failure-free interconnections • maintainable, repairable, replaceable • partially functional if damaged, fault tolerant • means of calibration • output signal compatible with downstream amplification and signal processing to allow closed loop sense–perceive–act	• all components stretchable • thin • self-healing • self-powering • compatible with energy harvesting, wireless power • greener and more sustainable, non-toxic, biodegradable, compatible with green electronics • include local signal processing (for arrays) • cleanable or sterilizable * • feels good when touched *

impacts, which could last only 0.5 msec [214], the sensors require a high speed of response [214].

Often requirements must be traded off. There is a 'goal conflict' between high resolution and high frequency readout [214], for example. Likewise, high sensitivity and extraordinary stretchability or large area may be difficult to achieve simultaneously.

There are, however, some universal requirements, such as a small number of electrical leads. Wires not only serve as antennas for the introduction of electromagnetic noise, but they also provide potential points of failure and may hinder the motion of the system [210]. Another common requirement is low cross-sensitivity to interference, whether from ambient conditions, primarily temperature and humidity, or from signals generated by other sensors in the e-skin [57, 63]. Challenges to realization, and required future work, are discussed next, in section 1.5.

1.5 Challenges to realization of soft, continuous tactile e-skins

It was said in 2013 that,

> *The integration of artificial skin into robotic systems has long been foreseen. For the last decades the introduction was always just a couple of years away.* [164]

While a great deal of research has been done since then, the statement still holds true today, and it applies as well to non-robotics applications. For example, fabric-based e-skins for monitoring knee bending and posture were prototyped in the late 1990s yet did not reach the market, and wearable tattoos, which debuted 10 years ago, are still called 'promising'. Challenges in implementing tactile imaging have been discussed for over three decades [87]. Below we overview some of the impediments to implementing soft, continuous e-skins for tactile imaging into systems, as well as some suggestion for overcoming the challenges. The issues are divided into sensing, application, and systems levels, following table 1.2, although all are inter-related. Progress toward EIT tactile imaging specifically is deferred to chapter 2.

1.5.1 Sensor-level

Research on e-skins has been strongly focused on sensor-level improvements, often on one or two metrics, such as sensitivity, resolution, or ultimate strain. These efforts have been successful, although they may have come at the cost of design and fabrication complexity (section 1.3) or performance on other metrics. Sensors have not typically been evaluated across a full range of requirements (such as given in table 1.2). As a result, it has been noted that some prototypes have little chance of ever being successfully integrated into a system [164].

The requirement for sensor softness comes with a significant cost: material memory. Viscoelastic behaviors and hysteresis lead to first-cycle effects, slow recovery after contact, non-monotonic signals, and signal spikes upon removal of contact (see e.g. [215–217]). Polymer chain entanglement, uncoiling and re-coiling, and reptation allow large strains but lead to long relaxation times, and even to multiple time constants as different physical mechanisms become dominant. Due to baseline offsets and slow recovery, the AC performance of elastomeric sensors can be better than their DC performance. These memory issues have been considered highly undesirable [22, 28] because it increases demands on signal processing. However, given the difficulty of designing soft materials without memory effects, while also meeting all the other performance demands, these issues may nevertheless best be handled in software, particularly with rapid advances in learning algorithms. (For EIT-based sensors, see section 2.6.4.) Moreover, learning is the approach taken by biological systems: our tissue has hysteresis, yet our neural networks handle it. ML is now able to compensate for complex behaviors due to pressure or strain histories [118], as can event-driven signal output [17]. ML is also being put to use in handling nonlinear signals, non-uniform materials (due to imperfect mixing, anisotropy, bubbles, damage, and other imperfections, which may be difficult to measure and model), and strains induced by the tactile contacts themselves or by bending of a robot limb. Relaxing the requirements on the sensors may speed implementation of tactile systems. However, some issues may be only partially amenable by software, such as slow material response times.

Offloading sensor requirements to the surrounding physical system has also been used to good effect. For example, a layer of foam under the sensing layer makes the system robust to impact [164], and layers of foam can also increase the dynamic range [167]. The use of protective coverings [195, 218] relieves the requirement on the sensor to be damage-resistant.

Calibration of sensors is rarely discussed. A sensor may experience drift due to memory effects, humidity, temperature, and gradual degradation. Its readings may be influenced by variations in positioning, electrode placement, sensor layer thickness and homogeneity, stiffness of the underlying substrate, or thickness of overlying protective layers. Readings may change based on deformations or slip during robot motion. For arrays of sensors, there is inter-device variability. Initial and periodic calibration is therefore needed, preferably in some rapid and automated way, *in situ*, that does not require much human effort. Robot self-calibration of its sensors by touches at known locations was suggested in [219]. For wearable devices, calibration may need to be performed for each individual person.

More attention is needed on the following aspects of sensor performance:

- Lifetime. Testing, if done at all, is typically to an upper limit of only a few thousand cycles.
- Repeatability. Sensor-to-sensor and day-to-day variability are not typically measured.
- Environmental sensitivity. Changes in performance due to temperature and humidity are rarely studied [41].
- Dependability. This is a high-level requirement without clear tests or simple metrics.

1.5.2 Application-level

> *One possible reason for the comparatively slow progress in tactile sensing technology is the prevailing focus of the majority of the researchers on high spatial resolution and sensitivity, instead of a concentration on implementable sensor systems…* [164]

Implementation challenges arise from hardware issues that may initially seem mundane, as well as from signal analysis. As is evident from the large number of proposed skin designs, both the electro-mechanical interfaces and the output data formats take a large variety of forms, so each implementation risks being unique rather than generalizable. In addition, from a new user's perspective, devices that are at the research prototype stage are risky and involve a steep learning curve, the payoff of which is unclear. On top of that, the substantial effort of putting together a complex system, when weighed against the possible usefulness of the information that may be gained, has generally not been deemed worthwhile by roboticists. Devices that make their way onto robots more typically consist of off-the-shelf-components that can be applied using standard processes, like soldering. The adoption of e-skin technologies will require closer collaboration between developers and users, and consider users' current workflows, experience, and expertise.

Soft sensors, particularly polymer-carbon composites, are often cross-responsive to multiple stimuli: temperature and humidity can strongly affect their output [220–222]. While cross-sensitivity has been promoted as 'multifunctional', in practice there is a need to decouple or compensate confounding influences. Sensors combined together in a skin can also interfere with each other [52], mechanically and electrically. There has been little discussion of compensation, although ML has been proposed for handling complex inputs from a variety of stimuli [39]. The use of a reference sensor that remains unstrained can be effective for environmental compensation [223], and efforts to develop strain-independent pressure sensors have also been successful [131].

Power is a much-examined and critical consideration, especially for portable, wearable, and implantable systems [65]. Resistive sensors in particular draw power continuously, and signal processing and transmission can require significant power. For some devices, such as those that are skin-attached, power delivery can be wireless. While batteries are typically used in autonomous applications, energy harvesting is also being considered, as discussed in [30, 51], including photovoltaic and thermoelectric solutions, but the energy harvesting efficiency is low and needs to be improved [53, 57, 61]. Low-power circuit design is the focus of much work [61]. Power solutions strongly depend on the use case and environment. A human may not tolerate the bulk and weight of a power source used for a humanoid robot, and wireless energy may be infeasible for an autonomous system. In all cases, however, reduction of the required power during operation will be important for real-world implementations.

Relatively little attention has been paid to the electro-mechanical challenge of making robust connections between a soft sensor material and the metal wires going to the electronics system. It has been noted that electrical connections have been largely ignored and that wiring remains a key issue [2]. In the related field of e-textiles, connectors were described in [10, 183]: in that field also, connectors remained an open field of research with each solution customized to an application. Some more recent e-textile reviews have been mute on the issue [54, 184, 185], but the Institute of Printed Circuits (IPC) has a sub-committee working on IPC-8941, Guideline for Connectors for E-Textiles to cover connector types, materials, and processes [186]. Interconnects are a problem because conventional processes such as soldering are generally incompatible with stretchable substrates. Thus, alligator clips are often employed as a temporary expedient. Press-fit connections have also been employed, but they have been found to be unsatisfactory and too bulky. Silver epoxy is also used, although there may be a mechanical stiffness mismatch at the interface that can span orders of magnitude, leading to significant stress concentrations there and thus interconnect failure. Discontinuities in elastic modulus (which go from as little as 10 Pa for gels and 10^6 Pa for PDMS up to 10^{11} Pa for metals [4]) can lead to delamination even under low strain. Modulus gradients (see e.g. [224]) can ameliorate the stress concentrations but are not straightforward to produce. Liquid metals can accommodate strains at the interface, but they require encapsulation. The lack of general-purpose, off the shelf solutions to making connections, and also reversible disconnecting, remains a significant hurdle for applications.

As mentioned previously, for tactile skins, as for other systems, the characteristics of most importance are task or application-dependent [213]. In a typical product development process, the first steps include identification of a market need and ranking the requirements of the corresponding users and other stakeholders. This information provides the designer with a means to navigate among the numerous trade-offs that must be made. For example, tactile sensors made from non-woven fabrics show greater repeatability in imaging than woven fabrics [169], but high stretchability is also important and non-wovens can undergo little strain. Some of the vexing trade-offs include the following [51, 64, 91, 169, 213, 214]:

- sensitivity versus linearity;
- accuracy versus softness;
- sensor resolution versus number of electrodes, versus frame rate, versus area;
- coverage or density versus bandwidth, versus electrical cross-talk;
- technological capability versus fabrication cost, versus wearability;
- multi-functionality versus cross-sensitivity.

In some cases, conflicting goals must both be satisfied, for example for high sensitivity and collision tolerance [164]. The designer must therefore ask, for a given application what is 'good enough'? What is an acceptable tradeoff between manufacturability and performance for this specific envisioned product? For EIT sensors, for instance, is the advantage of the ease of fabricating an entirely soft resistive sensor with a relatively small number of electrodes at the perimeter worth the cost of relatively high power consumption and coarser resolution than another system?

Decisions must be made concerning how much capability is required to substantially improve performance over existing systems. As noted, achieving a multifunctional e-skin with large area and high resolution is challenging [62]. So, if the most important use of an e-skin is tactile imaging, should work focus on making a uni-functional skin, given that even those have not yet been commercialized? The tendency has instead been to put a large number of requirements on the sensor, resulting in complex fabrication. The field may have allowed the perfect to become the enemy of the good, keeping it from moving substantially forward. Alternatively, the balance between performance and cost may simply be unacceptable at the present state of technology development.

1.5.3 System-level

> *Despite the experimentation with a wide spectrum of transduction methods, materials, and innovative designs, touch sensing has not made much headway in robotic applications.* [213]

The need for a systems-level approach to move beyond laboratory prototypes has been clear for some time. In particular, Dahiya *et al* [2, 6, 7] have pointed out the substantial problems that must be solved for tactile skins to be able to imbue a 'sense of touch' to robots, prosthetics, and other devices. The solutions require a holistic or system-level approach and co-design with users. Development of e-skins requires collaboration across disciplines [52, 59], including material science, mechanical, electrical, and systems engineering, mathematics, robotics and mechatronics, and computer science, among others. The unresolved problems include wiring, power consumption, integration, handling large amounts of data in real time, and usefully processing the data, along with manufacturability, robustness, and maintainability of the overall system [213].

1.5.3.1 Integration

The performance of an e-skin is determined not only by its sensing elements, but also by the way they are combined [213], both with each other and with the system their information supports. Although applications of e-skins require less stringent device tolerances and lower speed than integrated circuits [60], large-scale integration is still a challenge [65]. One aspect is a 'packaging' problem. It involves electrical routing of a large number of connections to devices all over the surface, including over joints, so stretchability of the wire harnesses must be considered [22]. The skins and any protective layers need to be fitted onto the larger system, also over joints [99]. Sensors may give weak signals that require local amplification before transmission, and the signal may also benefit from local digitization, requiring an A/D converter. Expanding from one sensor to a network of them has repercussions on the performance. The large number of interconnects leads to signal cross-talk (interference) [17], which has been identified as the most significant and challenging problem [63]. Interconnections also introduce electromagnetic noise, since wires serve as antennas. Keeping noise at a minimum is critical for EIT, as discussed in chapter 6, to generate images without either artefacts or severe distortion. Shielding must therefore be considered. Just mounting all the hardware properly is thus a challenge.

A collection of sensors spread over the surface needs to be formed into an integrated network to be of use [225]. Their power needs and data generated must be managed alongside that of cameras and other sensors, and of motion controllers. The design of a successful scheme must consider system aspects such as distributed computing, networking, robustness, and maintainability [213]. It must also consider what the system will do with the tactile information it receives, whether communication, maneuvering, or learning how to perform a task.

1.5.3.2 Information processing and use

Once assembled, the system must processing large amounts of information, deciphering tactile signals from one or more e-skins. Simple determinations include detecting a signal peak that indicates a contact. Higher level tasks include classification of shapes, gestures, and poses [59] or discriminating human motion from environmental conditions [60]. Beyond that, processing data from spatially distributed e-skins can be used to construct a 'world model' [213], which might be created by machine learning through physical exploration. Achieving 'perception' was reviewed in [59], including the use of synaptic transistors and devices with memory, as well as conventional CMOS computation. Challenges were identified as: limited computational ability, immaturity of system-level integration, unreliability of sensor signals, and high power consumption.

Obtaining information from the streams of sensor data in such a way that it can be acted upon with low latency has been another issue. It was noted that the RI-MAN robot had a feedback control time of 20 ms, which was deemed insufficient [226]. Research is being done on algorithms to shorten tactile feedback response times [227].

As noted above, beyond the copious amounts of data coming from just the e-skin, additional data may also be needed from cameras, motors, and other hardware to gather information, carry out tasks, and make decisions. Sensor data fusion, combining signals from different sensory modalities, is another area that is seeing much work [62, 213]. There have been some calls for standardization of interfaces and data formats, which would require greater coordination between developers and users.

There has been much recent work on machine learning. The development of edge AI chips offer the possibility to realize the goal of artificial skin perception [59]. Transferability of ML models generated on various systems is therefore also now a consideration [62].

1.5.3.3 Robustness

E-skin may experience wear and tear. While self-healing has been demonstrated [65], this capability is atypical [52, 53]. Thus, at the system level damaged sensors or connectors need to identified and dealt with. Routing around them is an option, as is repair or exchange. If a sensor repair must be effected, the method should be straightforward and verifiable [223]. Otherwise, the system must be designed to permit facile replacement.

1.5.3.4 Manufacturing

There has been increasing recognition of the need for economic manufacturability of e-skins (see e.g. [34, 41, 52, 57, 60, 63, 65, 66, 228]). The primary commercialization challenges have been identified as high cost, complex designs, and fragility [229]. Scalable approaches are required to produce large-area soft devices with good yield and reliability. Nevertheless, research has often remained siloed, focused on single-metric device-level improvements, despite the fact that stretchability, resolution, and sensitivity have not been the limiting factors to adoption. Some of the approaches to improved performance, for example arrays of FETs, microstructured surfaces, or encapsulated liquids, have required laborious multi-step processing and assembly with custom-made materials and specialized equipment, with registration and uniformity required over large areas. Some devices, despite their performance, may be simply too complicated to see realization outside the lab. Thus, roboticists and other engineers who wish to deploy the sensors in system prototypes have not had access to enough of them, and co-development between end-users and manufacturers has not been systematically pursued.

1.6 Outlook for tactile e-skins

Many groups in diverse fields have been working toward the realization of tactile e-skins, using a wide range of approaches and leading to significant advances in capability [40, 41]. The basic requirements for e-skin, such as stretchability and imaging ability, have largely been met. Yet despite longstanding and enthusiastic declarations in the literature that there is an enormous demand for e-skins, and assertions of their importance for vaguely-posed applications, the 'killer app' that will drive commercialization has yet to be unidentified, although in the skin-wearables arena, health monitoring of cardiovascular conditions is mentioned most frequently. Despite a 2018 commercial report projecting the market value of e-skin to be nearly $500M in 2020 [230], and another projecting $35B by 2030 [229], tactile e-skins remain at the research stage [64] and there is still a dearth of available products. The application of tactile sensing that has reached the market is therapy robots, such as the pettable toy Paro. E-skins with more sophisticated capability have not seen widespread adoption, due largely to obstacles in going from small lab demonstrations to system deployment in the real world. Challenges still to be addressed include power and integration. The simplicity of EIT-based tactile imaging hardware, as will be discussed in chapter 2, could facilitate integration. Given the challenges identified above and because of difficulties in funding and publishing solutions to practical problems, the pull of a successful commercial product and collaboration between academia and industry is likely to be required to spur such work.

References

[1] Dargahi J and Najarian S 2004 Human tactile perception as a standard for artificial tactile sensing—a review *Int. J. Med. Robot. Comput. Assist. Surg.* **1** 23–35

[2] Dahiya R S, Metta G, Valle M and Sandini G 2010 Tactile sensing—from humans to humanoids *IEEE Trans. Robot.* **26** 1–20

[3] Rogers J A, Someya T and Huang Y G 2010 Materials and mechanics for stretchable electronics *Science* **327** 1603–7

[4] Wagner S and Bauer S 2012 Materials for stretchable electronics *MRS Bull.* **37** 207–17

[5] Benight S J, Wang C, Tok J B H and Bao Z A 2013 Stretchable and self-healing polymers and devices for electronic skin *Prog. Polym. Sci.* **38** 1961–77

[6] Dahiya R S, Mittendorfer P, Valle M, Cheng G and Lumelsky V J 2013 Directions toward effective utilization of tactile skin: a review *IEEE Sensors J.* **13** 4121–38

[7] Dahiya R S and Valle M 2013 Tactile sensing technologies *Robotic Tactile Sensing: Technologies and System* ed R S Dahiya and M Valle (Dordrecht, Netherlands: Springer) pp 79–136

[8] Hammock M L, Chortos A, Tee B C K, Tok J B H and Bao Z A 2013 25th anniversary article: the evolution of electronic skin (e-skin): a brief history, design considerations, and recent progress *Adv. Mater.* **25** 5997–6037

[9] Lucarotti C, Oddo C M, Vitiello N and Carrozza M C 2013 Synthetic and bio-artificial tactile sensing: a review *Sensors* **13** 1435–66

[10] Castano L M and Flatau A B 2014 Smart fabric sensors and e-textile technologies: a review *Smart Mater. Struct.* **23**

[11] Chortos A and Bao Z 2014 Skin-inspired electronic devices *Mater. Today* **17** 321–31

[12] Silvera-Tawil D, Rye D, Soleimani M and Velonaki M 2015 Electrical impedance tomography for artificial sensitive robotic skin: a review *IEEE Sensors J.* **15** 2001–16

[13] Silvera-Tawil D, Rye D and Velonaki M 2015 Artificial skin and tactile sensing for socially interactive robots: a review *Robot. Auton. Syst.* **63** 230–43

[14] van den Brand J, de Kok M, Koetse M, Cauwe M, Verplancke R, Bossuyt F, Jablonski M and Vanfleteren J 2015 Flexible and stretchable electronics for wearable health devices *Sol. State Electron.* **113** 116–20

[15] Wang X, Dong L, Zhang H, Yu R, Pan C and Wang Z L 2015 Recent progress in electronic skin *Adv. Sci.* **2** 1500169

[16] Yogeswaran N *et al* 2015 New materials and advances in making electronic skin for interactive robots *Adv. Robot.* **29** 1359–73

[17] Chortos A, Liu J and Bao Z A 2016 Pursuing prosthetic electronic skin *Nat. Mater.* **15** 937–50

[18] Dagdeviren C, Joe P, Tuzman O L, Park K-I, Lee K J, Shi Y, Huang Y and Rogers J A 2016 Recent progress in flexible and stretchable piezoelectric devices for mechanical energy harvesting, sensing and actuation *Extreme Mech. Lett.* **9** 269–81

[19] Natale L and Cannata G 2017 Tactile sensing *Humanoid Robotics: A Reference* ed A Goswami and P Vadakkepat (Dordrecht, Netherlands: Springer) pp 1–24

[20] Wang X, Liu Z and Zhang T 2017 Flexible sensing electronics for wearable/attachable health monitoring *Small* **13** 1602790

[21] Heo J S, Eom J, Kim Y-H and Park S K 2018 Recent progress of textile-based wearable electronics: a comprehensive review of materials, devices, and applications *Small* **14** 1703034

[22] Ibrahim A, Pinna L, Seminara L and Valle M 2018 Achievements and open issues toward embedding tactile sensing and interpretation into electronic skin systems *Material-Integrated Intelligent Systems: Technology and Applications* ed S Bosse, D Lehmhus, M Busse and W Lang (Weinheim: Wiley-VCH Verlag GmbH & Co. KGaA) pp 571–93

[23] Liu H *et al* 2018 Electrically conductive polymer composites for smart flexible strain sensors: a critical review *J. Mater. Chem.* C **6** 12121–41

[24] Wallin T J, Pikul J and Shepherd R F 2018 3D printing of soft robotic systems *Nat. Rev. Mater.* **3** 84–100

[25] Wang S, Oh J Y, Xu J, Tran H and Bao Z 2018 Skin-inspired electronics: an emerging paradigm *Acc. Chem. Res.* **51** 1033–45

[26] Xu F, Li X, Shi Y, Li L, Wang W, He L and Liu R 2018 Recent developments for flexible pressure sensors: a review *Micromachines* **9** 580

[27] Almansoori M T, Li X and Zheng L 2019 A brief review on e-skin and its multifunctional sensing applications *Curr. Smart. Mater.* **4** 3–14

[28] Chen J, Yu Q, Cui X, Dong M, Zhang J, Wang C, Fan J, Zhu Y and Guo Z 2019 An overview of stretchable strain sensors from conductive polymer nanocomposites *J. Mater. Chem.* C **7** 11710–30

[29] Dahiya R 2019 E-skin: from humanoids to humans *Proc. IEEE* **107** 247–52

[30] García Núñez C, Manjakkal L and Dahiya R 2019 Energy autonomous electronic skin *npj Flex. Electron* **3** 1

[31] Iskarous M M and Thakor N V 2019 E-skins: biomimetic sensing and encoding for upper limb prostheses *Proc. IEEE* **107** 2052–64

[32] Jiang C, Cheng X and Nathan A 2019 Flexible ultralow-power sensor interfaces for e-skin *Proc. IEEE* **107** 2084–105

[33] Kumar K S, Chen P Y and Ren H L 2019 A review of printable fexible and stretchable tactile sensors *Research* **2019** 3018568

[34] Li J-a, Ma Z, Wang H-t, Gao X-x, Zhou Z, Tao R-w, Pan L-j and Shi Y 2019 Skin-inspired electronics and its applications in advanced intelligent systems *Adv. Intell. Syst.* **1** 1900063

[35] Miao P, Wang J, Zhang C, Sun M, Cheng S and Liu H 2019 Graphene nanostructure-based tactile sensors for electronic skin applications *Nano-Micro Lett.* **11** 71

[36] Park H, Lee D, Park G, Park S, Khan S, Kim J and Kim W 2019 Energy harvesting using thermoelectricity for IoT (internet of things) and e-skin sensors *J. Phys.: Energy* **1** 042001

[37] Takei K, Gao W, Wang C and Javey A 2019 Physical and chemical sensing with electronic skin *Proc. IEEE* **107** 2155–67

[38] Wang B and Facchetti A 2019 Mechanically flexible conductors for stretchable and wearable e-skin and e-textile devices *Adv. Mater.* **31** 1901408

[39] Xie M, Hisano K, Zhu M, Toyoshi T, Pan M, Okada S, Tsutsumi O, Kawamura S and Bowen C 2019 Flexible multifunctional sensors for wearable and robotic applications *Adv. Mater. Technol.* **4** 1800626

[40] Yang J C, Mun J, Kwon S Y, Park S, Bao Z and Park S 2019 Electronic skin: recent progress and future prospects for skin-attachable devices for health monitoring, robotics, and prosthetics *Adv. Mater.* **31** 1904765

[41] Xu K, Lu Y and Takei K 2019 Multifunctional skin-inspired flexible sensor systems for wearable electronics *Adv. Mater. Technol.* **4** 1800628

[42] Chen W and Yan X 2020 Progress in achieving high-performance piezoresistive and capacitive flexible pressure sensors: a review *J. Mater. Sci. Tech.* **43** 175–88

[43] dos Santos A, Fortunato E, Martins R, Águas H and Igreja R 2020 Transduction mechanisms, micro-structuring techniques, and applications of electronic skin pressure sensors: a review of recent advances *Sensors* **20** 4407

[44] Ganesh R S, Yoon H-J and Kim S-W 2020 Recent trends of biocompatible triboelectric nanogenerators toward self-powered e-skin *EcoMat* **2** e12065

[45] Lee Y, Park J, Choe A, Cho S, Kim J and Ko H 2020 Mimicking human and biological skins for multifunctional skin electronics *Adv. Funct. Mater.* **30** 1904523

[46] Liu K, Wu Y, Wang S, Wang H, Chen H, Chen B and Yao J 2020 Artificial sensitive skin for robotics based on electrical impedance tomography *Adv. Intell. Syst.* **2** 1900161

[47] Liu H, Guo D, Sun F, Yang W, Furber S and Sun T 2020 Embodied tactile perception and learning *Brain Sci. Adv.* **6** 132–58

[48] Shih B, Shah D, Li J, Thuruthel T G, Park Y-L, Iida F, Bao Z, Kramer-Bottiglio R and Tolley M T 2020 Electronic skins and machine learning for intelligent soft robots *Sci. Robot* **5** eaaz9239

[49] Tallman T N and Smyl D J 2020 Structural health and condition monitoring via electrical impedance tomography in self-sensing materials: a review *Smart Mater. Struct.* **29** 25

[50] Zhang S, Li S, Xia Z and Cai K 2020 A review of electronic skin: soft electronics and sensors for human health *J. Mater. Chem.* B **8** 852–62

[51] Bunea A-C, Dediu V, Laszlo E A, Pistriţu F, Carp M, Iliescu F S, Ionescu O N and Iliescu C 2021 E-skin: the dawn of a new era of on-body monitoring systems *Micromachines* **12** 1091

[52] Chen J, Zhu Y, Chang X, Pan D, Song G, Guo Z and Naik N 2021 Recent progress in essential functions of soft electronic skin *Adv. Funct. Mater.* **31** 2104686

[53] Guo Y, Wei X, Gao S, Yue W, Li Y and Shen G 2021 Recent advances in carbon material-based multifunctional sensors and their applications in electronic skin systems *Adv. Funct. Mater.* **31** 2104288

[54] Komolafe A *et al* 2021 E-textile technology review—from materials to application *IEEE Access* **9** 97152–79

[55] Li D, Yao K, Gao Z, Liu Y and Yu X 2021 Recent progress of skin-integrated electronics for intelligent sensing *Light: Adv. Manuf.* **2** 39–58

[56] Oh H S, Lee C H, Kim N K, An T and Kim G H 2021 Review: sensors for biosignal/health monitoring in electronic skin *Polymers* **13** 2478

[57] Pierre Claver U and Zhao G 2021 Recent progress in flexible pressure sensors based electronic skin *Adv. Eng. Mater.* **23** 2001187

[58] Scaffaro R, Maio A and Citarrella M C 2021 Ionic tactile sensors as promising biomaterials for artificial skin: review of latest advances and future perspectives *Eur. Polym. J.* **151** 110421

[59] Wang M, Luo Y, Wang T, Wan C, Pan L, Pan S, He K, Neo A and Chen X 2021 Artificial skin perception *Adv. Mater.* **33** 2003014

[60] Wang L, Jiang K and Shen G 2021 Wearable, implantable, and interventional medical devices based on smart electronic skins *Adv. Mater. Technol.* **6** 2100107

[61] Chen Y, Gao Z, Zhang F, Wen Z and Sun X 2022 Recent progress in self-powered multifunctional e-skin for advanced applications *Exploration* **2** 20210112

[62] Gao S, Dai Y and Nathan A 2022 Tactile and vision perception for intelligent humanoids *Adv. Intell. Syst.* **4** 2100074

[63] Li W-D *et al* 2022 Recent advances in multiresponsive flexible sensors towards e-skin: a delicate design for versatile sensing *Small* **18** 2103734

[64] Lin J-C, Liatsis P and Alexandridis P 2022 Flexible and stretchable electrically conductive polymer materials for physical sensing applications *Polym. Rev.* **63** 67–126

[65] Nie B, Liu S, Qu Q, Zhang Y, Zhao M and Liu J 2022 Bio-inspired flexible electronics for smart e-skin *Acta Biomater.* **139** 280–95

[66] Zarei M, Lee G, Lee S G and Cho K 2022 Advances in biodegradable electronic skin: material progress and recent applications in sensing, robotics, and human–machine interfaces *Adv. Mater.* **35** 2203193

[67] Zhao S and Ahn J-H 2022 Rational design of high-performance wearable tactile sensors utilizing bioinspired structures/functions, natural biopolymers, and biomimetic strategies *Mat. Sci. Eng.* R **148** 100672

[68] Luo Y *et al* 2023 Technology roadmap for flexible sensors *ACS Nano* **17** 5211–95

[69] Mengüç Y, Park Y-L, Pei H, Vogt D, Aubin P M, Winchell E, Fluke L, Stirling L, Wood R J and Walsh C J 2014 Wearable soft sensing suit for human gait measurement *Int. J. Robot. Res.* **33** 1748–64

[70] Wang P, Liu J, Yu W, Li G, Meng C and Guo S 2022 Flexible, stretchable, breathable and sweatproof all-nanofiber iontronic tactile sensor for continuous and comfortable knee joint motion monitoring *Nano Energy* **103 Part A** 107768

[71] Shi G, Zhao Z, Pai J-H, Lee I, Zhang L, Stevenson C, Ishara K, Zhang R, Zhu H and Ma J 2016 Highly sensitive, wearable, durable strain sensors and stretchable conductors using graphene/silicon rubber composites *Adv. Funct. Mater.* **26** 7614–25

[72] Carpi F and Rossi D D 2005 Electroactive polymer-based devices for e-textiles in biomedicine *IEEE Trans. Inf. Technol. Biomed.* **9** 295–318

[73] Araki T, Nogi M, Suganuma K, Kogure M and Kirihara O 2011 Printable and stretchable conductive wirings comprising silver flakes and elastomers *IEEE Elect. Dev. Lett.* **32** 1424–6

[74] Chossat J B, Tao Y W, Duchaine V and Park Y L 2015 Wearable soft artificial skin for hand motion detection with embedded microfluidic strain sensing *IEEE Int. Conf. Robotics and Automation (ICRA) (Seattle, WA, May 26–30)* pp 2568–73

[75] Hammond F L, Menguc Y and Wood R J 2014 Toward a modular soft sensor-embedded glove for human hand motion and tactile pressure measurement *2014 IEEE/RSJ Int. Conf. Intelligent Robots and Systems (IROS 2014)* 4000–7

[76] Carneiro M R and Tavakoli M 2021 Wearable pressure mapping through piezoresistive C-PU foam and tailor-made stretchable e-textile *IEEE Sensors J.* **21** 27374–84

[77] Yang J, Liu S, Meng Y, Xu W, Liu S, Jia L, Chen G, Qin Y, Han M and Li X 2022 Self-powered tactile sensor for gesture recognition using deep learning algorithms *Appl. Mater. Interfaces* **14** 25629–37

[78] Kim D H *et al* 2011 Epidermal electronics *Science* **333** 838–43

[79] Schwartz G, Tee B C K, Mei J G, Appleton A L, Kim D H, Wang H L and Bao Z N 2013 Flexible polymer transistors with high pressure sensitivity for application in electronic skin and health monitoring *Nature Commun.* **4** 1859

[80] Kramer R K, Majidi C and Wood R J 2011 Wearable tactile keypad with stretchable artificial skin *IEEE Int. Conf. Robotics and Automation (ICRA) (Shanghai, 9–13 May)* pp 1103–7

[81] Büscher G H, Kõiva R, Schürmann C, Haschke R and Ritter H J 2015 Flexible and stretchable fabric-based tactile sensor *Robot. Auton. Syst.* **63** 244–52

[82] Wagner J, Morath H, Zhang J, Wieczorek F, Lüneburg L, Fitzek F H P and Nguyen G T 2022 Tactile electronics meets softwarised networks *IEEE 19th Ann. Consumer Communications & Networking Conf. (CCNC) (Las Vegas, NV, 8–11 Jan)* pp 961–2

[83] Ko S H and Rogers J 2021 Functional materials and devices for XR (VR/AR/MR) applications *Adv. Funct. Mater.* **31** 2106546f

[84] Xu J, Li X, Chang H, Zhao B, Tan X, Yang Y, Tian H, Zhang S and Ren T-L 2022 Electrooculography and tactile perception collaborative interface for 3D human–machine interaction *ACS Nano* **16** 6687–99

[85] Gerratt A P, Michaud H O and Lacour S P 2015 Elastomeric electronic skin for prosthetic tactile sensation *Adv. Funct. Mater.* **25** 2287–95

[86] Sareh S, Jiang A, Faragasso A, Noh Y, Nanayakkara T, Dasgupta P, Seneviratne L D, Wurdemann H A and Althoefer K 2014 Bio-inspired tactile sensor sleeve for surgical soft

manipulators *IEEE Int. Conf. Robotics and Automation (ICRA) (Hong Kong, China, 31 May–7 June)* pp 1454–9
[87] Nicholls H R (ed) 1992 *Advanced Tactile Sensing for Robotics* vol 5 (Singapore: World Scientific)
[88] Walt Disney Pictures 2014 Big Hero 6 (based on characters published by Marvel Comics)
[89] Roncone A, Hoffmann M, Pattacini U and Metta G 2015 Learning peripersonal space representation through artificial skin for avoidance and reaching with whole body surface *2015 IEEE/RSJ Int. Conf. Intelligent Robots and Systems (IROS) (Hamburg, 28 Sept–2 Oct)* pp 3366–73
[90] Nicholls H R and Lee M H 1989 A survey of robot tactile sensing technology *Int. J. Robot. Res.* **8** 3–30
[91] Yoshikai T, Fukushima H, Hayashi M and Inaba M 2009 Development of soft stretchable knit sensor for humanoids' whole-body tactile sensibility *9th IEEE-RAS International Conference on Humanoid Robots (Paris, 7–10 Dec)* pp 624–31
[92] Ye Z, Pang G, Xu K, Hou Z, Lv H, Shen Y and Yang G 2022 Soft robot skin with conformal adaptability for on-body tactile perception of collaborative robots *Robot. Auton. Lett.* **7** 5127–34
[93] Arents J, Abolins V, Judvaitis J, Vismanis O, Oraby A and Ozols K 2021 Human–robot collaboration trends and safety aspects: a systematic review *J. Sens. Act. Networks* **10** 48
[94] Ackerman 2018 Moxi prototype from diligent robotics starts helping out in hospitals *IEEE Spectr.* (Sept. 18)
[95] Ackerman 2020 Meet Moxie, a social robot that helps kids With social-emotional learning *IEEE Spectr.* (Apr 28)
[96] Miyagawa M, Kai Y, Yasuhara Y, Ito H, Betriana F, Tanioka T and Locsin R 2020 Consideration of safety management when using Pepper, a humanoid robot for care of older adults *Intel. Control Autom.* **11** 15–24
[97] Elkmann N, Fritzsche M and Schulenburg E 2011 Tactile sensing for safe physical human–robot interaction *ACHI 2011: 4th Int. Conf. Advances in Computer-Human Interactions (ACHI) (Gosier, Guadeloupe, Feb. 23–28)*
[98] Sekitani T and Someya T 2010 Stretchable, large-area organic electronics *Adv. Mater.* **22** 1–19
[99] Bhattacharjee T, Jain A, Vaish S, Killpack M D and Kemp C C 2013 Tactile sensing over articulated joints with stretchable sensors *World Haptics Conf. (WHC) (Daejeon, Korea, 14–17 April)* pp 103–8
[100] Armleder S, Dean-Leon E, Bergner F and Cheng G 2022 Interactive force control based on multimodal robot skin for physical human–robot collaboration *Adv. Intell. Syst.* **4** 2100047
[101] Ohmura Y and Kuniyoshi Y 2007 Humanoid robot which can lift a 30kg box by whole body contact and tactile feedback *2007 IEEE/RSJ Intl. Conf. Intelligent Robots and Systems (IROS 2007) (San Diego, CA, Oct. 29–Nov. 2)* pp 1136–41
[102] Yoshikai T, Hayashi M, Ishizaka Y, Sagisaka T and Inaba M 2007 Behavior integration for whole-body close interactions by a humanoid with soft sensor flesh *2007 7th IEEE-RAS International Conference on Humanoid Robots (29 Nov.–1 Dec. 2007)* pp 109–14
[103] Yoshikai T, Hayashi M, Ishizaka Y, Fukushima H, Kadowaki A, Sagisaka T, Kobayashi K, Kumagai I and Inaba M 2012 Development of robots with soft sensor flesh for achieving close interaction behavior *Adv. Artif. Intell.* **2012** 157642

[104] Pugach G, Melnyk A, Tolochko O, Pitti A and Gaussier P 2016 Touch-based admittance control of a robotic arm using neural learning of an artificial skin *IEEE/RSJ Int. Conf. Intelligent Robots and Systems (IROS) (Daejeon, Korea, 9–14 Oct)* pp 3374–80

[105] Ilievski F, Mazzeo A D, Shepherd R F, Chen X and Whitesides G M 2011 Soft robotics for chemists *Angew. Chem. Int. Ed.* **50** 1890–5

[106] Kim S, Laschi C and Trimmer B 2013 Soft robotics: a bioinspired evolution in robotics *Trends Biotechnol.* **31** 287–94

[107] Majidi C 2013 Soft robotics: a perspective - current trends and prospects for the future *Soft Robot.* **1** 5–11

[108] Rus D and Tolley M T 2015 Design, fabrication and control of soft robots *Nature* **521** 467–75

[109] Trivedi D, Rahn C D, Kier W M and Walker I D 2008 Soft robotics: biological inspiration, state of the art, and future research *Appl. Bionics Biomech.* **5** 520417

[110] Tondu B, Ippolito S, Guiochet J and Daidie A 2005 A seven-degrees-of-freedom robot-arm driven by pneumatic artificial muscles for humanoid robots *Int. J. Robot. Res.* **24** 257–74

[111] Amend J, Cheng N, Fakhouri S and Culley B 2016 Soft robotics commercialization: jamming grippers from research to product *Soft Robot.* **3** 213–22

[112] Kellaris N, Gopaluni Venkata V, Smith G M, Mitchell S K and Keplinger C 2018 Peano-HASEL actuators: muscle-mimetic, electrohydraulic transducers that linearly contract on activation *Sci. Robot.* **3** eaar3276

[113] Bauer S, Bauer-Gogonea S, Graz I, Kaltenbrunner M, Keplinger C and Schwödiauer R 2014 25th anniversary article: a soft future: from robots and sensor skin to energy harvesters *Adv. Mater.* **26** 149–62

[114] Mosadegh B, Polygerinos P, Keplinger C, Wennstedt S, Shepherd R F, Gupta U, Shim J, Bertoldi K, Walsh C J and Whitesides G M 2014 Pneumatic networks for soft robotics that actuate rapidly *Adv. Funct. Mater.* **24** 2163–70

[115] Marchese A D, Katzschmann R K and Rus D 2015 A recipe for soft fuidic elastomer robots *Soft Robot.* **2** 7–25

[116] Niiyama R, Sun X, Sung C, An B, Rus D and Kim S 2015 Pouch motors: printable soft actuators integrated with computational design *Soft Robot.* **2** 59–70

[117] Hines L, Petersen K, Lum G Z and Sitti M 2017 Soft actuators for small-scale robotics *Adv. Mater.* **1603483**

[118] Weerakoon L, Ye Z, Bama R S, Smela E, Yu M and Chopra N 2021 Adaptive tracking control of soft robots using integrated sensing skin and recurrent neural networks *IEEE Int. Conf. Robotics and Automation (ICRA) (Xi'an, China, 30 May-5 June)* pp 12170–6

[119] Argall B D and Billard A G 2010 A survey of tactile human–robot interactions *Robot. Auton. Syst.* **58** 1159–76

[120] Mukai T, Onishi M, Odashima T, Hirano S and Luo Z 2008 Development of the tactile sensor system of a human-interactive robot 'RI-MAN' *IEEE Trans. Robot.* **24** 505–12

[121] Tapus A, Mataric M and Scassellati B 2007 Socially assistive robotics [grand challenges of robotics] *Robot. Autom. Mag.* **14** 35–42

[122] Sharkey A and Wood N 2014 The Paro seal robot: demeaning or enabling *40th Ann. Conv. Society for the Study of Artificial Intelligence and the Simulation of Behaviour (AISB) (London, Apr 1–4) vol 36 p 2014*

[123] Wada K, Shibata T, Saito T and Tanie K 2002 Analysis of factors that bring mental effects to elderly people in robot assisted activity *IEEE/RSJ Int. Conf. Intelligent Robots and Systems* vol 2 *(Lausanne, 30 Sept.–4 Oct.)* pp 1152–7

[124] Petersen S, Houston S, Qin H, Tague C and Studley J 2017 The utilization of robotic pets in dementia care *J. Alzheimers Dis.* **55** 569–74

[125] Shibata T 2011 Life innovation with therapeutic robot, Paro *Innovation. Perspectives for the 21st Century* (Seville: BBVA) pp 351–63

[126] The Edge CNBC 2018 This robotic therapy seal is revolutionizing elderly care (https://www.cnbc.com/video/2018/10/02/robotic-therapy-seal-paro-is-revolutionizing-elderly-care.html)

[127] Stiehl W D, Lieberman J, Breazeal C, Basel L, Lalla L and Wolf M 2005 Design of a therapeutic robotic companion for relational, affective touch *IEEE Intl. Workshop on Robot and Human Interactive Communication (ROMAN 2005) (Nashville, TN, 13–15 Aug)* pp 408–15

[128] Block A E and Kuchenbecker K J 2017 Physical and behavioral factors improve robot hug quality *26th IEEE International Symposium on Robot and Human Interactive Communication (RO-MAN) (Lisbon, Aug 28–Sept 1)*

[129] Block A E and Kuchenbecker K J 2019 Softness, warmth, and responsiveness improve robot hugs *Int. J. Soc. Robot.* **11** 49–64

[130] Park K, Yuk H, Yang M, Cho J, Lee H and Kim J 2022 A biomimetic elastomeric robot skin using electrical impedance and acoustic tomography for tactile sensing *Sci. Robot* **7** eabm7187

[131] Nagakubo A, Alirezaei H and Kuniyoshi Y 2007 A deformable and deformation sensitive tactile distribution sensor *IEEE Int. Conf. Robot. Biomimetics (ROBIO) (Sanya, China, Dec. 15–18)* pp 1301–8

[132] Tawil D S, Rye D and Velonaki M 2011 Touch modality interpretation for an EIT-based sensitive skin *2011 IEEE Int. Conf Robotics and Automation (ICRA) (Shanghai, 9–13 May)* pp 3770–6

[133] Silvera-Tawil D, Rye D and Velonaki M 2014 Interpretation of social touch on an artificial arm covered with an EIT-based sensitive skin *Int. J. Soc. Robot.* **6** 489–505

[134] Takeda T, Hirata Y and Kosuge K 2007 Dance partner robot cooperative motion generation with adjustable length of dance step stride based on physical interaction *IEEE/RSJ Int. Conf. Intelligent Robots and Systems (IROS) (San Diego, CA, 29 Oct.–2 Nov)* pp 3258–63

[135] Fitter N T and Kuchenbecker K J 2016 Equipping the Baxter robot with human-inspired hand-clapping skills *25th IEEE Int. Symp. Robot and Human Interactive Communication (RO-MAN)* (New York: IEEE Press) pp 105–12

[136] Castro A, Silva F and Santos V 2021 Trends of human–robot collaboration in industry contexts: handover, learning, and metrics *Sensors* **21** 4113

[137] He B, Liu H, Xu C, Wang Y, Lu P and Zhou Y 2022 Whole-body compliant control of robot arms based on distributed flexible tactile electronic skin *Int. J. Human. Robot* https://doi.org/10.1142/S0219843622500141

[138] Hakozaki M, Oasa H and Shinoda H 1999 Telemetric robot skin *Proc. 1999 IEEE Int. Conf. Robotics and Automation* vol 2 *(Detroit, MI, 10–15 May 1999)* pp 957–61

[139] Cannata G, Maggiali M, Metta G and Sandini G 2008 An embedded artificial skin for humanoid robots *IEEE Int. Conf. Multisensor Fusion and Integration for Intelligent Systems (Seoul, 20–22 Aug)* pp 434–8

[140] Ohmura Y, Kuniyoshi Y and Nagakubo A 2006 Conformable and scalable tactile sensor skin for curved surfaces *Proc. IEEE Int. Conf. Robotics and Automation (ICRA) (Orlando, FL, 15–19 May)* pp 1348–53

[141] Vidal-Verdú F, Barquero M J, Castellanos-Ramos J, Navas-González R, Sánchez J A, Serón J and García-Cerezo A 2011 A large area tactile sensor patch based on commercial force sensors *Sensors* **11** 5489–507

[142] Yoshikai T, Hayashi M, Ishizaka Y, Fukushima H, Kadowaki A, Sagisaka T, Kobayashi K, Kumagai I and Inaba M 2012 Development of robots with soft sensor flesh for achieving close interaction behavior *Adv. Artif. Intell.* **2012** 157642

[143] Hoshi T and Shinoda H 2006 Robot skin based on touch-area-sensitive tactile element *Proc. IEEE Intl. Conf. Robotics and Automation (ICRA 2006) (15–19 May 2006)* pp 3463–8

[144] Lacasse M-a and Duchaine V 2010 Characterization of the electrical resistance of carbon-black-filled silicone: application to a flexible and stretchable robot skin *IEEE Conf. on Robotics and Automation (ICRA) (Anchorage, AL, May 3–8)* pp 4842–8

[145] Kim J, Park D, Moon S, Park C, Thiyagarajan K, Choi S, Hwang H and Jeong U 2022 Omnidirectional tactile profiling using a deformable pressure sensor array based on localized piezoresistivity *Adv. Mater. Technol.* **7** 2100688

[146] Vu C C and Kim J 2020 Simultaneous sensing of touch and pressure by using highly eastic e-fabrics *Appl. Sci.* **10** 989

[147] Takei K, Takahashi T, Ho J C, Ko H, Gillies A G, Leu P W, Fearing R S and Javey A 2010 Nanowire active-matrix circuitry for low-voltage macroscale artificial skin *Nat. Mater.* **9** 821–6

[148] Hughes D and Correll N 2015 Texture recognition and localization in amorphous robotic skin *Bioinspir. Biomim.* **10** 055002

[149] Portaro M, Brittany R and Harnett C 2022 Characterizing the pressure response of microstructured materials for soft optical skins *MRS Adv.* **7** 538–42

[150] Yao S and Zhu Y 2015 Nanomaterial-enabled stretchable conductors: strategies, materials and devices *Adv. Mater.* **27** 1480–511

[151] Hong S, Lee S and Kim D H 2019 Materials and design strategies of stretchable electrodes for electronic skin and its applications *Proc. IEEE* **107** 2185–97

[152] Park H, Jeong Y R, Yun J, Hong S Y, Jin S, Lee S-J, Zi G and Ha J S 2015 Stretchable array of highly sensitive pressure sensors consisting of polyaniline nanofibers and Au-coated polydimethylsiloxane micropillars *ACS Nano* **9** 9974–85

[153] Lipomi D J, Vosgueritchian M, Tee B C-K, Hellstrom S L, Lee J A, Fox C H and Bao Z 2011 Skin-like pressure and strain sensors based on transparent elastic films of carbon nanotubes *Nature Nanotech.* **6** 788–92

[154] Lacour S P, Wagner S, Huang Z Y and Suo Z 2003 Stretchable gold conductors on elastomeric substrates *Appl. Phys. Lett.* **82** 2404–6

[155] Graz I M, Cotton D P J and Lacour S P 2009 Extended cyclic uniaxial loading of stretchable gold thin-films on elastomeric substrates *Appl. Phys. Lett.* **94** 071902

[156] Lacour S P, Jones J, Wagner S, Li T and Suo Z G 2005 Stretchable interconnects for elastic electronic surfaces *Proc. IEEE* **93** 1459–67

[157] He J, Zhou R, Zhang Y, Gao W, Chen T, Mai W and Pan C 2022 Strain-insensitive self-powered tactile sensor arrays based on intrinsically stretchable and patternable ultrathin conformal wrinkled graphene-elastomer composite *Adv. Funct. Mater.* **32** 2107281

[158] Sun Y G and Rogers J A 2007 Structural forms of single crystal semiconductor nanoribbons for high-performance stretchable electronics *J. Mater. Chem.* **17** 832–40
[159] Cheng M Y, Tsao C M, Lai Y Z and Yang Y J 2011 The development of a highly twistable tactile sensing array with stretchable helical electrodes *Sens. Actuators* A **166** 226–33
[160] Balakrisnan B, Nacev A, Burke J M, Dasgupta A and Smela E 2012 Design of compliant meanders for applications in MEMS, actuators, and flexible electronics *Smart Mater. Struct.* **21** 075033
[161] Ding Y, Xu T, Onyilagha O, Fong H and Zhu Z 2019 Recent advances in flexible and wearable pressure sensors based on piezoresistive 3D monolithic conductive sponges *Appl. Mater. Interfaces* **11** 6685–704
[162] Mannsfeld S C B, Tee B C K, Stoltenberg R M, Chen C V H H, Barman S, Muir B V O, Sokolov A N, Reese C and Bao Z N 2010 Highly sensitive flexible pressure sensors with microstructured rubber dielectric layers *Nat. Mater.* **9** 859–64
[163] Choong C L *et al* 2014 Highly stretchable resistive pressure sensors using a conductive elastomeric composite on a micropyramid array *Adv. Mater.* **26** 3451–8
[164] Strohmayr M W, Worn H and Hirzinger G 2013 The DLR artificial skin, Step I: uniting sensitivity and collision tolerance *2013 IEEE Int. Conf. Robotics and Automation (ICRA) (Karlsruhe, May 6–10)* pp 1012–8
[165] Oh J, Yang J C, Kim J-O, Park H, Kwon S Y, Lee S, Sim J Y, Oh H W, Kim J and Park S 2018 Pressure insensitive strain sensor with facile solution-based process for tactile sensing applications *ACS Nano* **12** 7546–53
[166] Pan L J, Chortos A, Yu G H, Wang Y Q, Isaacson S, Allen R, Shi Y, Dauskardt R and Bao Z N 2014 An ultra-sensitive resistive pressure sensor based on hollow-sphere microstructure induced elasticity in conducting polymer film *Nat. Commun.* **5** 3002
[167] Chen Y, Yu M, Bruck H A and Smela E 2018 Characterization of a compliant multi-layer system for tactile sensing with enhanced sensitivity and range *Smart Mater. Struct.* **27** 065005
[168] Barnett E M, Lofton J J, Yu M, Bruck H and Smela E 2017 Targeted feature recognition using mechanical spatial filtering with a low-cost compliant strain sensor *Sci. Rep.* **7** 5118
[169] Elsanadedy A 2012 Application of electrical impedance tomography to robotic tactile sensing *MS Thesis* Mechanical Engineering, Carleton University, Ottawa, Ontario, Canada
[170] Cochrane C, Koncar V, Lewandowski M and Dufour C 2007 Design and development of a flexible strain sensor for textile structures based on a conductive polymer composite *Sensors* **7** 473–92
[171] Sekitani T, Nakajima H, Maeda H, Fukushima T, Aida T, Hata K and Someya T 2009 Stretchable active-matrix organic light-emitting diode display using printable elastic conductors *Nat. Mater.* **8** 494–9
[172] Chen Y, Yu M, Bruck H A and Smela E 2018 Compliant multi-layer tactile sensing for enhanced identification of human touch *Smart Mater. Struct.* **27** 125009
[173] Cuasay L O M, Salazar F L M and Balela M D L 2022 Flexible tactile sensors based on silver nanowires: material synthesis, microstructuring, assembly, performance, and applications *Emerg. Mater.* **5** 51–76
[174] Wang Y, Gregory C and Minor M A 2018 Improving mechanical properties of molded silicone rubber for soft robotics through fabric compositing *Soft Robot.* **5** 272–90
[175] Chen Y, Deng Z, Ouyang R, Zheng R, Jiang Z, Bai H and Xue H 2021 3D printed stretchable smart fibers and textiles for self-powered e-skin *Nano Energy* **84** 105866

[176] Dai H B and Thostenson E T 2019 Large-area carbon nanotube-based flexible composites for ultra-wide range pressure sensing and spatial pressure mapping *ACS Appl. Mater. Interfaces* **11** 48370–80
[177] Alirezaei H, Nagakubo A and Kuniyoshi Y 2009 A tactile distribution sensor which enables stable measurement under high and dynamic stretch *IEEE Symp. 3D User Interfaces (Lafayette, LA, 14–15 March)* pp 87–93
[178] Bera T K, Mohamadou Y, Lee K, Wi H, Oh T I, Woo E J, Soleimani M and Seo J K 2014 Electrical impedance spectroscopy for electro-mechanical characterization of conductive fabrics *Sensors* **14** 9738–54
[179] Lee H, Park K, Kim J and Kuchenbecker K J 2021 Piezoresistive textile layer and distributed electrode structure for soft whole-body tactile skin *Smart Mater. Struct.* **30** 085036
[180] Avloni J and Henn A 2007 Development of new conductive and microwave lossy materials involving conducting polymer coatings *Polymers in Defence and Aerospace Applications (Toulouse, Sept 18–19)* (ChemTec) pp 16–9
[181] Grancarić A M, Jerković I, Koncar V, Cochrane C, Kelly F M, Soulat D and Legrand X 2017 Conductive polymers for smart textile applications *J. Indust. Textiles* **48** 612–42
[182] Pressure Profile Systems 2017 Application Blog, http://www.pressureprofile.com/application-blog/?category=TactArray#breast-cancer-apphttp://www.pressureprofile.com/tact-array-sensors
[183] Zeng W, Shu L, Li Q, Chen S, Wang F and Tao X-M 2014 Fiber-based wearable electronics: a review of materials, fabrication, devices, and applications *Adv. Mater.* **26** 5310–36
[184] Homayounfar S Z and Andrew T L 2020 Wearable sensors for monitoring human motion: a review on mechanisms, materials, and challenges *SLAS Technol.* **25** 9–24
[185] Zhou Z, Chen N, Zhong H, Zhang W, Zhang Y, Yin X and He B 2021 Textile-based mechanical sensors: a review *Materials* **14** 6073
[186] Zaman S U, Tao X, Cochrane C and Koncar V 2022 Smart e-textile systems: a review for healthcare applications *Electronics* **11** 99
[187] Cheng S, Narang Y S, Yang C, Suo Z and Howe R D 2019 Stick-on large-strain sensors for soft robots *Adv. Mater. Interfac.* **6** 1900985
[188] Majidi C, Kramer R and Wood R J 2011 A non-differential elastomer curvature sensor for softer-than-skin electronics *Smart Mater. Struct.* **20** 105017
[189] Park Y L, Chen B R and Wood R J 2012 Design and fabrication of soft artificial skin using embedded microchannels and liquid conductors *IEEE Sensors J.* **12** 2711–8
[190] Hammond F L, Kramer R K, Wan Q, Howe R D and Wood R J 2014 Soft tactile sensor arrays for force feedback in micromanipulation *IEEE Sensors J.* **14** 1443–52
[191] Judd E, Digumarti K M, Rossiter J and Hauser H 2020 NeatSkin: a discrete impedance tomography skin sensor *3rd IEEE Int. Conf. Soft Robotics (RoboSoft) (New Haven, CT, 15 May-15 July)* pp 33–8
[192] Oh J, Kim S, Lee S, Jeong S, Ko S H and Bae J 2021 A liquid metal based multimodal sensor and haptic feedback device for thermal and tactile sensation generation in virtual reality *Adv. Funct. Mater.* **31** 2007772
[193] Cho D, Bhuyan P, Sin D, Kim H, Kim E and Park S 2022 Stretchable, soft, and variable stiffness elastomer foam with positive and negative piezoresistivity enabled by liquid metal inclusion *Adv. Mater. Technol.* **7** 2101092

[194] Tawil D S, Rye D and Velonaki M 2011 Improved image reconstruction for an EIT-based sensitive skin with multiple internal electrodes *IEEE Trans. Robot.* **27** 425–35

[195] Tawil D S, Rye D and Velonaki M 2012 Interpretation of the modality of touch on an artificial arm covered with an EIT-based sensitive skin *Int. J. Robot. Res.* **31** 1627–41

[196] Yoshimoto S, Kuroda Y and Oshiro O 2020 Tomographic approach for universal tactile imaging with electromechanically coupled conductors *IEEE Trans. Ind. Electron.* **67** 627–36

[197] Wu H, Zheng B, Wang H and Ye J 2022 New flexible tactile sensor based on electrical impedance tomography *Micromachines* **13** 185

[198] Alirezaei H, Nagakubo A and Kuniyoshi Y 2007 A highly stretchable tactile distribution sensor for smooth surfaced humanoids *Humanoids '07: 7th IEEE-RAS Int. Conf. Humanoid Robots (Pittsburgh, PA, Nov. 29–Dec. 1)* pp 167–73

[199] Vandeparre H, Watson D and Lacour S P 2013 Extremely robust and conformable capacitive pressure sensors based on flexible polyurethane foams and stretchable metallization *Appl. Phys. Lett.* **103** 204103

[200] Li S, Liu G, Wen H, Liu G, Wang H, Ye M, Yang Y, Guo W and Liu Y 2022 A skin-like pressure- and vibration-sensitive tactile sensor based on polyacrylamide/silk fibroin elastomer *Adv. Funct. Mater.* **32** 2111747

[201] Hu W L, Niu X F, Zhao R and Pei Q B 2013 Elastomeric transparent capacitive sensors based on an interpenetrating composite of silver nanowires and polyurethane *Appl. Phys. Lett.* **102** 083303

[202] Liu Y *et al* 2022 Skin-integrated, stretchable, transparent triboelectric nanogenerators based on ion-conducting hydrogel for energy harvesting and tactile sensing *Nano Energy* **99** 107442

[203] Park H, Oh S-J, Kim D, Kim M, Lee C, Joo H, Woo I, Bae J W and Lee J-H 2022 Plasticized PVC-gel single layer-based stretchable triboelectric nanogenerator for harvesting mechanical energy and tactile sensing *Adv. Sci.* **9** 2201070

[204] Ahn Y, Song S and Yun K S 2015 Woven flexible textile structure for wearable power-generating tactile sensor array *Smart Mater. Struct.* **24** 075002

[205] Charalambides A and Bergbreiter S 2016 Rapid manufacturing of mechanoreceptive skins for slip detection in robotic grasping *Adv. Mater. Technol.* **2** 1600188

[206] Shih B, Christianson C, Gillespie K, Lee S, Mayeda J, Huo Z and Tolley M T 2019 Design considerations for 3D printed, soft, multimaterial resistive sensors for soft robotics *Front. Robot. AI* **6** 30

[207] Hamidi A and Tadesse Y 2020 3D printing of very soft elastomer and sacrificial carbohydrate glass/elastomer structures for robotic applications *Mater. Design* **187** 108324

[208] Guo S-Z, Qiu K, Meng F, Park S H and McAlpine M C 2017 3D printed stretchable tactile sensors *Adv. Mater.* **29** 1701218

[209] Ntagios M 2022 Embedded sensing for advanced robotic applications *PhD Thesis* College of Science and Engineering, University of Glasgow

[210] Tawil D S 2012 Artificial skin and the interpretation of touch in human–robot interaction *PhD Thesis* School of Aerospace, Mechanical and Mechatronic Engineering, University of Sydney, Australia

[211] Tawil D S, Rye D and Velonaki M 2011 Improved EIT drive patterns for a robotics sensitive skin *Australasian Conf. Robotics and Automation (ACRA) (Sydney, Dec. 2–4)* 425–35

[212] Mukai T, Hirano S, Yoshida M, Nakashima H, Guo S J and Hayakawa Y 2011 Whole-body contact manipulation using tactile information for the nursing-care assistant robot RIBA *IEEE/RSJ Int. Conf. Intelligent Robots and Systems (San Francisco, CA, Sept. 25–30)*

[213] Dahiya R S, Metta G, Cannata G and Valle M 2011 Guest editorial: special issue on robotic sense of touch *IEEE Trans. Robot.* **27** 385–8

[214] Strohmayr M W and Schneider D 2013 The DLR artificial skin, Step II: scalability as a prerequisite for whole-body covers *2013 IEEE/RSJ Int. Conf. Intel. Robots and Systems (IROS) (Tokyo, Nov 3–7)* pp 4721–8

[215] Elsanadedy A, Mamatjan Y, Ahmadi M and Adler A 2012 Characterisation of conductive polymer for EIT based sensor *Int. Conf. Electrical and Computer Systems (Ottawa, Aug 16–18)* 117

[216] Yang C L, Mohammed A, Mohamadou Y, Oh T I and Soleimani M 2015 Complex conductivity reconstruction in multiple frequency electrical impedance tomography for fabric-based pressure sensor *Sensor Rev.* **35** 85–97

[217] Jeong Y J, Oh T I, Woo E J and Kim K J 2017 Integration of piezo-capacitive and piezo-electric nanoweb based pressure sensors for imaging of static and dynamic pressure distribution *39th Ann. Int. Conf. IEEE Engineering in Medicine and Biology Society (EMBC) (Jeju, Korea, 11–15 July)* pp 21–4

[218] Sun L, Jiang S, Xiao Y and Zhang W 2020 Realization of flexible pressure sensor based on conductive polymer composite via using electrical impedance tomography *Smart Mater. Struct.* **29** 055004

[219] Cannata G, Denei S and Mastrogiovanni F 2010 Towards automated self-calibration of robot skin *IEEE Int. Conf. Robotics and Automation (ICRA) (Anchorage, AL, May 3–7)* pp 4849–54

[220] Wissman J *et al* 2013 New compliant strain gauges for self-sensing dynamic deformation of flapping wings on miniature air vehicles *Smart Mater. Struct.* **22** 085031

[221] Sauerbrunn E, Chen Y, Didion J, Yu M, Smela E and Bruck H A 2015 Thermal imaging using polymer nanocomposite temperature sensors, EIT *Phys. Stat. Sol.* A **212** 2239–45

[222] Bragaglia M, Paleari L, Lamastra F R, Puglia D, Fabbrocino F and Nanni F 2021 Graphene nanoplatelet, multiwall carbon nanotube, and hybrid multiwall carbon nanotube–graphene nanoplatelet epoxy nanocomposites as strain sensing coatings *J. Reinf. Plast. and Compos.* **40** 632–43

[223] Cuellar C, Watson K and Smela E 2023 Fabrication, characterization, and repair of nanocarbon-loaded aircraft paint-based sensors for real-world SHM: studies at the laboratory scale *Struct. Health Monit.* https://doi.org/10.1177/14759217231198015

[224] Byun J, Oh E, Lee B, Kim S, Lee S and Hong Y 2017 A single droplet-printed double-side universal soft electronic platform for highly integrated stretchable hybrid electronics *Adv. Funct. Mater.* **27** 1701912

[225] Visentin F, Fiorini P and Suzuki K 2016 A deformable smart skin for continuous sensing based on electrical impedance tomography *Sensors* **16** ARTN 1928

[226] Mukai T, Onishi M, Odashima T, Hirano S and Luo Z 2008 Development of the tactile sensor system of a human-interactive robot 'RI-MAN' *IEEE Trans. Rob.* **24** 505–12

[227] Youssefi S, Denei S, Mastrogiovanni F and Cannata G 2015 A real-time data acquisition and processing framework for large-scale robot skin *Rob. Autom. Syst.* **68** 86–103

[228] Yoon S H, Huo K, Zhang Y, Chen G, Paredes L, Chidambaram S and Ramani K 2017 iSoft: a customizable soft sensor with real-time continuous contact and stretching sensing

Proc. 30th Ann. ACM Symp. User Interface Software and Technology (Québec City, QC, Canada: Association for Computing Machinery) pp 665–78

[229] *Emergen Research 2022 E Skin Market Size, Share, Trends, By Product (Electronic skinsuit and Electronic patches), By Component (Stretchable Circuits, Photovoltaics System, and Others), By Sensor Type, By Application, and By Region Forecast to 2030*

[230] Kumar R and Mutreja S 2018 *Electronic Skin Market by Application (Personal Healthcare Monitoring, Wearable Technology, and Others)—Global Opportunities Analysis and Industry Forecast, 2020–2025* Report No. A04210

Chapter 2

Use of electrical impedance tomography for tactile imaging

The absence of internal electrodes allows electrical impedance tomography (EIT)-based tactile sensors to be entirely stretchable, and the sophistication of the image reconstruction allows the sensors to be exceptionally simple and the number of electrical connections to be relatively small. Thus, the use of EIT is promising for system integration of tactile imagers. After introducing the reasons for using EIT, this chapter gives a synopsis of how it works.

EIT was developed for imaging the human body for medical diagnostics. Its application to tactile imaging has significantly different requirements, however. For example, the resistance of a sensor can be tailored, which is advantageous, but the potentially large range of resistance changes and the need to make immediate decisions based on the images present distinct challenges. It is therefore worthwhile to examine EIT from this perspective, which is done here.

A comprehensive survey of the literature is presented, which shows the performance achieved in sensing tactile inputs and the applications that have been demonstrated. The latter have included interactions with humans, pressure mapping, control of systems, and structural health monitoring. The review also examines experimental conditions. Sensor materials have primarily been conductive elastomers and fabrics although a few other approaches have been devised, such as liquid-filled containers. Targets for detection have chiefly comprised human fingers, weights, and probes. Diverse electrical connection methods have been tried, with varying success, as have different boundary conditions; these two topics require further attention in order to advance from prototypes to real-world applications. Data collection has regrettably often employed a measurement configuration known to be one of the worst. Turning next to reconstruction, this has usually been by one-step Tikhonov methods using the EIDORS software, although recently attention has begun to turn from EIT to machine learning (ML).

doi:10.1088/978-0-7503-5402-8ch2

2.1 Overview

By 'EIT' we mean the use of a continuous resistive sensor that is effectively two-dimensional (2D) and has only peripheral electrodes, combined with a physics-based inverse solution method to generate tactile images, and by 'tactile imaging' we mean spatially representing the characteristics of transient contacts, such as their strengths, positions, and shapes. We follow the convention in the tactile imaging field in treating the terms EIT and electrical resistance tomography (ERT) as interchangeable. Several in-depth reviews of EIT and its uses for tactile imaging have been published [1–3].

The foremost selling point of EIT-based sensors is the absence of internal electrodes [4]. This permits the sensors themselves to be entirely stretchable and to be applied conformally over complex 3D surfaces and bending joints. Since the sensor is inherently 2D, in contrast with the 3D human bodies encountered in medical EIT, the sensor behaves largely the same way when wrapped or stretched as it does when flat [1]. Another attractive feature of EIT is the relatively small number of required electrical connections, which facilitates system integration. The sensor architecture itself can also, in many cases, offer the advantage of exceptional simplicity, consisting in its most elementary form of a material or coating that directly transforms spatial deformations into voltage signals. EIT exchanges the local amplification, routing, and signal processing hardware of sensor arrays for an external board with switches that can be controlled by a microprocessor. EIT-based tactile skins are thus thought to have the potential to be manufacturable at relatively low cost. Endeavors such as giving humanoid robots embodied tactile imaging, as discussed in chapter 1, have been hindered by the presence wires in the contact area and by the complex fabrication of sensing elements [5, 6], both of which are addressed by EIT e-skins.

The placement of electrodes solely at the perimeter comes at a cost, however: the foremost disadvantage of EIT is its sensitivity to noise (see chapter 6), which, if not kept low, results in poor imaging performance [7, 8] and which is most pronounced at the center of the sensor (see chapter 5). In addition, EIT images are of lower quality than those obtained by more complicated array approaches [9], although richer than that of row-column architectures having the same number of wire leads [10]. Furthermore, EIT must contend with image artefacts (see chapter 7), which are spurious image features that are unassociated with tactile contacts, having various origins, including noise, electrode motion, and stress at electrodes. Temporal resolution, or imaging speed, is another consideration: tens of Hz is routine. Frame rates are limited by the number of voltage readings the speed of the switching circuitry, and the time required to compute the image. With a one-step reconstruction method, much of the computation is done only once, in advance. This reduces the computational load but it yields less accurate images than more time-consuming iterative approaches. While computational cost goes approximately as the square of the number of electrodes, in practice systems rarely have more than 16 electrodes (see section 2.6.2), and as shown in chapter 7, it may in fact be advantageous to reduce the number to 12 or 13.

Given time constraints on image formation and its inherent spatially-dependent sensitivity, EIT-based sensing is promising for applications requiring spatial resolution on the order of 10% of the sensor diameter and temporal resolution up to approximately 50 Hz [6]—in other words, for large-area tactile imaging rather than for small end effectors for object manipulation [6].

2.2 Introduction to EIT

To start, what is EIT? Tomography refers to imaging the internal properties of a body from measurements made on its surface using penetrating electromagnetic energy. EIT is a technique for obtaining the internal impedance (or admittance) distribution of a body from current injection and voltage measurements (or vice versa) made at its perimeter. Stated more generally, EIT can be used for imaging contrasts in a body's electrical properties [11]. When the injected current is DC, as is common in tactile imaging (section 2.6.2), the terms ERT and electrical resistivity imaging (ERI) are also used.

EIT was developed for medical applications in the 1970s [12, 13]. It has relatively recently been adapted, beginning in 2007, to tactile sensing over an area [1–3]. We refer to this as *tactile imaging* to distinguish it from sensing pressure or strain at a single point. In tactile imaging, the body being mapped is an effectively two-dimensional continuous sensor that locally changes resistance upon experiencing pressure or strain.

2.2.1 Reasons for using EIT for tactile imaging

Why should one consider using EIT for tactile imaging? Tactile imagers should show the spatial locations of one or more contacts as well as their strengths and sizes. As discussed below, EIT is well suited for applications such as human-device interfaces that may be large area, continuous, stretchable, or curved, but that do not need high resolution or high frame rates. It is well suited because, firstly, electrodes are placed exclusively at the sensor's perimeter, allowing the sensing area to remain entirely soft. Secondly, EIT requires relatively few electrical leads to produce a useful image; typically 16 or fewer are employed. While the spatial resolution is on the order of 15%–20% of the sensor diameter or 4% of the sensor area, comparable to that of a 4×4 array of row and column sensors having the same number of electrical connections, EIT provides richer information about the number, position, area, shape, and strength of touches, as illustrated in figure 2.1. This is because the electrodes are used repeatedly in different combinations and because the imaging algorithms make use of well-known physics. Thirdly, EIT can be readily implemented. The hardware for data collection is relatively simple and can be run by a microcontroller, and there is open source software for converting the voltage data to images, the most often used being EIDORS (electrical impedance and diffuse optical tomography reconstruction software, which is Matlab-based) [14–17]. Also, images can be produced in real time, at rates of tens of Hertz. Thus, there is a growing interest in this technique for electronic skins, or 'e-skins'.

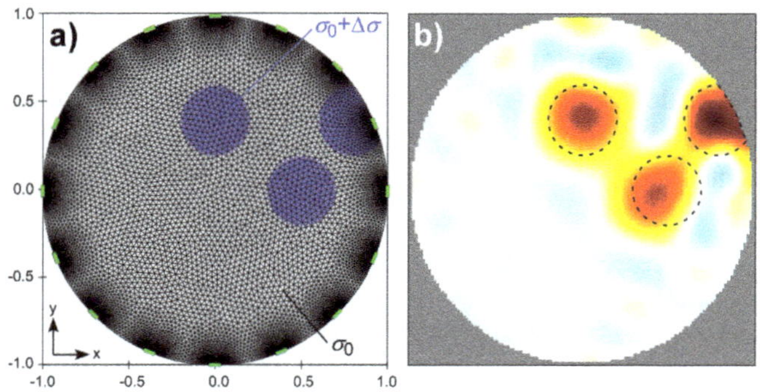

Figure 2.1. Example simulated conductivity distribution to be measured and the image that was reconstructed using EIT with perimeter measurements. (a) 2D simulation of a circular sensor of dimensionless radius 1 with uniform conductivity σ_0 and a three-circle target of conductivity change $\Delta\sigma$ (indicated in blue), each circle of radius $r_T = 0.2$. (For a discussion of units in EIDORS, see chapter 3.) Here the contrasts $\Delta\sigma$ are areas of uniformly higher resistivity (lower conductivity) relative to the background σ_0. The mesh is also shown. (b) Example EIT reconstruction (target indicated by the dashed lines). Colors correspond to estimated changes in conductivity, from red (largest increase in resistivity) to blue (decreases in resistivity), with white indicating no change. The dependence of the reconstructed image quality on various parameters is discussed in subsequent chapters of this book.

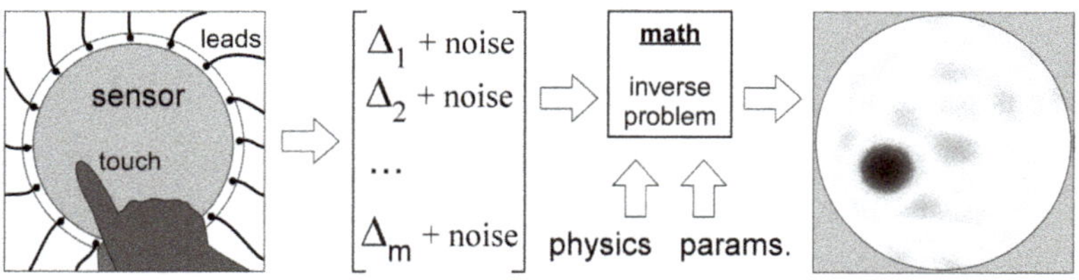

Figure 2.2. The EIT process (left to right) from the touch experiment to the resulting voltage difference data, required physics, and model choices, to the algorithm and final reconstruction.

Compared with using an array of point electrodes, EIT changes the problem from signals coming from a large number of individual sensors to, in essence, a visual recognition task with tactile 'cameras'. Dealing with images is advantageous because image processing is an advanced field.

2.2.2 Synopsis of the EIT process

A high-level overview of the EIT method is illustrated in figure 2.2. A series of voltage measurements is made at the outer edge of the sensor giving a vector $\mathbf{\Delta}$ of m voltage differences Δ_i, which are noisy. An EIT algorithm converts $\mathbf{\Delta}$ into an image, which in difference EIT [13], also called time difference EIT [18], represents the difference in conductivity between a reference state and the touched state. The heart of the method

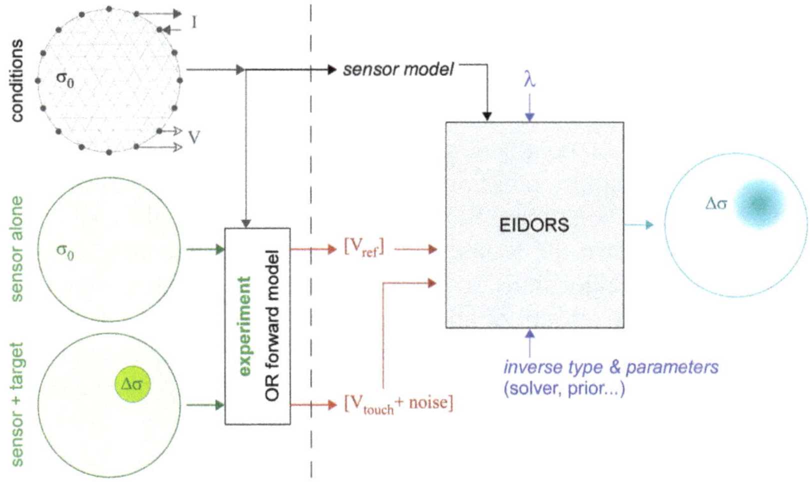

Figure 2.3. Information flow in EIT when the data are analyzed with EIDORS. The reference state has conductivity σ_0, and a tactile contact induces an unknown conductivity change $\Delta\sigma(x,y)$, resulting in a set of boundary voltages $\mathbf{V}_{\text{ref}}$ and $\mathbf{V}_{\text{touch}}$, which contain noise. (Voltages can also be obtained from a simulation using a forward model.) The voltages and measurement conditions are input to the program, along with choices for solving the inverse problem to estimate the conductivity change.

is an algorithm to perform an inverse problem, going from perimeter voltages to an interior conductivity distribution, known as reconstruction.

The information flow for performing EIT is summarized in figure 2.3, exemplified by the EIDORS software used in the majority of the tactile imaging work. (The author's work utilized v3.10-ng, 2019.) The experiment or simulation (left side) employs certain conditions, such as injected currents, specification of voltage-measuring electrodes, and initial sensor conductivity, σ_0, which are input, as sensor model information, to the inversion algorithm. The conductivity of the reference state σ_0 is usually assumed to be known and uniform. Constant current is typically injected into two of the electrodes and voltage differences measured across pairs of all the other electrodes. The current injecting electrodes are then rotated by one position and another set of voltage measurements is made, resulting, after rotation around the whole perimeter, in roughly 200 voltage measurements. Tactile imaging usually uses difference imaging, in which a set of baseline voltages $[V_{\text{ref}}] = \mathbf{V}_{\text{ref}}$ is first obtained without any tactile contacts; then voltages $[V_{\text{touch}}] = \mathbf{V}_{\text{touch}}$ are obtained at later times, which may indicate a contact, and which are compared to the baseline. The differences $\mathbf{\Delta} = \mathbf{V}_{\text{touch}} - \mathbf{V}_{\text{ref}}$ are input to the algorithm.

The collected data can be processed in different ways (right side of figure 2.3). Most work on EIT for tactile imaging uses a *sensitivity matrix* approach to image reconstruction (see chapter 4), although there are other methods that carry out reconstruction differently, such as the originally used Sheffield back-projection method [19] or the D-bar method [20]. Briefly, the sensitivity matrix $\mathbf{J}$, also called the

Jacobian, linearly relates changes in voltages at locations i on the perimeter of the sensor to changes in conductivity at locations k within the area of the sensor,

$$J\,\sigma = \Delta \tag{2.1}$$

where $\boldsymbol{\sigma}$ is the vector of conductivity changes and $\boldsymbol{\Delta}$ is the vector of voltage differences[1]. The linear approximation is valid for small changes in conductivity.

Based on Maxwell's equations, EIT attempts to find the unknown conductivity difference $\Delta\sigma(x,y)$ between the touched state and the baseline conductivity $\sigma_0(x,y)$ using a specified solver (algorithm), so-called prior, and hyperparameter λ. The latter two specify the type and amount of image smoothing, respectively, done to mitigate the effects of noise on the voltage signal. As discussed in later chapters, EIT is highly sensitive to noise, so the best method of handling noise is a central issue in image reconstruction.

2.3 Requirements for tactile imaging in comparison with medical imaging

Because EIT was developed for medical imaging, starting in the 1970s [12, 13], a section devoted to comparing the requirements of the two fields is in order. Much has been learned about EIT from the medical arena [11, 22–25] as summarized in [13]. Examples of medical applications include measuring the amount of air in the lungs and the detection of breast cancer. The adoption of EIT for use with tactile imaging is much more recent, as reviewed in section 2.4.

The experimental conditions, the characteristics of the sensed region, the target attributes, and the performance requirements can be considerably different for tactile imaging [1] than for medical imaging, as summarized in table 2.1. Primarily, in tactile imaging the number, locations, sizes, shapes, and strengths of contacts are not only unknown but also highly variable: the expected conductivity changes have high dynamic range, and touches can appear anywhere on the sensor area at any time. In addition, whereas the sensed region in medical imaging is substantially

[1] Put another way, if $\mathbf{V}$ is the vector of measured voltages, one can write:

$$\mathbf{V} = \mathbf{U}(\boldsymbol{\sigma}) + e,$$

where $\mathbf{U}(\boldsymbol{\sigma})$ is the noise-free 'perfect' set of voltage differences that would come from the physics-based forward model, $\boldsymbol{\sigma}$ is the conductivity distribution over the sensor, and e is the noise that appears on top of that signal, treated as additive. (Note that this $\boldsymbol{\sigma}$ differs from the definition used in equation (2.1).) A Taylor expansion of $\mathbf{U}$ around the reference state conductivity distribution $\boldsymbol{\sigma}_0$ can be written [21]:

$$\mathbf{U}(\sigma) = \mathbf{U}(\boldsymbol{\sigma}_0) + \mathbf{J}\Delta\boldsymbol{\sigma} + \text{higher order terms},$$

where $\mathbf{J}$ is the sensitivity matrix, which relates changes in boundary voltages to changes in conductivity around the reference state conductivity,

$$\mathbf{J} = \partial\mathbf{U}/\partial\boldsymbol{\sigma}|_{\sigma 0}$$

and $\Delta\boldsymbol{\sigma} = \boldsymbol{\sigma}-\boldsymbol{\sigma}_0$ is the conductivity change (the $\boldsymbol{\sigma}$ in equation (2.1)).

Table 2.1. Differences between EIT imaging for medical and tactile imaging applications.

Item	Medical	Tactile
goal	diagnosis of a condition	take action based on environmental awareness, interpretation of touch
electrodes	manually placed, positions variable; relative positions change with patient motion and body shape; contact impedance at electrode-body interface may be high	positions fixed during manufacture; can be low contact impedance; strain at interfaces between rigid (metal) electrodes and stretchable sensor must be prevented to avoid artefacts
injected current frequency	usually AC	usually DC
injected current amplitude	limited by safe patient exposure	limited only by power consumption and heating considerations
sensed area conductivity	fixed by biology	can be tailored via the sensor material
sensed region	3D body, size varying among patients; some regions may not change or be of interest	2D sensor area of fixed size, entire area is of interest
conductivity distribution	varies across body due to anatomy (e.g. lung vs. bone), but may be fairly uniform within a region of interest (ROI); can be anisotropic	typically uniform across sensor, but can be strongly anisotropic (e.g. fabric)
change in conductivity	limits known and fixed by biology, changes of interest often small	unknown a priori, changes may be large, have large dynamic range
# targets	there may be a fixed ROI	unknown a priori, can be multiple simultaneous contacts
timing of targets	sometimes a predictable timing of contrast changes	sporadic contacts (most of the time no contacts)
target position	depends on application whether: within an ROI, known or estimated by anatomy (e.g. lungs), or unknown a priori (e.g. breast cancer)	unknown a priori – can be anywhere on the sensor
target size		unknown a priori, but may range from smaller than image resolution up to significant fraction of sensor area
target shape		unknown a priori; typically oval if from finger touches
number of images used for decisions	can be many	decisions may need to be based on a single image
false positives (artefacts)	averaging can ameliorate	generally cannot be tolerated for real-time operation
false negatives (poor detectability)	critical to avoid; averaging can ameliorate	depending on the application missed faint touches may be acceptable

unchangeable, fixed by biology and anatomy, in tactile imaging the conductivity and sensitivity of the sensor can be engineered. Furthermore, in order to allow real-time decision-making, to take action based on environmental awareness or to interpret a touch sequence, tactile imaging requires rapid data collection and image processing [1], and decisions may need to be made on the basis of a single image. Thus, artefacts due to noise (chapter 6 and section 7.1) cannot be tolerated. Advantageously, the inverse problem to be solved is simplified in 2D compared with 3D [26]. Thus, it is worthwhile to re-examine EIT from the tactile imaging perspective, which is the topic of this book.

2.4 EIT for tactile imaging literature

Prior reviews of tactile sensors utilizing EIT [1–3] have covered the basics of their operation and have collected example configurations and applications. The reader is referred to these as a starting point and we therefore take a slightly different approach in this chapter. A guide to the literature on EIT-based tactile sensors is given in table 2.3, which highlights the main findings and novel contributions of each study. Since our aim is introducing EIT to experimentalists, specifics about the sensors are provided, as well as the experimental or simulation conditions, and finally the reconstruction method. Although this collection of papers is focused on standard EIT—peripheral electrodes and conventional inversion algorithms—also included are occasional examples of devices with interior electrodes and closely related applications that are non-tactile. Table 2.2 provides previously undefined acronyms and terms that are used in table 2.3.

The first work on tactile imaging using EIT was done in the early 1990s. Changes in boundary voltages of conductive rubber sheets under pressure demonstrated feasibility [26, 29] and were confirmed by simulation [30]. Then after a decade of dormancy, the field took off in 2007 with the bold, pioneering work of Nagakubo, Alirezai *et al* [33–35], intended for eventual application in artificial skins for robotics, as well as fundamental work by Kato, Mukai *et al* [10, 36, 37], who were also from the robotics field. Significantly, Nagakubo made use of the EIDORS software, the introduction of which led to its subsequent wide adoption. Ensuing work has included applications, characterization, new geometries and materials, hardware improvements, and imaging advances.

It should be noted that pressure strain field sensing, which was an early proposed application of tactile imaging EIT, formed a branch into structural health monitoring (SHM), as reviewed in [55]. The work described in this chapter and that in SHM are related but are sufficiently different, for example in electrode placements and injection-measurement (I–M) patterns, that SHM applications were not included here. (For examples of EIT for SHM, see appendix A.)

2.5 Capabilities and applications of EIT for tactile imaging

2.5.1 Demonstrations of capability

After the earliest work to demonstrate basic feasibility of using EIT for tactile imaging [26, 29, 30], the seminal work showed the capability to use stretchable sensors, measure load, detect multiple simultaneous contacts, distinguish types of tactile interactions, and handle irregularly shaped sensing areas and varying electrode placements, as well as to apply the sensors on curved surfaces and detect the bending angle of a joint [5, 33–35, 44]. Standard evaluation of sensors and algorithms includes detecting forces applied over single and multiple points of varying position and size. EIT tactile imagers are able, for example, to tell number of contacts in a sensor stretched over a hemisphere, can recognize edges and gaps on contacting shapes, and can distinguish an L-shaped object from an O-shaped

Table 2.2. Acronyms and material names frequently employed in EIT sensors.

Name	Definition or information
	Material components
ABS	Acrylonitrile butadiene styrene
C	Carbon
CB	Carbon black
CNT	Carbon nanotube
PANI	Polyaniline
PCB	Printed circuit board
PDMS	Poly(dimethyl siloxane)
PET	Polyethylene terephthalate
PSS	Poly(styrene sulfonate)
PU	Polyurethane
PVA	Poly(vinyl alcohol)
TPU	Thermoplastic polyurethane
	Commercial products
321 Less EMF	Silver-coated nylon, loose knit, stretchable (Less EMF), 0.5 Ω m^{-2}
EeonTex LR-SL-PA-10E5	Carbon coated nylon, tight knit, stretchable (Eeonyx Corp.), 10^5 Ω sq^{-1}
EeonTex NW170-SL-PA-1500	Carbon-coated non-woven, non-stretchable (Eeonyx Corp.), 1500 Ω m^{-2}
EeonTex NW170-SL-PA-2000	Polypyrrole-coated knit fabric, stretchable (Eeonyx Corp.), 2.8 kΩ sq^{-1}
MedTex180	Stretchable metalized fabric (Statex (now Shieldex)), 660 mS sq^{-1}
NW170-SLPA-20K	(Eeonyx) 3.5 kΩ cm^{-1}
Velostat or Linqstat	Carbon-loaded elastomer (polyolefin or other) (3M); Velostat, 500 Ω m^{-1} or 31 kΩ sq^{-1}, 0.1 mm thick
	Sensor types
PSCR	Pressure sensitive conductive elastomer, carbon-loaded rubber (PCR Technical)
PSCR2	Pressure sensitive conductive rubber *, positive GF for pressure and strain (Tokai Rubber Industries, Ltd., now Sumitomo Riko)
SCRS	Stacked contact resistance sensor

* Filler unspecified in any of the publications using it in table 2.3; figures show sensors are black in color. Current products from Sumitomo Riko have a different appearance and are metal-filled.

one [5]. Static [43] and time-varying [37] pressures obtained from EIT experimentally have been validated. With a clever sensor design, it was possible to correctly measure pressure distributions even if the sensor was undergoing dynamic and complex deformations [38]. Adding a model for movement

Table 2.3. Survey of studies using EIT for tactile imaging: summary of key findings, sensor configuration, forward problem conditions, and reconstruction information, in chronological order and, within a given year, alphabetically by first author. The symbol '‡' indicates the author's own estimate from figures in the publication, a calculation based on values given in the publication, an assumption based on other work by the cited group, or a conclusion drawn by the author from the results presented; information not provided in the table was unobtainable. For studies employing machine learning (ML) approaches see table 2.5.

Reference	Year	Findings	Sensor	Conditions	Reconstruction
	Key	• **Summary of new contribution** • Some findings, particulars	• **Materials**, details, conductivity • Shape, size, thickness • Boundary conditions (BCs) • Electrical connections	• *Simulations/ experiments* • Number of electrodes • I–M pattern • Electrical input • Conductivity, contrast • Target	• Reconstruction method • Prior, regularization • Other information
[26]	1990	• **Show feasibility of reconstructing conductivity profile from boundary measurements** • Boundary voltages change with load • Proposed application is for sensing pressure distributions of patients on beds	• **C-black loaded rubber**	• *Simulations* • 16 electrodes • Square sensor • Target = conductivity profile	• Algorithm of [28], 5 iterations
[29]	1992	• **Prototype sensor to measure distributed pressure** • (***no imaging***) • different loads and positions tested • output voltages change under loads • electrodes attached by glue are unreliable	• 2 Types of commercial **conductive rubber** sheet: one R varies with force, one switches on/off with force • Rectangle, ‡4 × 10.5 cm • Brass screws clamped to sample, soldered to wires	• *Experiments* • 16 electrodes • I–M = ADJ–ADJ • AC current • 0.2 or 1 kg load, $d_T = 1.3$ cm	• Forward voltages found, no imaging

[30]	1993	• **Simulate response to pressure distribution** • Method has low tolerance to noise • Internal electrodes lower sensing errors • Proposed application is for patient pressure sensing		• *Simulations* • 32 Electrodes (alternatively 28 at perimeter + 4 **internal**) • 4 current injection patterns • Noise added • Target = conductivity distribution	• Gauss–Newton algorithm based on [28]
[31, 32]	2007	• **Apply EIT to map conductivity of sensor** • (***Not tactile imaging***) • Map film conductivity, validate • Conductivity changes with strain, etching the film, and pH	• **Thin film**, layer by layer deposited CNTs in PSS + either PVA or PANI, on glass (*not stretchable*), 150 S cm^{-1} • Square, 2.5 × 2.5 cm^2, or rectangle, 2.5 × 6 cm^2 • Ag paste to equidistant Cu header pins, soldered to wires	• *Experiments* • 32 Electrodes • I–M = ADJ–ADJ • AC current • Target = etched pattern	• Regularized Gauss–Newton, iterative method
[33]	2007	• (*in Japanese*) • **Stretchable tactile sensor based on EIT** • **Demonstrate load-sensing experimentally** • **Detect multiple contacts on surface; detect tactile interactions: pinch, rub, grab** • **Consider irregular shaped sensing areas, electrode placements, and internal electrodes**	• **PSCR**, solid and with array of holes (mesh-like) (0.76 and 14.6 kΩcm) • Circle, d_S = ‡15 cm diameter, also rectangle ‡15 × 25 cm^2 and irregular shape • Free edges, placed on surface or edges taped onto dummy face or elbow • Alligator clip electrodes or ‡pins	• *Experiments* • ‡16 Electrodes • Target = fingers (d_T = ‡1 cm)	• EIDORS

(*Continued*)

Table 2.3. (*Continued*)

Reference	Year	Findings	Sensor	Conditions	Reconstruction
[34]	2007	• Stretchable tactile sensor based on EIT • **Simulate arbitrary shapes** • **Test asymmetric electrode placement** • **Test 4 sensor materials, combinations** • Detect multiple pressure contacts on surface; detect tactile interactions: pinch, rub, grab • **Wrap sensor on complex 3D curved surface** • **Pressure sensing even under strain** • Consider irregular shaped sensing areas, electrode placements, and internal electrodes • Knits have low hysteresis; fast load removal has large hysteresis compared to slow load removal • Minimal detectable area is 10% in center	• 4 Sensors: (1) 2 **PSCR** sheets (A = 0.76, B = 14.6 kΩcm), B with 5×5 mm^2 conductive paint patches; works as **SCRS**, (2) **PSCR** B with array of 5 mm diameter holes at 7.2 mm pitch, on 2 cm thick foam, (3) conductive knit **fabric** coated with carbonic paint, (4) 3 layers of **fabric** (conductive knit +insulating loose weave + Ag-plated nylon mesh) • Circle, d_S = ‡15 cm, also rectangles 1.5×5 cm^2 or ‡1.5×25 cm^2 and irregular shape, t = ‡1 mm • Free edges, placed on surface or edges taped onto dummy face or elbow • Alligator clip electrodes or ‡pins	• *Simulations and experiments* • 16 electrodes • I–M = ADJ–ADJ • DC current • Target = fingers, fist, weights of various sizes	• Customized EIDORS with GUI that imports custom CAD sensor designs
[35]	2007	• Same as [34] plus: • **Detect bending angle of joint**	• Same as [34]	• Same as [34]	• Same as [34]

[36]	2007	• Use PSCR with positive GF • **Positive value constraint on resistivity in inverse problem stabilizes the solution** • Detect multiple finger pressure points • Imaging 10 frames s^{-1}	• ‡**PSCR2**, ρ increases with pressure, strain • Circle, d_S=20 cm, t = 1 mm • Mounted in frame ‡over Cu sheet • Cu strip electrodes vulcanization glued with conductive rubber, to alligator clips	• *Experiments* • 16 Electrodes • I–M = ADJ–ADJ • AC 1.6 kHz 2 V_{pp} • Target = fingers	• Instead of regularization use non-negative least squares algorithm to stabilize solution; calculate sensitivity matrix in advance
[37]	2008	• Same as [36] plus • **Measure time-varying pressure, validate with force gauge** • Imaging ‡3 frames s^{-1}	• Same as [36] + • **PSCR2** • Sensor mounted in frame • Electrodes applied by vulcanization gluing + soldered wires	• Same as [36] • AC 3.7 kHz 4.5_{pp} V • Force gauge tip, $d_T = 0.1d_S$	• Same as [36]
[10]	2008	• Same as [36, 37] • ‡ Sensor has marked memory effects • **Suggest reducing computational load by reconstructing only when sensor output changes**	• Same as [36]	• Same as [36]	• Same as [36]
[38]	2009	• Introduce **stretch-insensitive** pressure sensor; **stably measure pressure under different strains** • Sensor based on reducing contact resistance • Detection of multiple finger pressure points on flat, curved, and balloon surfaces • Detect dynamic, complex deformations • Highly nonlinear response to pressure	• Stretchable **SCRS**: high, constant R conductive yarn net + array of disconnected conductive squares, strains to 140% • Rectangle, 9 × 16 cm^2 • BCs same as [34] + sometimes edges clamped by frame • ‡Alligator clips	• *Experiments* • 16 Electrodes • I–M = ADJ–ADJ • Target = fingers	• Newton's iteration method • Laplace prior, regularization used

(*Continued*)

Table 2.3. (*Continued*)

Reference	Year	Findings	Sensor	Conditions	Reconstruction
[39]	2009	• Internal reference electrode improves resolution, lowers noise sensitivity • Metrics: resolution, position error, ringing • **I = POL pattern worst, ADJ worst with noise, other patterns similar**		• Simulations • 16 or 17 electrodes • I, M = ADJ to POL or **internal** • DC 110 mA • $\sigma_0 = 1$ S cm^{-1}, $\Delta\sigma = +10\%$ • Target = mesh elements	• GN one-step • Hyperparameter λ, selected by optimizing metrics • 200 reconstructions per FEM mesh element
[40]	2009	• Suggestion to use EIT for sensing skin • (*No EIT imaging done*) • Made whole-body stretchable knit skin for humanoid robot • Sensor had anisotropic, nonlinear response with memory	• Six layers of insulating and conductive **stretchable** knit **fabrics** • Thin copper wire or brass buttons touching the fabric		
[41]	2011	• Same as [39] plus • **NOSER and Gaussian regularization give slightly better resolution** • **The best current injection pattern depends on the prior, but I = 8 is always worst** • 60 Hz imaging	• **SCRS**: knit carbon-loaded fabric (Eeonyx Corp., $\sigma_0 = 12.5$ mS sq^{-1}) + array of conductive fabric squares (Less EMF, Inc., $\sigma_0 = 660$ mS sq^{-1}) + foam covering • Rectangle, 20 × 32 cm^2, $t = 0.6$ mm • ‡Free edges, placed on surface • Cr-plated brass eyelet electrical connections ‡clamped to fabric	• *Experiments* + *simulations* • 16 to 19 electrodes (0–3 **internal**) • I–M = varied • DC 1.8 mA • Target = weight, $d_T = 2$ cm	• EIDORS, difference imaging, GN one-step • 3 priors studied (Laplacian, Gaussian, NOSER) plus total variation, **W = I**, hyperparameter selected by optimizing resolution • 150 reconstructions per FEM mesh element

[42]	2011	• **Six modalities of human touch studied** (35 participants) • Classifier (LogitBoost algorithm for supervised ML) used to identify touch modality; five attributes employed • Accuracy comparable to human touch recipient • 60 Hz imaging	• Same as [41]	• *Experiments* • 17 Electrodes (1 **internal**) • I = ADJ, M = dif. to center electrode • DC 1.8 mA • target = weight, $d_T = 2$ cm and finger and hand contacts	• EIDORS + custom software • Tikhonov regularization, NOSER prior, λ chosen empirically
[43]	2012	• **Pressure information from images quantified; change in conductivity is nonlinear with pressure** • Sensor performance characterized: images suffered from hysteresis, nonlinearity; memory of prior contacts retained in subsequent images • Image metrics: resolution, position error; sensor metric: hysteresis	• **PSCR** (CS57–7RSC) + conductor (2 x 2 cm^2 Cu sheet) under pressure point, works as **SCRS** • Square, 5 × 5 cm^2, $t = 5$ mm • Edges fixed in frame • Penetrating Cu electrodes in fixture	• *Experiments* • 16 Electrodes • I–M = ADJ–ADJ • AC current • target = Cu sheet 2 × 2 cm^2 with weights added	• EIDORS, difference imaging, one-step inversion • Laplace prior, λ found by L-curve • Complete electrode model • Image ROI used to determine pressure
[5]	2012	*(Thesis)* • [43] plus: • **EIT performed on a curved surface** (hemisphere): position, number, and shape of objects recognized	• [43] plus: • **PSCR**, 2. two non-woven **fabric** layers with different R, 3. woven conductive fabric 4. two woven conductive fabric layers • Also circular mounted in a frame, $d_S = 21$ cm	• *Simulation and experiments* • [43] plus: • AC current 12.5 or 50 kHz • Target = fingers	• EIDORS, difference imaging, one-step solver • Laplace prior, $\lambda = 0.032$ or 0.15 • Complete electrode model • Image ROI used to determine pressure

(Continued)

Table 2.3. (*Continued*)

Reference	Year	Findings	Sensor	Conditions	Reconstruction
		• Quality of voltage data depends on excitation frequency • **Developed reconstruction model for 2D surface meshes in 3D space, included in EIDORS** • Non-conductive fabric sewn to boundary to prevent strain at electrodes: **electrode mounting is critical**—position accuracy is reduced by electrode motion artefacts, press-mounting gives more noise, artefacts found around perimeter • Single and two-layer fabric have hysteresis and poor pressure sensing • Position errors due to image artefacts • Additional sensor metric used: drift • Neural network for hysteresis-compensation suggested	• Mounted in fixture with Cu sheet electrodes or free edges with button (snap) electrodes		
[44]	2012	• [42] Plus: • **Irregular shaped skin mounted on curved surface** (mannequin arm) without stretching	• Same as [41] plus • Protective suede cover on sensor • Sensor has irregular shape	• *Experiments* • 17 peripheral electrodes + 2 **internal** electrodes • DC current	• EIDORS + custom software

		• **8 Human touch modalities studied** (40 participants), anywhere between shoulder and wrist using either hand • 71% accuracy, compared to 90% for human • Robot requires means to ascribe meaning to data • 45 Hz imaging		• Target = weight, $d_T = 2$ cm and finger and hand contacts	• Generalized Tikhonov regularization, Gaussian prior, λ chosen empirically
[45]	2012	*(Thesis)* • [39, 41, 42, 44] plus • **Tactile imaging for HRI** • Gaussian prior has better performance (resolution, distance error) than Laplace, NOSER, total variation in both rectangular, circular domains • **I = pseudo-polar has best noise performance with peripheral electrodes** • Internal electrodes improve amplitude and amplitude uniformity • Interpretation of social touch demonstrated • 22 mW power consumption	• Same as [39, 41, 42, 44]	• *Experiments* • Contrast = +10%	• Same as [39, 41, 42, 44]

(*Continued*)

Table 2.3. (*Continued*)

Reference	Year	Findings	Sensor	Conditions	Reconstruction
[46]	2012	• Detect multiple pressure points; quantization is difficult, images were blurred • Pressure can create deformation close to the electrodes • 60 Seconds per image (‡0.02 Hz)	• Silver-coated **fabric** (Less EMF, $\rho = 1\ \Omega\ \text{sq}^{-1}$) • Circle, $d_S = 20$ cm • Loosely mounted to frame at periphery, ‡ laid over foam • ‡ Cu strip electrodes taped down	• *Experiments* • 16 Electrodes • I = ADJ • AC 10 mA, 2 kHz • Isotropic conductivity assumed • Weight with $d_T = 0.05 d_S$ and finger press, pull	• EIDORS, generalized Tikhonov regularization • NOSER prior, $\lambda = 10^{-3}$
[47]	2013	• **Switching circuit + microcontroller operated EIT** • Resistance decreases with pressure, conductive weights (‡ contact resistance sensor) • Weak response to insulating objects; use with conductive layer (‡ to form SCRS)	• Two tested: (1) **carbon-loaded rubber** (Velostat, 3M, 500 $\Omega\ \text{m}^{-1}$) for conductive objects; (2) Velostat + Al-laminated fabric for non-conductive objects • Rectangle, $19 \times 25\ \text{cm}^2$ • Free edges, placed on surface • Alligator clip electrodes	• *Experiments* • 16 Electrodes • I–M = ADJ–ADJ • AC and DC, 50–200 μA • Target = weight	• EIDORS, generalized Tikhonov regularization • Laplace prior or identity matrix
[48]	2013	• **Demonstration of sensing human pressure** • Positions of small weights detected • Hysteresis present • Rectangular sensors showed artefacts near corners • Humans standing on sensor detected	• Two **fabric** systems: • 1) Stretchable fabric (EeonTex LR-SL-PA-10E5, $10^5\ \Omega\ \text{m}^{-2}$), circular d_S = ‡15 cm, mounted in frame over foam; • 2) Non-woven (NW170-SL-PA-1500, Eeonyx, 1500 $\Omega\ \text{m}^{-2}$) square, ‡$10 \times 10\ \text{cm}^2$ and ‡$40 \times 40\ \text{cm}^2$	• *Experiments* • 1) 16 and 2) 32 electrodes • I = ADJ • AC 10 mA 2 kHz • Target = weight, d_T = ‡4 cm, and human feet	• Generalized Tikhonov regularization, difference imaging

			• Edges clamped in frame, laid over foam • ‡ Clamped Cu strip electrodes, going to alligator clips		
[49]	2014	• **Interpretation of human social touch for HRI** • Context of touch must be considered	• Same as [44]	• Experiments • Same as [44]	• Same as [44] + • Complete electrode model
[50]	2014	• **Effect of C loading on performance: low fill fractions have higher sensitivity to strain, but also greatest variability**, non-uniform resistivity postulated as the reason • Images of target at different C vol%	• **Carbon nanofiber (CNF) loaded PU** (ReoFlex 20, Smooth-On) (7.5–15 vol%) • Square, 2.5 × 2.5 cm^2, t = ‡2.5 mm • Ag paste electrodes fixed on vertical edge	• *Experiments* • 28 Electrodes • I–M = ADJ–ADJ • DC 2.5 mA • Target = 1.2 kg mass resting on 3 marbles	• Generalized Tikhonov regularization, iterative method • Laplace prior
[9]	2015	• **Ionic liquid (IL) based array sensor** • (*Sensor not continuous*) • Design, manufacture of sensor • Model for hyperelastic pressure sensing; simulate deformation • Proof of concept for using IL sensor for contact location and force (the latter nonlinear); validated with force gauge	• **IL** (1-ethyl-3-methylimidazolium ethyl sulfate (EMISE), ρ = 2.5 Ωm) ionic **liquid** encapsulated in silicone (Ecoflex) microchannels (350 μm × ‡1000 μm) • Square ‡4 × 4 cm^2, t = ‡1–2 mm • Free-standing film • Electrodes Ni strands + Ni-coated C fibers in silicone (ρ = 8000 Ωm)	• *Experiments and simulations* • 12 Electrodes • I–M = ADJ–ADJ • Current AC 1 kHz • $\sigma_0 = 0.4$ S m^{-1} • Target = force gauge probe tip $d_T = 0.6$ cm	• EIDORS for simulations • Weighted filtered back projection for experiments

(*Continued*)

Table 2.3. (*Continued*)

Reference	Year	Findings	Sensor	Conditions	Reconstruction
[1]	2015	• **Review**: EIT for robot skin • See table 1.1			
[51]	2015	• [50] Plus • **Sensor material response:** mechanism of resistance change depends strongly on C nanofiber vol% • Imaging < 0.1 Hz	• Same as [50]	• Same as [50]	• Same as [50]
[52]	2015	• Imaging of finger contacts with fabric sensor • Imaging of noise	• **Fabric** (‡MedTex180) • Circle, d_S=20 cm • Unconstrained edges • Alligator clip electrodes	• *Experiments* • 8 Electrodes • I–M = ADJ–ADJ • DC 100 mA • Target = finger	• EIDORS, GN one-step • NOSER prior, λ found by tuning
[53]	2015	• **Image real and imaginary parts of signal;** real part decreases with frequency f, at $f > 100$ kHz imaginary part is more reliable • Capacitance changes with pressure • Impedance measurements on fabric compared to saline tank • GREIT metrics used to evaluate images • Response to load is nonlinear, has hysteresis	• Non-stretchable conductive **fabric** (EeonTex NW170-SL-PA-1500) • Circle d_S=‡20 cm • Peripherally clamped, over foam • Cu plate electrodes clamped to fabric	• *Experiments* • 16 electrodes • I–M = ADJ–ADJ • AC 5 mA 1–250 kHz • Target = weights up to 4 kg, d_T = ‡4 cm	• KHU Mark2 EIT system • Generalized Tikhonov regularization, $\lambda = 0.02$

[54]	2016	• Demonstration of stretchable fabric pressure sensor • Weight detected	• Medtex 130 knit **fabric** (Ag-coated nylon, < 1 Ω sq^{-1}) • Circle, d_S=10 cm • Free edges, placed over foam • Stainless steel button electrodes (snaps) piercing fabric	• *Experiments and simulations* • 8 electrodes • I–M = ADJ–ADJ • DC 14 mA • Target = 250 g weight, $d_T = 0.3d_S$	• EIDORS, one-step regularized Tikhonov regularization, difference imaging • $\lambda = 0.5$
[55]	2016	• (*No tactile imaging*) • **Reduce computational requirements for reconstruction with new algorithm**: constrain resistivity change to be sum of 2D sine waves, recover coefficients of the sine waves by inverting a small, sparse matrix • Solution is independent of σ_0, **J** • Images had more noise than EIT images	• 3 Systems: • CNF/epoxy coupon (*rigid*) • CB filled composite (*rigid*) • (3) same as [50], 11 wt% (decrease in ρ with pressure)	• *Simulations and experiments* • For system (3), same as [50]	• New EIT reconstruction algorithm • Regularization used on forward problem inversion
[56]	2016	• Force detection for sensor on curved surface • Develop low-cost hardware • Positions, number of objects detected, but not shape	• Same as [52] plus • Attached to various curved surfaces over stretchable foam	• *Experiments* • Same as [52] • Probes with d_T = 30–50 mm	• EIDORS, GN one-step • NOSER prior • Parameters determined empirically based on image errors
[57]	2016	• Waterproof sensor can be washed • Demonstrate pressure sensing • Resistance is linear with strain, pressure	• **Carbon-loaded latex** (CNTs) film transferred onto woven **fabric** + adhesive layer • Rectangle, ‡20 × 20 cm^2 • Cu tape electrodes	• *Experiments* • 28 Electrodes • M = ADJ • DC current • Target = rod	• GN iterative algorithm

(*Continued*)

Table 2.3. (*Continued*)

Reference	Year	Findings	Sensor	Conditions	Reconstruction
[58]	2017	• **Piezo-capacitive and piezoelectric sensors** • PVDF, PU nanowebs formed by electro-spinning • Strong hysteresis present; sensor layer delamination a problem • Imaged pressure locations • Imaging 10 Hz	• 5–7 layer sensors of conductive **fabric** (NW170-SLPA-20K) + adhesive + PVDF and/or PU • Square, 10 × 10 cm^2, $t = 0.3$ mm • Cu tape electrodes	• *Experiments* • 16 Electrodes • I–M = ADJ–ADJ • AC 1 mA 10 kHz • Target =- fingers	• KHU Mark2.5 EIT system, GREIT reconstruction algorithm
[59]	2017	• **Printed, molded sensors with anisotropic response**, linear with strain to 40%, GF = 1.6 • Sensor characterized • **Determine stretch direction by anisotropic EIT** • **Used to control robot three-finger gripper** • Imaging 2 Hz	• **Carbon-loaded silicone** (CNTs in EcoFlex0030, Smooth-On), 2.5 wt%, 2.6 kΩ-mm • Dome-shaped (oval base 7 × 14 cm^2) and flat (square, 5 × 5 cm^2, $t = 5$ mm) • Unconstrained edges • Ag paste to connect wires	• *Experiments* • 16 Electrodes • I–M = ADJ–ADJ • Current injection • Target = indenter, fingers	• Difference imaging, generalized Tikhonov regularization • Anisotropic EIT: separate images created for current injection and voltage measurements in parallel or perpendicular
[60]	2017	• **Repairable sensor**, by adding paste to damaged area and curing • Imagining during hammer impact	• **Carbon-loaded silicone** (CNTs) • Square, ‡5 × 5 cm^2 • Unconstrained edges	• *Experiments* • 32 Electrodes • I–M = 5–2 • Target = finger, hammer	• Resistivity reconstruction method (EIT)

[61]	2017	• **Study 3 I–M patterns** • Metrics: size and position errors, ringing • Voltage collection 70 Hz	• Conductive **fabric** (Eeonyx, polypyrrole-coated) • Circle d_S = ‡15 cm • Clamped at edges in frame • Cu strip electrodes clamped to fabric	• *Simulations and experiments* • 16 electrodes • I–M = ADJ–ADJ, PP–ADJ, PP–PP • DC current • Target = finger	• EIDORS, generalized Tikhonov regularization, difference imaging • NOSER prior; ‡large λ • Thresholds f used to define ROIs varied with I–M pattern
[62]	2017	• High-speed EIT system by measuring voltages concurrently from all electrodes • **Low power consumption** of 10 mW • ‡ Artefacts seen at electrodes • Voltage collection 78 Hz	• Same as [61]	• *Experiments* • 16 electrodes • I–M = ADJ–ADJ • DC 32 μA • Target = fingers	• EIDORS • Difference imaging • Threshold $f = 0.1$
[63]	2017	• **Methodology to ascertain displacement field** from EIT images, elastic modulus, Poisson ratio; use 3D mesh • Use nanocomposite resistivity model • Results similar to ANSYS results	• Same as [50] with 10.5 vol%, $\sigma_0 = 1$ S m^{-1} • Rectangle, ‡2.5 × 2.5 cm^2, t = 2.5 mm	• *simulations and experiments* • 28 electrodes • I–M = ADJ–ADJ • Target = 1.2 kg mass resting on 3 marbles	• Generalized Tikhonov regularization, one-step process, difference imaging • Laplace prior, L-curve used to select λ • Apply as constraint non-negative $\Delta\sigma$

(*Continued*)

Table 2.3. (*Continued*)

Reference	Year	Findings	Sensor	Conditions	Reconstruction
[64]	2017	• **To compensate memory effects, apply dynamic baseline update for EIT** triggered by contacts and motion with capacitance sensing and time derivative; show continuous contact sensing; shifts in reference baseline distort contact localization • **Toolkit developed (iSoft) for arbitrary sensor geometries, best electrode placements** • Single-layer sensor with multiple sensing modalities; contact and stretch sensing • Microcontroller with custom shield • Uni-directional stretch sensing based on resistance change over whole area; **contacts localized during stretch** • **In central 80% of sensor, 8 and 16 electrodes showed same accuracy**, errors occurred near electrodes • First cycle effects seen up to 50 stretch cycles • **Accuracy of detecting human interactions** evaluated • **Applications demonstrated: device control, interactive sticker** • 35 Hz EIT imaging	• **Carbon loaded silicone** (Elastosil LR 3162,Wacker, 11 Ωcm) sandwiched between heat-stabilized films; settling time > 10 sec. • Multiple shapes and sizes, 10×10 cm^2 to 20×20 cm^2 • Free; clamped on 2 edges for stretching; sensor fixed on surface for interactive objects • Metal ribbon crimp ends soldered to wires	• *Simulations and experiments* • 16 Electrodes • I–M = ADJ–ADJ • DC < 0.5 mA • Target = fingers	• Custom toolkit for forward problem that interfaces with EIDORS, GN one-step • NOSER prior, $\lambda = 0.01$

[65]	2017	• **Touch sensing based on current shunting by human body (Electrick)**: body draws current to ground from conductor **(electric field tomography)** • **ML with classification model** (using Weka)**, regression models** (SMOReg, RBF) to **handle arbitrary geometries, fabrication variability, discrete and continuous touch** • Investigate numerous conductive materials, identify optimal surface resistivity range; investigate number of electrodes, sensor size, surface geometry; Velostat most accurate (most uniform resistivity) • System performance tested with multiple users • Show single contact localization, tracking; surface topography does not affect accuracy • **Accessible to hobbyists; demonstrations** with game controller, soft toys, interactive objects; also works with salt-filled JellO and Playdoh, C fiber loaded silicone	• 3 Materials: printed and molded **carbon-loaded ABS** (Zen Toolworks), **Velostat**, **C-loaded paint** (MG Chemicals) • Various sizes, 15 × 15 to 60 × 60 cm^2, t = 1–3 mm • Unconstrained edges • Cu tape electrodes soldered to wire	• *Experiments* • 8, 16, 32 electrodes • I–M = ADJ–ADJ • AC max 0.4 mA 200 kHz • Target = fingers	• EIDORS, GN one-step • Alternative ML system used

(*Continued*)

Table 2.3. (*Continued*)

Reference	Year	Findings	Sensor	Conditions	Reconstruction
[66]	1. 2018	• **Sensed force range extended using 2 layers of foam with different stiffness** • Human touch strength, modalities identified • Linear response to force • Imaging 1 Hz	• **Carbon loaded latex** (graphite nano-platelets, 25 wt%) painted onto a latex membrane, 5 mS sq^{-1}, GF = 8 • Circle, $d_S = 20$ cm, $t = 0.3$ mm • Clamped at edge, laid over foam layers (each 13 mm thick) • Carbon yarn electrodes attached with C-loaded latex	• *Experiments* • 16 Electrodes • I = ADJ–ADJ • DC 3 mA • $\sigma_0 = 1$ S sq^{-1} for imaging • Target = fingers, hand	• EIDORS, ‡GN one-step reconstruction • Laplace prior, $\lambda = 0.3$
[67]	2018	(*Thesis*) • [66] + • Sensor characterized, has low sensitivity to pressure; response to at least 100 Hz; first cycle baseline offset • **Find number of artifacts as a function of λ**, find optimal λ vs noise at different σ_0 • **Correct amplitude errors due to λ** • For quantitative results, **include any non-uniform background σ_0** in forward model • **Memory effects handled by updating background conductivity**	• same as [66]	• *Simulations and experiments* • Same as [66] • $\sigma_0 = 10^{-2}$ S $s^{-1}q^{-1}$, $\Delta\sigma = -40\%$	• Same as [66] • Vary λ, σ_0, noise

[68]	2018	• **Transparent tactile sensor** • Detects contact with insulators • ‡ artefacts at the electrodes	• **CNT film** spray-coated (150 coats) onto silicone **elastomer** (PDMS) sheet • Square, 3 × 3 cm^2, $t = 1$ mm • Mounted in frame • Cu alligator clip electrodes	• *Experiments* • 16 Electrodes • I–M = ADJ–ADJ • DC 20–80 μA • Target = glass rod, $r_T = 0.13$	• GN iterative
[69]	2018	• **Pressure-insensitive tensile strain sensor** • Nonlinear response to strain (‡quadratic) • Sensor characterized; tested 10k cycles to 30% strain • Resistance change under tension due to micro-crack formation in CNT network • Study roles of porosity, thickness, C loading • Imaging 30 Hz	• Porous **carbon coated silicone** (CNTs, PDMS), 0.7–1 wt%; for 0.7 wt% at 0.7% strain, GF = 56 in tension, 0 in compression • Square, 11 × 11 cm^2, $t = 1$ mm • Unconstrained edges • **Embedded Ag-coated nylon mesh electrodes** (Shieldex, 1 Ω sq^{-1})	• *Experiments* • 24 electrodes • Target = fingers	• EIDORS, difference imaging
[70]	2018	• **Two-layer stretchable sensor (MultiSoft) using EIT for contact localization, ML for classification and magnitudes** • Use voltage data as SVM input • **Maintain contact localization during stretch** • Sensor relaxation time 2–5 sec	• **Carbon loaded silicone foam** (Wacker) 11 Ωcm **coated on silicone** (Dragon Skin) • Square, 15 × 15 cm^2, $t = 1$–3 mm • Unconstrained edges • Metal ribbon crimp ends soldered to wires	• *Experiments* • 16 Electrodes • I–M = ADJ–ADJ • DC 0.5 mA; read capacitance after voltage measurements • Target = fingers, force gauge probe	• EIDORS, GN one-step, difference imaging • Support vector machine (SVM) using a Weka toolkit, nonlinear classifier

(*Continued*)

Table 2.3. (*Continued*)

Reference	Year	Findings	Sensor	Conditions	Reconstruction
		• Rigid electrodes are problematic; fabrication uniformity is challenging • Applications demonstrated • 23 Hz imaging			
[71]	2019	• Flexible but not stretchable pressure sensor • Able to image loads, multiple points • Nonlinear (cubic) sensor response with memory	• **Carbon-coated non-woven fabric filled with elastomer** (CNTs, Ecoflex) • Square, 13 × 13 cm^2, $t = 0.8$ mm • Unconstrained edges • Ag paint, Ag epoxy electrodes	• *Experiments* • 32 Electrodes • I = ADJ, M = voltages with respect to preselected ground • DC 10 mA • Target = weights, circular $r_T = 2$ cm, also other areas	• Generalized Tikhonov regularization • Noise figure = 1 used to set λ (= 0.1)
[72]	2019	• **ML** (neural network) **to reduce systematic EIT image artefacts** due to electrode motion (errors and hysteresis still remain) • Model inputs were contacts over all areas, raw and desired image pairs; images were thresholded to $f = 0.55$, blobs < 15 pixels removed, edge suppression applied • 50 Hz imaging reduced to 1 Hz by slow mechanical response of fabric	• Conductive **fabric** (LTT-SLPA, Eeonyx, 10^4–10^7 Ω sq^{-1}) • Circle d_S=‡20 cm • Edges clamped in frame • Cu strip electrodes clamped to fabric	• *Simulations and experiments* • 16 Electrodes • DC current • Target = fingers	• KHU Mark 2.5, difference imaging, spatiotemporal total variation algorithm • Complete electrode model • Deep convolutional NN trained on point contacts (U-net, Tensorflow)

[73]	2019	• Images have errors and low resolution • Voltage collection 78 Hz, imaging 30 Hz	• Eeonyx stretchable **fabric** (30 kΩ surface resistance) • Circle d_S = ‡15 cm • Clamped at edge in frame • Cu strip electrodes on frame	• *Experiments* • 16 Electrodes • DC current • Target = fingers	• EIDORS
[74]	2019	• **Application: engine inspection**; sensor data used to determine aero-engine blade position and direction	• **CNT loaded PDMS** • hemispherical shell structure (o.d. = 1.8 cm, t = 1 mm) with protrusions	• *simulations and experiments* • 8 Electrodes • Target = engine blade	
[75]	2020	• **Multi-frequency EIT** • Reconstructed image depends on material type of contacting object; could be distinguished using principal component analysis	• **Velostat** • Circle, d_S = 20 cm • Unconstrained edges • Alligator clip electrodes	• *Experiments* • 16 electrodes • I–M = ADJ–ADJ • AC 100 μA 1–250 kHz • Target = various objects touched at the same location and pressure	• EIDORS • Difference imaging
[76]	2020	*(thesis, Ch. 6)*	• same as [72]	• *Simulations and experiments* • Same as [72]	• Same as [72]
[27]	2020	• Metrics: amplitude, position error, resolution, shape deformation • Pressure reduced resistance, increased capacitance • Relate applied pressure to impedance change • Imaging 10 Hz	• Three-layer sensor with conductive elastic **fabric** (170-SLPA-2000, EeonTex, 2.8 kΩ sq^{-1}, t = 0.5 mm) sandwiching custom PU **nanoweb** (t = 100 μm), adhesive (Hotmelt NP373, Chemitec) • Square, 10 × 10 cm^2, or rectangle, 5 × 15 cm^2, t = 1.1 mm • Mounted to flexible PCB with eyelets	• *experiments* • 16 electrodes • I–M = ADJ–ADJ • AC 1 mA, 11 kHz • Target = weight, d_T = 1 cm, load cell	• GREIT algorithm • 1000 solutions of EIT with forward problem data for training

(Continued)

Table 2.3. (*Continued*)

Reference	Year	Findings	Sensor	Conditions	Reconstruction
[2]	2020	• **Review**: EIT for robot e-skin • see table 1.1			
[77]	2020	• Pressure sensors and electrodes screen printed • **Use a sensitivity map to correct the EIT image amplitude**	• 4.5 wt% **CB loaded TPU**, 20 μm thick screen printed onto PET sheet, covered with protecting PET sheet, total t = 100 μm • Square, 10 × 10 cm^2 • Unconstrained edges • Printed Ag paste electrodes	• *Simulations and experiments* • 8 Electrodes • I–M = ADJ–ADJ • DC 0.8 mA • Target = iron weights, d_T = 20 mm, 50 g, and other objects	• EIDORS, GN one-step, difference imaging • Tikhonov regularization
[3]	2020	• **Review**: EIT applied for structural health and condition monitoring • See table 1.1			
[78]	2020	• Alternative to traditional EIT: **uses contact resistance between 2 conductive layers; voltage measured between drive layer and electrodes at perimeter of probe layer** • Contact area varies with pressure • Weight correction done for non-uniform layer conductivities • Optimal λ depends on object shape	• Two-layer **SCRS**; conductive **paint** (PTP-EG1210OG, Plascoat, 20 Ω surface resistance) for probing and conductive **fabric** (MK-KTN260, Tanimura Corporation, 0.05 Ω) for driving layers • Square, 3, 6, 10 cm on a side and fingertip-shaped sensor • Free edges, on rigid surface • ‡ Conductive epoxy to Cu strips	• *Experiments* • 16 Electrodes • DC 3.3 V • Target = force sensor and cylindrical object	• Generalized Tikhonov regularization • Tikhonov prior, λ found using L-curve, λ^2 = 1000

[79]	2020	• Liquid based sensor; **pressure reduces the liquid under that region**, increases it elsewhere • Main source of error is electrode placement	• **Water** (liquid conductor) surmounted by a layer of air and an elastic membrane, inside a vertical frame • Circular, ds = ‡20 cm • Wire electrodes in water, alligator clips	• *Experiments* • 16 electrodes • I–M = ADJ–ADJ • 6–18 mA • Target = fingers	• Generalized Tikhonov regularization • Discrete Laplacian regularization, λ selected empirically
[80]	2021	• **Correction of amplitude regularization error** using a scaling matrix, based on radial position and λ	• Same as [67] • $\sigma_0 = 10^{-2}$ S m^{-1}	• *Simulations and experiments* • 16 electrodes • I = ADJ • DC 3 mA • $\Delta\sigma = -40\%$, $d_T = 0.2d_S$ • Target = force transducer with PTFE indenter d_T = 10 mm, 5 mm displacement • Noise-free simulations	• Same as [67] • For simulations $\lambda = 2 \times 10^{-8}$, 0.005, 0.05, 0.3; for experiments $\lambda = 0.2$ chosen based on no image artifacts
[81]	2021	• **Improve tracking** of object motion on a surface by **addition of hidden Markov models** for the trajectory		• Simulations • 16 electrodes • I–M = OPP–ADJ • $\sigma_0 = 1$ S m^{-1}, $\Delta\sigma = +1000\%$ • Gaussian noise, 5 levels	• PyEIT, one-step generalized Tikhonov regularization, difference imaging • NOSER prior with p = 0.5, $\lambda = 10^{-2}$ • HMM: Viterbi algorithm

(*Continued*)

Table 2.3. (*Continued*)

Reference	Year	Findings	Sensor	Conditions	Reconstruction
[82]	2021	• Average conductivity changed with pressure up to 10 kPa, then plateaued • Smaller FEM elements reduced position error	• Smartfoam (15DC-3G, Nanocomposite Products) spray-coated with latex-PSS-MWCNT layer. • Rectangle, 11 × 13 cm^2 • Unconstrained edges • Cu tape electrodes supplemented with Ag paste	• *Experiments* • 18 electrodes • I = ADJ • DC current • Target = weights, $d_T = 12$ mm	• Iterative GN • Tikhonov regularization
[83]	2021	• **New sensitivity matrix that makes the sensitivity more uniform across the sensor** • **Image fusion** based on wavelet transform to fuse images from different sensitivity matrices **to increase accuracy**	• Pressure-sensitive conductive foam; flexible but not stretchable • Square, 20 × 20 cm^2 • Freely moving sensor • Metal snap electrodes connecting sensor to flexible PCB	• *Simulations and experiments* • 16 electrodes • I–M = ADJ–ADJ • AC, 100 mA, 50 kHz for experiments, 1 A for simulations • For simulations $\sigma_0 = 0.001$ S m^{-1}, $\sigma_T = 0.1$ S m^{-1} • Target = loads (rubber blocks) for experiments	• COMSOL used for modeling
[84]	2022	• **Detect shape of balloon catheter** • Application: detecting athero-sclerosis, lumen shape during angioplasty • Used measurements from elec-trodes on central catheter shaft • Noise was a problem in reconstructions	• Two rings of electrodes on outer surface of catheter enclosed by a silicone balloon filled with **saline solution** • $\sigma_0 = 1.6$ S m^{-1}	• *Simulations and experiments* • 16 electrodes, nonpla-nar placement around catheter • I = radial pattern, M = ADJ or OPP • AC 140 μA, 11 kHz	• EIDORS, GN, both abso-lute and difference imaging • NOSER prior, $\lambda = 10^{-2}$ chosen by cross-validation

				• Target = tubes with different cross-sections, elasticity	
[85]	2022	• **Conductive liquid-filled porous elastic polymer sensor** • **ML post-processing for image segmentation** to improve images—remove artefacts and improve spatial resolution, uniformity	• **salt-water** filled porous PU **foam** (125–300 µS cm^{-1}) encased in Ecoflex substrate • Square, 20 × 20 cm^2, t = 5 mm • ‡ Unconstrained edges • Ag electrodes connected to wires	• *experiments* • 16 Electrodes • Not bipolar • AC voltage, 40 kHz • Target = load cell indenter d_T = 15 mm	• NOSER prior • PyTorch framework: pyramid scene parsing network (PSPNet) based on MobileNet, Adam optimizer, learning rate 0.001, 100 epochs • Training: 780 reconstructed images of multi-point touches
[86]	2022	• Material modeled to estimate strain; pressure map created • Mechanical perturbations caused large changes in electrode impedance, noise • Stress relaxation was significant; sensor conductivity was inhomogeneous	• **Carbon** (8%–10% CB, Vulcan XC 75R) **loaded** silicone **rubber** (Dragon skin 10 NV Smooth-On) • Circle, d_S = 10 cm, t = 4 mm • ‡ Unconstrained edges	• *Experiments* • 16 Electrodes • I–M = ADJ–ADJ • DC 15–100 µA • Target = plastic cylinder $d_T = 0.2d_S$ (20 mm)	• EIDORS
[87]	2022	• **Use the onset of artefacts as a criterion for evaluating image quality**	• σ_0 = 0.01 • Circle, d_S = 1	• *Simulations* • 16 Electrodes • I–M = PP–ADJ • DC 10^{-3} (1 mA)	• EIDORS, GN one-step • Laplace prior, λ = varied • Noise = varied

(*Continued*)

Table 2.3. (*Continued*)

Reference	Year	Findings	Sensor	Conditions	Reconstruction
		• Noise level at which artefacts first appear, N_{th}, related to hyperparameter, λ • Artefact-based μs match *L*-curve μs • **Automated regularization recommended**		• Contrast = −10% or −40% • Target = circular or triangular $d_T = 0.2d_S$	
[88]	2022	• All 36 bipolar I–M patterns evaluated • I–M performance determined at small λ by symmetry, at large λ by sensitivity at the center • **Avoid high symmetry patterns and ADJ positions** • **The 3–3 pattern gives a good compromise** among performance measures, which include **uniformity of the metrics** as well as noise susceptibility • **Consider using 13 electrodes instead of 16**	• $\sigma_0 = 0.01$ • Circle, $d_S = 1$	• *Simulations* • 13, 15, 16 Electrodes • I–M = varied, all bipolar • DC 10^{-3} (1 mA) • Contrast = −10% • Target = circular $d_T = 0.2d_S$	• EIDORS, GN one-step • Laplace prior, λ = varied • Noise = noise-free and at N_{th}

[89]	2022	• Sensor is salt-water-filled container + membrane • Positions of weights imaged, forces quantified; 1 Hz tapping detected; sensitive to low force (0.06 N); minimal hysteresis • 3 Frames s^{-1} imaging	• **Salt-water**-filled tub surmounted by an **elastic membrane** (latex) • Circle, $d_S = 17.4$ cm, *depth* = 10 mm • Membrane clamped at edge, placed over rigid surface • Bolt electrodes	• *Experiments* • 16 Electrodes • I = ADJ • AC 50 kHz, 6 mA • Target = weights $d_T = 20$ mm	• EIDORS, generalized Tikhonov regularization, difference imaging • Laplace prior, $\lambda = 10^{-5}$
[90]	2022	• Current between electrodes on sheet 1 is altered by closer contact with sheet 2 • **Sensor mounted on printed circuit board** • **Use OpenCV to locate object in EIT image** • Characterization of sensor under different number of objects, positions, weights, areas • $\Delta\sigma$ was linear with weight; accuracy reduced at periphery	• **SCRS**: stack of 2 piezoresistive sheets (Velostat) • Circle, $d_S = 10$ cm, $t = 0.2$ mm • Held in place by electrodes on printed circuit board (PCB) • Ag paste electrodes to PCB	• *Experiments* • 16 Electrodes • I–M = ADJ–ADJ • DC current • Target = cylindrical weights	• PyEIT Python EIT toolkit, Newton-Raphson back-projection • Difference imaging • OpenCV to find centroid

improved the ability to track motion over the sensor [81]. Using ML techniques, an artificial skin could, in simulation, recognize the shape of a contacting object at any size or orientation [91].

2.5.2 Applications of EIT for tactile imaging

EIT-based tactile imaging has from the start been employed for applications. As mentioned above, detection of human tactile interactions has been a main driver for the field. The earliest papers showed the ability to distinguish pinch, rub, grab, and simultaneous multi-finger contacts [33–35] and wrapped the sensors around curved surfaces with the aim of mounting the system on a robot, and even creating a whole-body skin [40]. Using a classifier with different attributes on a series of tactile images, it was possible to identify touch modality with good accuracy [42] and start to ascribe meaning to the data for 'social' applications [44, 45, 49]. The range of forces for touch recognition was expanded using a multi-layer tactile sensing architecture [66]. Future directions include moving from arm-scale demonstrations to full-body robot e-skins.

One of the first suggested uses of EIT was for detection pressure distributions for prevention of pressure sores in patients [26, 30], and pressure mapping has since been realized. A sensing mat for human weight distribution on the feet while standing was shown [48]. EIT tactile imaging has also been used to detect the shape of a balloon catheter with the aim of detecting atherosclerosis and the lumen shape during angioplasty [84]. It has also been implemented for inspection: imaging data were used to determine the position and direction of an aero-engine blade [74].

Information from EIT tactile imagers has also been used to control system behavior. For instance, manual contact with an oval sensor has been used to control a three-fingered robot gripper, using the resistivity change in three locations to control the speed of each finger [59]. By employing joint torque data, a robot arm could learn to control its motion under external perturbations [92]. A number of example applications were demonstrated in [64, 70]: controlling the brightness of a lamp based on the bending of its arm, controlling a music player with an interactive sticker, controlling television volume and channel with a pillow, and controlling a smart watch with a wristband.

As mentioned previously, SHM is a related field. SHM involves continuous measurement to detect deformation or damage in composite aircraft panels, cement structures such as bridges, and the like as reviewed in [3]. Appendix A surveys papers on the use of tactile EIT for SHM.

2.6 EIT tactile imaging configurations, conditions, reconstructions

There has been considerable work on increasing the fidelity of the EIT image to the input stimulus. Below we survey the literature via an examination of the various sensor configurations, experimental or simulation conditions, and reconstruction approaches that have been used. Of the 68 papers, 62% were experimental, 9% simulation only, 25% both experimental and simulation, and 4% reviews.

2.6.1 Sensor configurations

2.6.1.1 Sensor materials

Sensor materials must among other things (table 1.2), have reasonable uniformity of conductivity and mechanical properties, a large gauge factor (sensitivity), and the possibility to be produced at large size. Sensors that minimize cross-sensitivities to environmental and other mechanical stimuli are also advantageous.

The materials that have been used for EIT tactile sensors are summarized in figure 2.4(a). Sensors have been dominated by, and roughly equally divided between, various conductive elastomers and fabrics; this mix has not changed significantly over time. They have been used to measure both pressure and strain.

Conductive elastomer sensors have consisted of various elastomers (rubbers, silicones, latex, ABS printer filament, TPU) loaded with various nanocarbons (C black, nanofiber, nanotubes, nano-platelets). Commercial conductive rubbers used in early work suffered from relatively low stretchability, nonlinearity, large hysteresis and memory [10, 43], and sensitivity to both pressure and stretch. The amount of carbon loading (or fill fraction) was investigated, showing that non-uniformity of the C distribution lead to problems, particularly at low loadings where sensitivity was highest [50]. Some of the more recent sensors have shown reasonable linearity with strain and pressure [57, 59, 66], although they still have significant memory, displaying first-cycle effects, baseline offsets, stress relaxation, and spikes upon unloading. If the material does not return to its original state after a tactile contact, the reference images are no longer valid, as pointed out in [5]. Such memory effects can, however, be at least partially compensated, as shown in [64]. Many of the recent materials have been custom-made, since it is relatively straightforward to mix nanocarbons into silicone, latex, or other elastomers. A repairable carbon-loaded silicone sensor was demonstrated [60]. Fabrication of sensors with uniform properties is, however, still challenging [70, 86]. An issue that has been little addressed in this literature is the strong dependence of the resistivity of filled polymers on temperature and humidity, which has been established in other sensing contexts (see e.g. [93–95]).

As noted in section 1.3.2.4.2, the commercial availability and integration simplicity of fabric-based sensors makes them highly attractive. Fabric-based sensors are typically coated with metal or a conjugated polymer and consist of either stretchable woven fabrics or flexible (but not stretchable) non-wovens (e.g. felts). Like the conductive elastomers, woven fabrics also suffer from memory effects. In addition the wovens are anisotropic, both mechanically and electrically. However, conductive fabrics have, in principle, tremendous advantages: they can be sewn and washed, and they are robust to handling and storage (they can retain their properties for decades). Unfortunately, suitable stretchable conductive fabrics are not readily available (some listed in table 2.3 have been discontinued, as have some we purchased several years ago), with fabrics that are available having too high a conductivity (requiring high current to produce reasonable voltage outputs), too little stretchability, or too much anisotropy (having stretchability in only one direction or 10 times higher conductivity in one direction), posing a problem for researchers who are interested in making soft sensors but do not

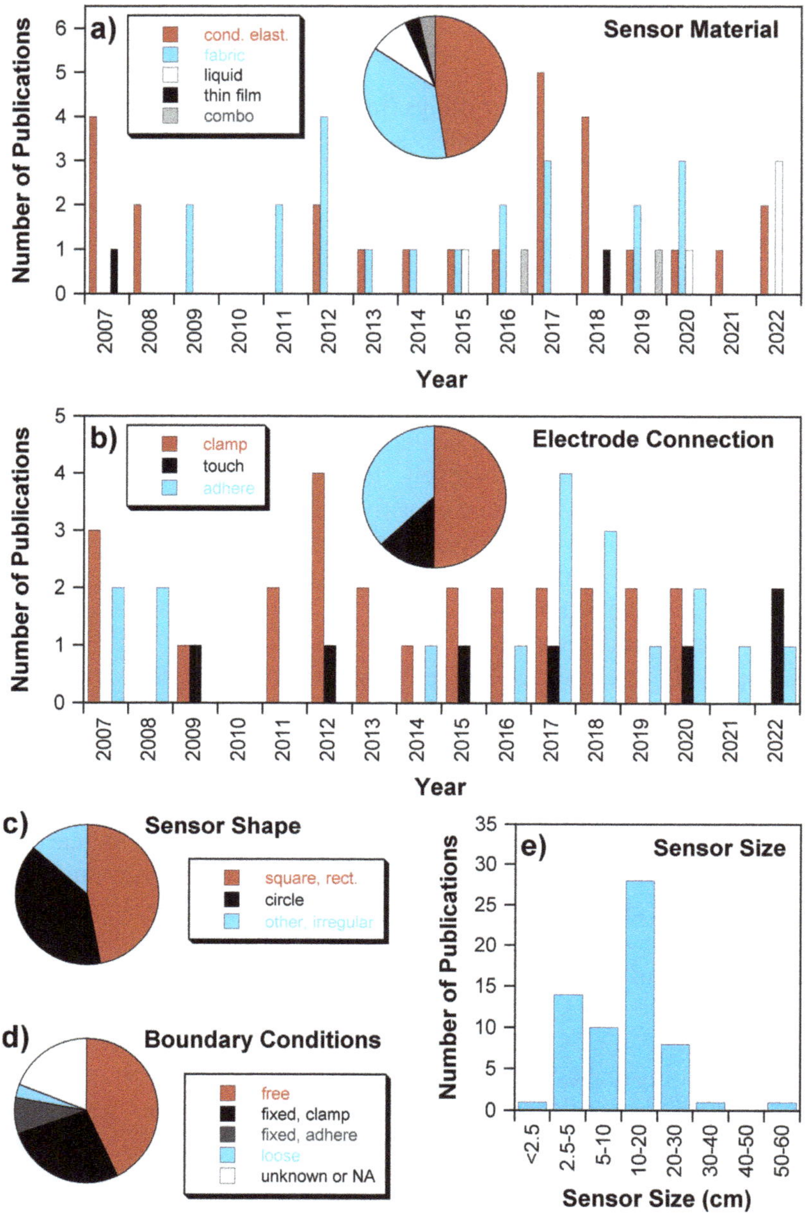

Figure 2.4. Summary of sensor configurations that have been employed in the tactile imaging EIT literature.

have access to looms to weave their own. A hybrid sensor has been shown, comprising a non-woven fabric filled with an elastomer [71].

Dissatisfaction with the early conductive elastomers and fabrics lead to work with contact-resistance based sensors. In one example of a stacked contact resistance sensor (SCRS), a top layer consisted of a stretchable net made from wavy yarns that straightened under strain while the resistance remained constant; this layer was supported on an insulating stretchable fabric base [38]. The second layer consisted of a conductive material cut into small disconnected pieces, also mounted on a stretchable base. Pressure changed the contact resistance between the yarn and the conductive pieces, lowering the resistance measured at the boundaries of the yarn net. The complexity of this sensor was high, but it delivered stretch-insensitive pressure sensing. However, multiple layers of fabric can introduce memory effects [5].

A delightful study by Zhang *et al* [65] investigated numerous conductive materials, including salty JellO. The sensing mechanism differed from the typical bulk resistivity or contact resistance change: it was based on the human body's shunting of current from the conductive material. Demonstration applications included interactive objects and toys, with ML applied to handle arbitrary geometries. The optimum surface resistivity range was identified. Also, in 2017, a pair of creative papers by Ramani *et al* [64] and Harrison *et al* [65] added to the sensing modalities and the number of materials. In addition, the authors created toolkits for handling arbitrary sensor shapes and fabrication variability. Numerous applications were demonstrated, illustrating how this technology can bring interactivity to diverse objects.

Several liquid-base sensors have been constructed, which operate similarly to EIT saline tanks (used to validate EIT simulations). They consist of containers filled with liquid, typically salt water but in one case an ionic liquid [9]; the containers have at least one elastomeric face [79, 84, 89]. A contact on an elastomeric face displaces the water underneath, leading to a local increase in resistance due to the decreased conductor thickness. Liquid based sensors in general have the disadvantages of being relatively heavy and prone to leaks, but can have advantages of simplicity and isotropy (unless the liquid is encapsulated in channels). One interesting approach contained the liquid in a foam encased within the elastomer skin [85].

2.6.1.2 Electrical connections

It has been known since the earliest studies [29] that attention must be paid to the method of applying electrodes. The connection issue has both mechanical and electrical aspects. Mechanically, deformations during tactile interactions can lead to fatigue or even delamination at that connection [5], and the much stiffer metal electrodes can damage an elastomeric sensor [29], particularly at sharp corners or if they are tightly clamped. Also, EIT is known to be sensitive to variations in electrode position and size [65]: inaccurate electrode placement can be a significant source of image errors [79]. Electrically, because voltage differences induced by tactile contacts on the sensor surface are small, images can be strongly distorted by changing contact resistance [72, 86] or electrode movement [70, 76, 77]. Furthermore, poor contacts can be a source of noise [86]. Nevertheless, the focus in the literature has been more on abstract electrode considerations than on the practical details of exactly how the connections have been, or should be, made.

Electrical connections to non-liquid sensors have primarily been made by clamping or adhesion, with the balance of these techniques not changing significantly over time (figure 2.4(b)). Clamps have included the ever-popular alligator clips as well as screws, bolts, eyelets, snaps, and crimps, as well as metal strips or wires clamped to the sensor using a frame. Adhesives have included silver paint, paste, or epoxy, or the sensing material itself. In one study of electrical connection methods, press-fit electrical contacts were found to be susceptible to noise and motion, and silver epoxy was found to be fragile, so piercing electrodes were recommended [5]. Metal strands or metal-coated yarns have been woven into fabric sensors, making strong connections by touch alone. Liquid sensors can also rely on simple metal-fluid contact.

The challenge of making robust electrical connections between soft materials (elastic moduli of 1–10 MPa) and metals (100 GPa) has been known for many years, for example in the fields of wearable devices and soft robots. In the EIT tactile imaging field, it has been noted that rigid electrodes are a problem [70]. Methods such as embedding thin serpentine shaped wires to allow some 'give' have been explored. For fabrics, button snaps have been used to provide a strong connections.

The introduction of noise at electrical contacts is problematic because EIT image reconstruction is highly sensitive to noise, as discussed in later chapters. EIT algorithms handle noise by eliminating high-spatial frequency image components, which smooths or defocuses the image, particularly in the center; the amount of smoothing is controlled by the hyperparameter λ and the type of smoothing by the prior (figure 2.3). With a small hyperparameter, the resolution can be ~5% of the sensor area for a 16 electrode system, but for a very large hyperparameter, a contact can appear to occupy the entire sensor area.

Further work on the issue of electrical connections is indicated. Performance should be evaluated both on the mechanical issues giving rise to stress and motion-induced artefacts and on the electrical issue of noise.

2.6.1.3 Boundary conditions

Closely related to the issue of electrical connection methods is that of perimeter boundary conditions. Because signals from near the boundary dominate those from the interior, as shown in later chapters, artefacts due to tugging, wrinkling [5], or other mechanical disturbances unassociated with contacts must be prevented. If clamping is used to bring electrodes into contact with the sensor, apart from the mechanical damage that may be caused, it can be difficult to achieve the same contact pressure at every electrode [29], and the contact resistance between soft materials and metal electrodes can be strongly pressure-dependent. Tactile pressure applied near the perimeter has been reported to deform the electrical contact area, affecting the image [46] or further amplifying contacts there [72]. To reduce strain at the electrode interface, non-stretchable fabric was sewn to the boundary [5]. In addition, motion artefacts occur [5, 72] and noise can be introduced [72] if the electrodes move during use. Artefacts can be seen at the electrodes [62, 68], at the perimeter [5], and at the corners of rectangular sensors [48]. For practical implementation, successfully managing the sensor boundaries can be vexing.

Reviewing how boundaries have been treated to date (figure 2.4(d)), roughly half of the publications that indicated how the sensor perimeter was handled had unconstrained, or free, sensor edges. This allows imaging without edge artefacts due to tugging, allowing proof of concept to be established for various ideas, but it is incompatible with integration of the technology into a system. Among the studies with fixed boundaries, most fixed the sensor in a rigid frame while some taped the edges, with electrical connections made outside the clamped region. For some of the liquid sensors, the question of fixing the sensor is not applicable; for a soft liquid-filled system the issue instead becomes preventing tactile interactions from distorting the sensor's shape.

The boundary condition on the bottom face of the sensor can be rigid in the case of a pressure sensor, and a few of the pressure sensors appear to have had their bottom faces adhered to a substrate. For a sensor based on strain, the underlying substrate must generally be soft, such as a layer of foam. As mentioned previously, the substrate can be arbitrarily shaped; provided that the sensor does not wrinkle, it remains effectively a 2D panel. Layers of materials above or below the sensor, in addition to providing mechanical protection, can also contribute to sensing performance. For example, a foam substrate can convert strain to a pressure or force signal, with the force range controlled by the stiffness of the foam [96]. Multiple layers of foam of different stiffness extend the sensing range to allow both high sensitivity to small forces and continued responsivity to high forces [66].

2.6.1.4 Sensor shape and size

Sensor shapes have been primarily circular and rectangular or square, which are standard shapes for EIDORS. Equal numbers of each have been reported (figure 2.4(c)). Rectangular sensors have sometimes shown artefacts at the corners [48]. A few groups have explored irregular shapes [34, 44], and even three-dimensional shapes, for which custom software is required to handle the reconstruction. Examples of irregular shapes include hourglass shapes for wrapping around a robot or mannequin arm, dome-shaped shells [59, 74], and star or dog-shaped personalized smart interfaces [64].

Typical sensor sizes are 10–20 cm in diameter or on a side (figure 2.4(e)), although an equal number have been smaller; not many have been larger. Despite the fact that many types of EIT sensors could be made arbitrarily large (see e.g. [66]), and that the impetus for much of the work is for whole-body tactile skins for robots [40], only a few large-scale systems have yet been realized. Among the largest were a 40×40 cm^2 fabric-based mat that detected the foot pressure of a human standing on it [48] and a 60×6 cm^2 panel for determining touch location and tracking accuracy [65].

2.6.2 Imaging conditions

2.6.2.1 Number of electrodes

A larger number of electrodes improves image resolution, although such improvements are incremental and not as large as one might expect. Improvements can even be non-existent when the level of noise necessitates the use of a large λ [88], as shown in section 5.4. (Specifically, the resolution is limited by the size of the smallest eigenpeaks available in the reconstruction, the size of which increase with λ.) A larger number of electrodes, in addition to adding system complexity, also requires significantly longer data collection times, which increases by approximately a factor of 4 for every doubling of the number of electrodes. It also increases image reconstruction time and computational resources.

Fully 2/3 of the papers in table 2.3 used 16 electrodes (figure 2.5(a)). Among those using other numbers, 8, 28, and 32 were each 8%–9%, with some papers testing

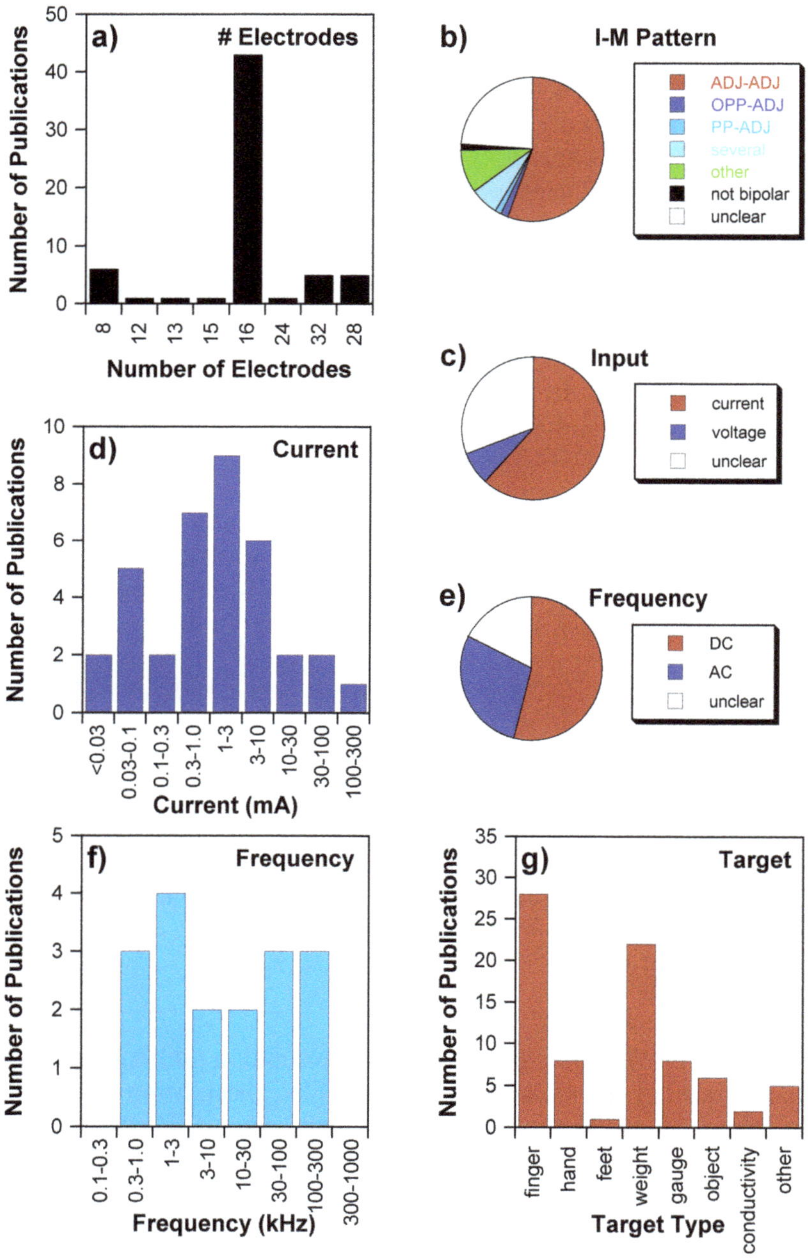

Figure 2.5. Summary of measurement conditions that have been employed in the tactile imaging EIT literature.

several of the arrangements. One publication noted that a 32-electrode configuration was not considered due to the low frame rate, and that for 80% of the sensor area in the center, 8 and 16 electrodes had the same accuracy [64]. Our work has shown that it may, in fact, be advantageous to reduce the number of electrodes from 16, for example down to 13 (chapters 5 and 7).

Several examples of work employing internal electrodes, which was done as early as 1993 [30], were included in the literature review of table 2.3. As can be understood from first principles, the resolution improves if internal electrodes are added. However, doing so negates the prime advantage of EIT, which is exactly the absence of internal electrodes.

2.6.2.2 Injection-measurement (I–M) patterns

For most of the papers included in table 2.3, the I–M pattern was, when specified, bipolar (figure 2.5(b)). (Perhaps surprisingly, nearly a quarter of the papers did not specify an I–M pattern.) Bipolar means that current is injected into two of the peripheral electrodes, and voltage differences are found between pairs of all the others. (In practice, the voltages of all the other electrodes are measured, either sequentially or simultaneously, with respect to ground, and the voltage differences are then obtained in software by subtraction.) Among the commonly used electrode pairs are ADJ, in which the electrodes are immediately adjacent to each other, OPP, in which they are located directly opposite each other on either side of the sensor, and PP, which stands for pseudo-polar and in which the electrodes are one position closer (or equivalently, further) than directly opposite. The injection (I) and measurement (M) patterns are specified with I first and M second, and these can be different. For example OPP–ADJ indicates that current is injected on opposite sides of the sensor and voltages are measured between every adjacent pair, excluding those in the injection pair.

The I–M pattern has been studied in the EIT literature since at least 1994, as well as in a few publications in tactile imaging EIT [39, 41, 61], but little of those conclusions has diffused over to experimental practice. The I–M pattern affects image metrics such as resolution, peak amplitude, and susceptibility to noise, as well as uniformity across the image. High symmetry patterns, such as OPP–OPP, have been reported to have notably poor performance, as does ADJ–ADJ at high noise. The reasons for this poor performance are discussed in detail in chapter 7. Nevertheless, 74% of the papers that specified a bipolar pattern in table 2.3 employed ADJ–ADJ. One 32-electrode system employed a 5–2 pattern (injection electrodes five positions apart and measurement electrodes two spaces apart). (Other bipolar patterns were used by systems with internal electrodes (e.g. [43]) or configurations such as electrodes placed in concentric rings in a balloon catheter [84].) One study noted that the best I–M pattern depended on the prior used during reconstruction [41]. Other considerations to be taken into account in choosing an I–M pattern are covered in chapter 7.

2.6.2.3 Powering the sensor

The systems in table 2.3 are resistive, with the exception of one piezoelectric sensor [58] and the previously-mentioned electric field tomography sensors [64]. Current can be injected and voltages measured at the other electrodes, or, vice versa, voltage can be applied to some of the electrodes and current measured between the others. Current injection is favored because it eliminates the influence of contact impedance between the electrodes and the sensor at the measurement electrodes, given the high input impedance of voltage-measuring instruments [56]. In addition, accurate programmable constant current sources are available, and voltage measurement is readily implemented. Thus, in 90% of the studies in which the input was specified, current was injected (figure 2.5(c)); a few studies employed a constant voltage input [36, 78]. Currents have varied by over 5 orders of magnitude, from 15 μA to 100 mA (figure 2.5(d)), with most being in the range of 1–3 mA.

As mentioned in section 1.3.2, a disadvantage of resistive sensors is their continuous power draw, particularly for battery-powered systems such as autonomous robots [97]. However, power consumption values as low as 22 [45] and 10 mW [62] have been achieved.

Both AC and DC current sources have been employed (figure 2.5(e)), with DC outnumbering AC by nearly 2:1 when the stimulation frequency was specified. AC stimulation allows measurement of the real and imaginary components of impedance, and it also eliminates polarization effects, but it requires more complex hardware [1, 77] and has a lower sampling rate [1]. Frequencies have ranged from 1 to 200 kHz (figure 2.5(f)), purportedly depending on the sensor impedance [75]. It has been found with a conductive rubber sensor that the quality of the raw voltage data depended on the frequency [5]. One study of a fabric sensor created images from both the real and imaginary parts of the signal, with the reliability of the former decreasing with frequency and the latter increasing [53]. Since the sensors themselves are resistive, the capacitive contribution presumably arises from various couplings between the sensor and its surroundings, which would be expected to depend on environmental factors. In one study using frequencies from 1 to 250 kHz, capacitance images were formed using a conducting fabric sensor, and the signal was found to change with applied pressure [53]. In another study in which the frequency was varied from 1 to 200 kHz, the images from a carbon-loaded elastomer obtained at different frequencies enabled principle component analysis to distinguish among six types of materials contacting the sensor (banana, wood, hand, etc) under well controlled laboratory conditions [75]. The value of this information, and its reliability in real-world situations, is still unclear.

2.6.2.4 EIT hardware

The big advantage of DC current injection is the miniaturizability of the hardware. A simple battery-powered programmable microcontroller board (such as an Arduino) controlling switches to a voltage-driven constant current source can be used to collect the data [47, 64]. These systems are thus readily portable and low cost [56], and data can be sent wirelessly to a cell phone for reconstruction.

2.6.2.5 Targets

For testing, loads such as static weights placed at known locations are often used as targets (24%) (figure 2.5(g)), as are pressure, force, or displacement gauges (9%), the latter allowing dynamic measurements. Given that a principal aim of tactile imaging is the detection of human interactions with a system, it is no surprise that fingers and hands have also frequently been targets (39%). In 12 publications (13%), the targets were moving: object tracking was performed or gestures such as pinching, rubbing, and tapping were recorded and classified. Occasionally other objects have been employed (7%) or other things used as targets, such as areas engineered to have different conductivity.

2.6.3 Reconstruction

Numerous algorithms have been developed for image reconstruction [21], not only for conductivity differences but also for absolute conductivity mapping. Some approaches make a linear approximation while others are nonlinear, some being one-step and others iterative. These approaches have largely been developed in the medical EIT literature and require advanced mathematical familiarity to sensibly evaluate. From an experimentalist's perspective, their various advantages may not be clear, nor which are appropriate for tactile imaging from perspectives such as hardware requirements and imaging rates. We begin with the tactile imaging work that has used tradition reconstruction before turning to the new ML approaches.

2.6.3.1 Traditional EIT

Information about reconstruction approaches used in the tactile imaging literature is shown in figure 2.6. The EIDORS software has been used for reconstruction in 70% of the studies that specified the system that was used, and PyEIT in 4%. In a quarter of the work done with EIDORS or PyEIT, custom software was used in addition, for example to allow importing of custom CAD sensor designs [34], to handle arbitrary sensor geometries [64], to classify touch modality [42], to improve target tracking [81], or to locate an object in the EIT image [90]. Custom reconstruction has been used to implement alternative algorithms with constraints on the resistivity change [36, 55].

Among the studies that specified whether the method was one-step or iterative, 70% used a one-step reconstruction. With a one-step algorithm, the regularized inverse of the sensitivity matrix is calculated once in advance, so that subsequent steps require only matrix multiplication. While the resulting images have lower accuracy, they offer—typically more important for tactile imaging—the advantage of speed. Real-time imaging is essential for applications that involve human–robot interactions. For example, tapping at 1 Hz is a typical human gesture [89]. Imaging speeds of 10 [58], 30 [69, 73], 35 [64], and even 60 Hz have been achieved [41]. However, an imaging speed of 50 Hz was reduced to an effectively 1 Hz response to stimuli by a slow sensor mechanical recovery [72], so the reconstruction and sensor speeds must be considered in conjunction with each other.

As mentioned previously, the main issue in reconstruction is handling noise. For reasons discussed in later chapters, the inverse problem to create an image from the boundary voltages is 'ill posed', and thus easily destabilized by noise. To create an

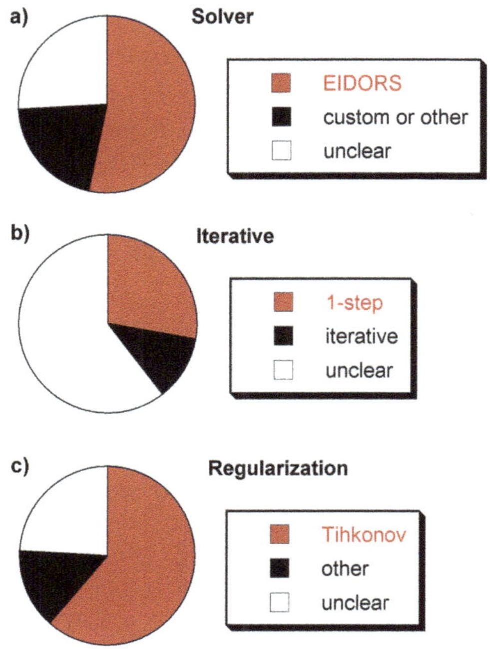

Figure 2.6. Summary of reconstruction approaches that have been employed in the tactile imaging EIT literature.

accurate image, 'regularization' is employed. Of the publications that specified the method, 80% employed Tikhonov regularization, which is detailed in chapter 4. This method employs a sensitivity matrix that is pre-calculated from the forward problem, thereby speeding computation. It also employs a smoothing filter (the prior) and a hyperparameter λ, which acts as a dial to adjust the amount of smoothing.

The tactile imaging literature, arising out of the sensor community and focused on showing proof of concept for sensor configurations, has largely focused on hardware improvements, on both the sensors and the data collection circuitry (forward problem issues, figure 2.3). Less attention has been paid to the effects on image quality of EIT reconstruction methods and parameters (the inverse problem). In fact, as seen from figure 2.6, these are often not specified. Yet, a study by Tawil *et al* that compared the priors used in Tikhonov regularized reconstructions demonstrated that such choices matter [41]. Critically for tactile imaging, Tikhonov regularization assumes a linear relationship between changes in conductivity and changes in perimeter voltage (given by the sensitivity matrix), which may not be valid for sensors under large deformations. Most critically, the extent of regularization, controlled by λ, has extensive effects on image quality (as discussed in chapter 5).

This lack of attention may be partly a result of the user-friendliness of software such as EIDORS, which can quickly generate reasonable images using its default settings, which may not be apparent to the user. It may also be partly due to the advanced mathematical treatment of EIT in the medical EIT literature, which can be largely incomprehensible to non-mathematicians, and the previous lack of a centralized in-depth review for the lay person. It is hoped that the later chapters of this book will clarify how forward and inverse problem parameters affect reconstruction quality.

Improvements and add-ons to the EIT algorithms for tactile imaging have been made. For example, putting a positive value constraint on the resistivity can be used instead of regularization to stabilize the solution of the inverse problem [36]. Skipping the reconstruction if sensor input is essentially unchanged from the prior set of measurements reduces the computational load [10], as does constraining the resistivity change to be sum of 2D sine waves [55]. By creating two images, one for voltage measurements made parallel to the current injection and one for measurements made perpendicular, called 'anisotropic EIT', the direction of stretch could be obtained [59]. As an example of an add-on, a toolkit to handle arbitrary sensor geometries was developed [64]. As another example, the displacements giving rise to the conductivity changes can be obtained by combining image information with knowledge of the sensor's mechanical properties and use of a 3D mesh [63]. It has also been shown that by dynamically updating the baseline data when there is a contact, sensor memory effects can be compensated to some extent [64]. It should also be noted that corrections to images can be made based on the known distorting effects of the hyperparameter [80].

Future studies on compensating for non-ideal sensor behavior, namely memory and anisotropy, which are the norm in sensor materials, would be welcome. In particular, add-ons for open-source software like EIDORS and PyEIT could be of value to the community. The other approach, rapidly gaining momentum, is to employ ML instead of EIT, as discussed in the next section.

2.6.4 Machine learning

ML has begun to be applied to tactile EIT; some of that literature is summarized in table 2.5; acronyms and terms used there are defined in table 2.4. Advanced EIT algorithms, including those based on ML, were reviewed in [2].

Initially, ML was used to improve the fidelity of, or further process information from, images first obtained by EIT. For example, ML has been used for touch localization or classification [42, 65] and to post-process images to aid in multi-point discrimination [85]. ML has also been applied to handle baseline offsets in the first several touch cycles due to sensor memory, and to maintain the ability to identify contacts upon stretching the sensor [70].

Work has also been done with ML to produce images directly from the voltage data. Artificial neural networks (ANNs) began to be investigated for EIT image

Table 2.4. Terms frequently employed in ML and robotics for tactile EIT.

Name	Definition or Information
Adam optimizer	Procedure to update network weights iteratively
Adalines	Adaptive linear elements
ANN	Artificial neural network, typically 1 hidden layer
CNN	Convolutional NN
DNN	Deep NN (typically more than one hidden layer)
MLP	Multi-layer perceptron
RBFNN	Radial basis function NN
ReLU	Rectified linear unit
SOM	Self-organized map; unsupervised learning, does not need information about the sensor

reconstruction as early as 1991 [98, 99]. The aims include reducing the computational load and speeding up image reconstruction by avoiding matrix inversion, as well as obtaining 'better' results, evaluated against various metrics. Generally the images look better: the geometry of the target and the amplitude of $\Delta\sigma$ is more accurate. This is not surprising, since the ML algorithm was trained to do exactly that.

ML has important advantages over conventional EIT for reconstruction. One is that there is no need to have a model for the potential fields in the sensor. Instead, the relationships between the impedance changes and conductivity variations are learned from examples during training. Of course, a corresponding disadvantage is that neglecting the simple physics puts the onus entirely on the training data to be sufficiently complete.

A pressing issue for traditional EIT has been that differences between the actual sensor and the sensor model result in degradation of the reconstruction. This is a problem because the conductivity of the sensor is often non-uniform due to imperfections, and the electrodes may not be perfectly positioned. For stretchable sensors, furthermore, the shape and relative electrode positions change under contact [100]. In addition, handling unconventional geometries is essential for tactile imaging [100]. While this was successfully demonstrated as early as 2007 [33, 34] and subsequently [64] with conventional EIT, with ML the geometry does not need to be specified [101], nor the initial conductivity of the sensor [102]: the training data alone from that particular sensor can be sufficient for the algorithm to be able to interpret the data. ML is also able handle non-idealities like electrode motion. Since the algorithms can be trained on the physical system with its non-idealities present, they can have high accuracy. A thorough and well-done study of a deep convolutional neural network (DCNN) showed that it could compensate for movements in electrode positions associated with a shape change of the sensor (such

Table 2.5. Survey of some publications on the use of machine learning instead of EIT for reconstruction of tactile sensor data.

Reference	Year	Findings	Sensor	Conditions	Reconstruction
	Key	• Some findings, particulars	• **Materials**, details, conductivity • Shape, size, thickness • Boundary conditions (BCs) • Electrical connections	• *Simulations/experiments* • Number of electrodes • I–M pattern • Electrical input • Conductivity, contrast • Target	• ML reconstruction method • training • Noise or SNR • Other information • Traditional EIT information
[98]	1991	• ***(Not tactile imaging)*** • Proof of concept demonstrated • Able to image patterns not used in training		• *Experiments* • Saline tank	• ANN with adalines receiving impedance differences • Training data: impedance changes from experiments, 320 patterns
[99]	1994	• ***(Not tactile imaging)*** • Linearly approximates the inverse problem • Resolution depends on radial position (as in EIT); resolution and noise rejection are traded off (as in EIT) • Good reconstructions when SNR is similar to training data, when geometry is similar to training data • Cannot handle large conductivity changes or interactions between multiple areas with conductivity change • Faster than back-projection (no longer used)		• *Simulations*	• ANN • Training data: impedance changes from forward problem simulations

(*Continued*)

Table 2.5. (*Continued*)

Reference	Year	Findings	Sensor	Conditions	Reconstruction
[101]	2015	• [47] plus • DNN used successfully with a sensor • Able to determine sensor's own shape • Survey of ANN approaches to image reconstruction of EIT data • ANN faster than iterative EIT (unfair comparison); similar position error • Could identify locations of 1–3 weights at the periphery with NN, • Had difficulty determining target shapes (note: the human arm also unable to discriminate shapes)	• **Velostat**, sensor has nonlinear change in resistance with pressure • Circle $d_S = 20$ cm	• *Experiments* • 16 Electrodes • DC current 200 μA • I–M = ADJ–ADJ • $R_0 = 23$ kΩ • Target = weight at different positions on sensor, $d_T = 25$ mm, $\Delta R = -3$ kΩ for conductive weight, +0.05 kΩ for insulating weight of 100 g	• ANN, SOM—Kohonen map • Training: voltage data from conductive target; # samples unknown • Noise unknown • EIT: EIDORS, iterative Tikhonov regularization
[92]	2016	• Learned what compliant forces to apply to a 2 DOF robot arm to control its motion when tactile signals are detected (human perturbations) • Identify joint torques during contact, learn tactile map of touch with SOM, learn sensorimotor loop • Operates at 40 Hz	• **Velostat** • rectangle 25 × 32 cm^2 wrapped around arm	• *Experiments* • 16 Electrodes • DC current 200 μA • 208 voltage measurements • Target = finger touches of varying force, position on sensor	• Same as [101] for supervised learning of sensor topology • 2nd NN based on Perceptron to learn compliant forces to apply, reinforcement learning, Widrow-Hoff learning rule • Training: voltage from touches + torque as a result of touch; # samples unknown • Noise unknown • EIT: NA

[107]	2017	• Used to estimate position of simulated target • Metrics: target area, position error • No need to select threshold for peak detection	• Circular sensor • $\sigma_0 = 6 \times 10^{-5}$ S m^{-1},	• *Simulations* • 16 Electrodes • 208 measurements • DC current • $\Delta\sigma$ = positive • Target = 3 sizes, $A_T = 1, 4, 9\%$ of A_S, varying position from 0 to $0.8r_S$	• ANN is an MLP, 2 neurons in 1 hidden layer, Levenberg–Marquardt algorithm • Supervised learning • Trained on simulated forward model differential voltage datasets • Training: # samples unknown • Gaussian noise, SNR 20 DB • EIT: unclear; threshold for ROI set manually depending on target size
[104]	2019	• ***(Not tactile imaging***, but 2D images) • Impedance data segmented, arranged in overlapping sub-meshes, represented as polynomial coefficients which are learned • Metrics: mean square error (MSE) in polynomial coefficient prediction, MSE of reconstruction • Best reconstructions with Levenberg–Marquardt networks of 10 neurons and cubic polynomials, but takes longest time to train	• Square sensor, 24 × 24	• *Simulations* • 16 Electrodes, M = ADJ, 208 voltage measurements • Target = square 8 × 8, 6 $\Delta\sigma$ levels; varying position	• Matlab ANN toolbox, Levenberg–Marquardt and scaled conjugate algorithms, variable number of hidden neurons, various architectures • Trained on 5–17k simulated forward model voltage datasets; 70:30 split • Noise unknown • EIT: NA

(*Continued*)

Table 2.5. *(Continued)*

Reference	Year	Findings	Sensor	Conditions	Reconstruction
[105]	2019	• DNN used for imaging with a sensor • Able to reconstruct targets not seen in training • Metric: MSE between target and reconstruction • NN had improved MSE compared to linear EIT; comparable to 10-iteration GN EIT but faster. • NN was robust to noise in simulations • NN had moderate accuracy with real sensor; results had to be smoothed to remove spikes; results are sensitive to training set • 50 Hz imaging	• **Fabric** (COM-14 112, Eeonyx) + silicone rubber, $\sigma_0 = 65$ µS m^{-1} • Square, 14 × 14 cm^2 • Conductive thread electrodes + Ag paste	• *Experiments* • 16 Electrodes • I–M = ADJ–ADJ • training target = 1 × 1-element square, 4 × 4 square, random positions of several 1 × 1 squares • reconstruction target = rectangle 4 × 8 and L-shape	• Deep neural network with fully connected network, ReLU function, Adam optimizer • Trained on 77k simulated forward model voltage datasets; 12k epochs; 90:10 • Gaussian noise, SNR down to 15 dB • EIT: EIDORS 10-iteration GN
[108]	2019	• Classification of touch position • Application on robot arm demonstrated • Training time and memory are reduced by using fewer independent measurements	• Three-layer **fabric** structure: conductive fabric (Less EMF), honeycomb mesh, high resistance fabric (Eeonyx) • Square, 13 × 13 or 17 × 17 cm^2 for testing; rectangle	• *Experiments* • 8 or 16 Electrodes • I–M = OPP–ADJ • Target = varying force, d_T=10 or 15 mm in 100 (10 × 10 array) or 49 (7 × 7) positions=classes	• ML classification algorithm, quadratic discriminant analysis (QDA), supervised learning • Two-algorithm training approach, 10-fold cross-validation

		• QDA faster to train than classification trees, SVM, KNN, and ensemble methods • Metrics: Euclidian error between classes, number of misclassifications • Error depends on the position of the target, worst in center • Multiple simultaneous inputs require further work • Errors larger in 8 electrode system than 16 • 78 Hz imaging	10×22 cm^2 for robot arm; t=1.5 mm • Alligator clip electrodes		• Training: 20 scans for each touch, 3.2k samples for each scan; 2400 datasets, 6 replicates (1 h total); samples divided into subsections of 160; test data of unknown pressure collected separately • Noise unknown • EIT: NA
[106]	2020	• COMSOL used for forward model to handle various sensor geometries, anisotropy • Sensor can detect a finger touch, simulations can detect 3 targets	• **Fabric** sensor (Carbotex 03–82, Sefar AG), $\sigma_0 = 3.1$ S cm^{-1} • Circular, $d_S = 25$ cm • Edges clamped in frame • Conductive Cu tape electrodes	• *Simulations and experiments* • 8 Electrodes • I = ADJ • DC current • $\Delta\sigma$ = positive • Experimental target = fingers • Simulated target = Gaussian $\Delta\sigma$ profile 0–20 S m^{-1}, d_T= 10–110 mm, varying position	• ANN with 1 hidden layer, 500 neurons, Matlab Neural Network Toolbox • Forward model implemented in COMSOL • Simulated forward model differential voltage datasets, 19k samples; 70:15:15, 20k epochs (19 h) • Gaussian noise std = 10^{-5} • EIT: NA

(*Continued*)

Table 2.5. (*Continued*)

Reference	Year	Findings	Sensor	Conditions	Reconstruction
[91]	2021	• Develop modular ML framework for robot recognition of objects by touch, recognize shapes even when rotated, scaled • Image reconstruction by low-order bivariate polynomials and radial basis function networks, segmentation using convolutional NN and transfer learning, + object recognition with subspace KNN ensemble classifier • Metrics: MSE in coefficient prediction for ANN, position error, resolution, and noise factor for image • Several types of ANN tested; 2nd order RBF had best performance • Compared to EIT with Laplace prior, reconstructions had lower MSE and PE, higher resolution	• Square sensor • Clamped boundary	• *Simulations* • 16 Electrodes • I–M = ADJ–ADJ • DC 1 mA • Target = 3 shapes, several sizes, positions, orientations, $\Delta\sigma$	• ANNs: multi-layer perceptrons, radial basis functions, and others; data represented as coefficients of polynomials • Impedance map decomposed into 4×4 patches, 16 Ml models learn one patch, patches stitched back together • Trained on simulated forward model differential voltage datasets, 6400 samples, 70:30 • White noise, SNR down to 5 dB • EIT: EIDORS, Tikhonov regularization with 4 priors, L-curve used to determine λ

[103]	2021	*(Thesis)* • Can compensate for electrode movement (traditional EIT cannot), even with noise • Features are blurry and that are close together are merged • Various electrode models discussed • Metrics: relative image error, image correlation coefficient • 278 Frames per second for reconstruction; bottleneck is data collection	• σ_0 =1 S cm^{-1}	• *Simulations* • 16 Electrodes, positions varied • I–M = ADJ–ADJ • targets = three shapes, 2 sizes each (0.15 to 0.4 of sensor length), $\Delta\sigma = -1\%$ or more, various locations; multiple targets also used	• Deep convolutional neural network (DCNN); regularization parameter (weight decay) tuned • Trained on simulated forward model differential voltage datasets, 48k samples • Gaussian white noise, SNR down to 20 dB • EIT: EIDORS, Tikhonov regularization, Laplace prior, λ tuned
[109]	2021	• Survey of literature on ML for EIT • Conductivity of the sensor depends nonlinearly on force • Metric: loss function spatial sensitivity aware MSE (SSA-MSE), position error (PE), resolution, sensitivity, two-point discrimination • DNN reconstruction has improved performance versus one-step and iterative GN: lower SSA-MSE and PE, higher resolution, sensitivity, and distinguishability, faster speed	• Two-layer **contact resistance** sensor: high conductivity **fabric** squares on foam over spray-coated resistive carbon black (3 mS m^{-1}) • Square, 20 × 20 cm^2 • Electrodes screwed into sensor + Ag paste; unconstrained edges except screws	• *Simulations and experiments* • 17 Electrodes, 1 **internal** • I, M = bipolar, RefC pattern • DC 3 mA • Experimental targets = 1 or 2 indenters, d_T = 20 mm; fingers and hands, various touch geometries • Simulation training = 1 × 1-element square, 2 × 2 to 24 × 24 square, random positions of several 1 × 1 squares, various positive and negative $\Delta\sigma$ levels	• DNN in Matlab, ReLU function, Adam optimizer • Trained on simulated forward model voltage datasets; 90:10 • Gaussian noise std = 0.5 mV • EIT: EIDORS, one-step and iterative GN

(Continued)

Table 2.5. (*Continued*)

Reference	Year	Findings	Sensor	Conditions	Reconstruction
		• Able to classify different finger and hand contacts • All methods were resilient to sensor damage (cuts made to base layer)			
[100]	2022	• COMSOL can model arbitrary geometries (in principle also anisotropy) • ANN reconstructions have higher fidelity to target • Multiple types of training data improve reconstructions • Reconstruction more accurate with a higher linear density of electrodes • Closely spaced touches overlap in the reconstruction	• **Stretchable inks** (Ag based for conductors, C based for sensing) printed and transferred onto cotton **fabric**, $\sigma_0 = 250$ S m^{-1} • Insole-shaped sensor (29 cm long)	• *Simulations and experiments* • 16 Electrodes • I–M = ADJ–ADJ • DC 0.25 mA • Experimental target = finger touch in 6 positions • Simulated target = Gaussian $\Delta\sigma$ profile, varying amplitude, position, size; also single square or circle with various size, position, $\Delta\sigma$	• ANN, Matlab Neural Network Toolbox, 800 neurons in 1 hidden layer, hyperbolic tangent functions, • Simulated forward model differential voltage datasets in COMSOL; 10k samples, 26k epochs • Gaussian noise std = 10^{-5} • EIT: Tikhonov regularization, one-step, NOSER prior, λ selected by iterative random optimization process
[102]	2022	• Sensor conductivity, electrode impedance do not need to be known; can use training data directly with ML • Requires little data (~ # electrodes)^2 measured with single-point indenter • Can handle inhomogeneous sensor due e.g. to imperfect mixing, air bubbles	• **Carbon** (6% MWCNT) **loaded silicone** (Ecoflex, Smooth-On) • Circle, $d_S = 6$ cm and irregular hourglass ‡6 × 8, $t = 2$ mm • Cu electrodes screwed into the sensor, attaching it to rigid substrate	• *Simulations and experiments* • 16 or 17 Electrodes • I–M = ADJ–ADJ • AC 1.5 mA, 6.3 kHz • Target = fingers, probe ($d_T = 12$ mm), model 2 DOF knee joint with curved surfaces • Training target = indenter, d_T=5 mm on 129 points separated by 5 mm	• Custom learning algorithm • Two-stage learning algorithm: (1) learn sensitivity matrix from tactile contact training data and the output voltages, (2) minimize deviation of reconstructed images from reference patterns

		• Applications for measurement of knee joint contact forces and tactile imaging • System less sensitive to forces at the center • ‡ Images comparable to EIT			
[110]	2022	• NN images have better fidelity to the target image, particularly for multiple contacts • Metrics: RMSE, image correlation coefficient • CNN is better than RBFNN • Landweber iterative reconstruction also tested • Filtering is needed (2D adaptive Wiener) to remove artefacts due to noise, interference • Pressure at multiple points can cause collapse, reducing image quality	• **Salt water** surmounted by an **elastic membrane** (PU), inside a vertical frame • Circle, $d_S = 10$ cm, *depth* = 11 mm • Flexible printed circuit with NI-Au-coated electrodes mounted on inner surface of elastomeric sidewall	• *Simulations and experiments* • 16 Electrodes • I–M unspecified • 1 mA, 60 or 100 kHz • Training target = 1–3 circles of $d_T = 20$ mm	• RBFNN and CNN • Training data: 15k samples from COMSOL, Matlab, 7:3 • Gaussian noise down to SNR 30 dB • EIT: Red Pitaya STEMLab 125–14, Tikhonov regularization
[8]	2022	• Bayesian learning can identify multi-point conductivity-change targets • Sparse Bayesian learning (SA-SBL) also tested • Metrics: position error (PE) and mean intersection over union (MIOU)	• **Conductive film** (Graphite128) spray painted onto paper • Square, 20 × 20 cm^2 • Stainless steel electrodes • ALSO • PU foam filled with conductive **liquid** in elastomeric shell (Ecoflex) • Square, ‡10 × 10 cm^2	• *simulations and experiments* • 16 Electrodes • I–M unspecified • Target = conductive weights OR probe with varying force	• Multi-frame constrained block sparse Bayesian learning (MFC-BSBL) • EIT: Tikhonov regularization, NOSER prior, unknown λ

(*Continued*)

Table 2.5. (*Continued*)

Reference	Year	Findings	Sensor	Conditions	Reconstruction
		• ‡ Images for EIT, ML appear to use different scales; actual improvements unclear	• ‡ Piercing Cu wires		
[111]	2022	• RBFNN and DNN for pressure mapping • DNN more accurate for small pressure hotspots, poor for distributed loads; RBFNN poor for small hotspots, better at distributed loads • ‡ All images poor	• **MWCNT-elastomer** (Kynar Aquatec latex) spray-coated onto **foam** (15DC-3G) on 3D printed support • 3 mm × 21 × 23 cm^2 • Cu tape and Ag epoxy to multi-strand wire electrodes	• *experiments* • 26 Electrodes • I–M = ADJ–ADJ • DC current • Target = polymer shapes of 10 mm dia to 45 × 100 mm with masses from 200–4000 g	• DNN: input layer with 598 neurons +4 hidden layers each with 2048 neurons + exponential linear unit activation functions + fully connected layer of 3,690 neurons • RBF: 1 fully connected layer of 100 neurons, Gaussian RBFs, kernel functions were centers of 100 clusters found using k-means, trained by solving least-squares problem without activation functions • Training data: training set of 75k cases, including noise, with uniform σ_0; Adam optimization algorithm, learning rate = 0.001, 30 epochs • EIT: total variation (TV) regularization

as elongation or shear), which traditional EIT could not [103]. Moreover, in the presence of noise the reconstructed images had higher resolution. Likewise, no assumptions about the stimuli need to be made, such as that conductivity changes are small.

For ML training, a relationship broadly similar to equation (2.1) is used, but rather than employing a sensitivity matrix **J** based on a physical model of the electric fields, the relationship between the spatial distribution of conductivity changes $\boldsymbol{\sigma}$ and the voltage difference data $\boldsymbol{\Delta}$ is learned by minimizing the difference between model predictions and a known set of $\boldsymbol{\sigma}$ provided by training data. The learned relationship may be based on features in the data and make use of a classifier, or, with 'deep learning', may operate on $\boldsymbol{\Delta}$ as a whole; deep learning generally requires more computational capability and training data. Both approaches can be implemented in Matlab.

In ML, the upfront work involves training and validating on a large data set, which can number thousands of examples [103–105]. Given the need for large datasets for training, most learning methods are based on forward problem simulations, for example using the forward model capability in EIDORS [104]. COMSOL has also been employed to create training data, which offers the advantage of handling sensors with anisotropy and arbitrary geometries [106]. While the training times can be long (in some cases many hours, depending on the approach), subsequent classification during use is fast. Reducing training time is important for applications that require fresh training for each user, such as for certain human-wearable devices, or for each new situation: it has been noted that deep learning models suffer from the poor generalizability and need to be retrained upon changes in the EIT hardware or measurement conditions [8]. The amount of training data can be reduced by employing some information about the physical system. For example, an interesting hybrid approach to the use of ML was introduced in [102]: the sensitivity map traditionally obtained from the physics of the forward problem was obtained by training an algorithm to learn the sensitivity map by contacting the sensor at a set of predetermined grid points. Only a small number of measurements was required, 129 instead of the more typical thousands, and the imaging was successful, the fidelity comparable to that from traditional EIT. This work used a linear mapping, valid for small conductivity changes, but a nonlinear mapping was suggested to accommodate larger changes due to heavier tactile contacts.

ML has been combined with other learning to advance robot capability. For example, with additional sensor data, specifically joint torques generated by tactile contacts, a robot arm learned to control its motion under touch perturbation [92]. In another study, a suite of ML techniques was sequentially applied, in simulation, to allow an artificial skin on a robot to recognize a shape in contact with the sensor, regardless of its size or orientation, directly from the voltage outputs [91]. This was done in three steps: image reconstruction, image segmentation, and object recognition. The reconstruction, based on the metrics of position error and resolution, was superior to that using a traditional Tikhonov regularization approach, demonstrating the feasibility of obtaining sophisticated 'actionable intelligence' from an e-skin.

When comparing ML results with EIT, much of the work has either not specified the comparison-case EIT reconstruction parameters or has used conditions known to give poor results. It is unclear whether some of these studies actually understood how EIT works. For example, it has been claimed that EIT may be unsuitable for real-time use because of the need for matrix inversion. Vague claims have also been made, such as that EIT does not have 'adequate perception,' without specifics about application requirements. Significantly, it remains unclear how, and in fact whether, ML can distinguish small signals that are at the level of the noise better than EIT can: head-to-head comparisons of reconstructions at various noise levels under fair conditions (such as a one-step reconstruction using one of the better I–M patterns, priors, etc) or with difficult signals (such as a small force adjacent to a large one), employing a complete set of performance metrics (including all the key image metrics, given in chapter 3, as well as computational requirements and imaging speeds), have not being shown. It can be argued that the ML algorithms have been given only 'softballs' and shown only proof of concept in simple experiments. It is clear that ML can pull out patterns on which it was trained from a noisy signal, since it is looking for those. For example, a system trained with a 25 mm diameter 100 g weight can readily see this target [101]. On the other hand, what if the target is smaller, lighter, more fleeting, or if it is next to a large, heavy weight? The whole problem with noise, as explained in later chapters, is that it can give the same voltage pattern as a real signal, so it remains undetermined how well the ML schemes can distinguish difficult and highly variable signals from noise.

Neither have various ML approaches been compared to each other. Although publications have raised the shortcomings of various other ML approaches, each has used a different set of training data; direct comparisons of the approaches on the same data have not been performed. A site for sharing such datasets, most of which are from simulations, but some of which are from experiments, could be helpful to newcomers. A standard training set that combine different types of targets would aid in evaluating new approaches. Also, standard metrics for comparing different approaches have not been put forward. Some that might be considered, aside from metrics concerning the reconstructed images, include the size of the required training data set, speed of training, speed of reconstruction, and computational requirements for training and reconstruction. An even-handed critical review of the ML approaches would also be welcome.

As of now, these ML tools are not as readily implementable by new users as EIDORS, but it is expected that this situation will change in the near future. Implementation on a cell phone has not yet been shown, either, although that may also soon be demonstrated. In the next few years it is possible that ML will completely replace traditional EIT for tactile image reconstruction.

2.7 Conclusions

EIT for tactile imaging, first suggested in the 1990s, has since 2007 been impressively and imaginatively demonstrated. Multiple sensor types of various shapes and materials have been shown on curved and compliant surfaces and with a range of tactile interactions. Work has included applications, characterization, new geometries and materials, hardware improvements, and imaging advances. The introduction of the EIDORS software running in Matlab opened the door to wide adoption of tactile EIT. Improvements to sensors has resulted in reduced memory effects, greater sensitivity, and response to only pressure or to only strain. There have also been advances that have simplified and miniaturized the EIT hardware; today EIT data collection is operated by microcontrollers and, because of the great increases in computing power, EIT algorithms can now be implemented on a cell phone.

In 2009, the outlook for the use of EIT for tactile imaging was confident, '*We are expecting the wide utilization of this technology in fields such as robotics, ergonomics and input-device engineering*' [38]. There are, however, still numerous challenges to address before this vision can be realized. EIT for tactile imaging requires familiarity with disparate areas: material science, electronic devices, signal processing, and linear algebra. The power requirements must be reduced, and no-stress electrical interfaces developed. Critically, the electronics must ensure the lowest noise possible. Signal processing, whether EIT, ML, or a combination of both, must handle sensor non-idealities, such as memory and non-uniform conductivity, as well as interfering signals. A familiarity with the mathematics of inverse problems and, more recently, machine learning, is also needed. The literature has shown progress in each of these areas.

References

[1] Silvera-Tawil D, Rye D, Soleimani M and Velonaki M 2015 Electrical impedance tomography for artificial sensitive robotic skin: a review *IEEE Sens.* J **15** 2001–16

[2] Liu K, Wu Y, Wang S, Wang H, Chen H, Chen B and Yao J 2020 Artificial sensitive skin for robotics based on electrical impedance tomography *Adv. Intell. Syst.* **2** 1900161

[3] Tallman T N and Smyl D J 2020 Structural health and condition monitoring via electrical impedance tomography in self-sensing materials: a review *Smart Mater. Struct.* **29** 25

[4] Dahiya R S, Mittendorfer P, Valle M, Cheng G and Lumelsky V J 2013 Directions toward effective utilization of tactile skin: a review *IEEE Sens.* J **13** 4121–38

[5] Elsanadedy A 2012 Application of electrical impedance tomography to robotic tactile sensing *MS Thesis* Mechanical Engineering, Carleton University, Ottawa, Ontario, Canada

[6] Liu H, Guo D, Sun F, Yang W, Furber S and Sun T 2020 Embodied tactile perception and learning *Brain Sci. Adv.* **6** 132–58

[7] Zhang Y, Lin Z, Huang X, You X, Ye J and Wu H 2020 A large-area, stretchable, textile-based tactile sensor *Adv. Mater. Technol.* **5** 1901060

[8] Ma G, Chen H, Wang P and Wang X 2022 Multi-frame constrained block sparse Bayesian learning for flexible tactile sensing using electrical impedance tomography *IEEE Trans. Comput. Imag* **8** 438–48

[9] Chossat J-B, Shin H-S, Park Y-L and Duchaine V 2015 Soft tactile skin using an embedded ionic liquid and tomographic imaging *J. Mech. Robot* **7** JMR-14-1234

[10] Kato Y, Hayakawa T and Mukai T 2008 Soft areal tactile sensor using tomography algorithm *J. Robot. Mechatron* **20** 628–33

[11] Adler A and Boyle A 2017 Electrical impedance tomography: tissue properties to image measures *IEEE Trans. Biomed. Eng.* **64** 2494–504
[12] Holder D S (ed) 2005 *Electrical Impedance Tomography: Methods, History and Applications* (Bristol: Institute of Physics Publishing)
[13] Adler A and Boyl A 2020 Electrical impedance tomography *Wiley Encyclopedia of Electrical and Electronics Engineering* ed J G Webster (New York: Wiley)
[14] Vauhkonen M, Lionheart W R, Heikkinen L M, Vauhkonen P J and Kaipio J P 2001 A MATLAB package for the EIDORS project to reconstruct two-dimensional EIT images *Physiol. Meas.* **22** 107–11
[15] Polydorides N and Lionheart W R B 2002 A Matlab toolkit for three-dimensional electrical impedance tomography: a contribution to the Electrical Impedance and Diffuse Optical Reconstruction Software project *Meas. Sci. Technol.* **13** 1871–83
[16] Adler A and Lionheart W R B 2006 Uses and abuses of EIDORS: an extensible software base for EIT *Physiol. Meas.* **27** S25–42
[17] Adler A 2019 EIDORS: Electrical Impedance Tomography and Diffuse Optical Tomography Reconstruction Software http://eidors3d.sourceforge.net/
[18] Grychtol B, Elke G, Meybohm P, Weiler N, Frerichs I and Adler A 2014 Functional validation and comparison framework for EIT lung imaging *PLoS One* **9** e103045
[19] Barber D C 2005 EIT: the view from Sheffield *Electrical Impedance Tomography: Methods, History and Applications of the series Series in Medical Physics and Biomedical Engineering* ed C G Orton, J H Nagel and J G Webster (Bristol: Institute of Physics Publishing) ch 11
[20] Hamilton S J, Lionheart R B and Adler A 2019 Comparing D-bar and common regularization-based methods for electrical impedance tomography *Physiol. Meas.* **40** ARTN 044004
[21] Liu D, Smyl D, Gu D and Du J 2020 Shape-driven difference electrical impedance tomography *IEEE Trans. Med. Imag* **39** 3801–12
[22] Lionheart W R B 2004 EIT reconstruction algorithms: pitfalls, challenges, and recent developments *Physiol. Meas.* **25** 125–42
[23] Bayford R H 2006 Bioimpedance tomography (electrical impedance tomography) *An. Rev. Biomed. Eng* **8** 63–91
[24] Gaggero P O 2011 Miniaturization and distinguishability limits of electrical impedance tomography for biomedical application *PhD Thesis* Nanomedecine Division, Centre Suisse d'Electronique et de Microtechnique (CSEM), University of Neuchâtel, Landquart, Switzerland
[25] Adler A, Grychtol B and Bayford R 2015 Why is EIT so hard, and what are we doing about it? *Physiol. Meas.* **36** 1067–73
[26] Knight R A and Lipczynski R T 1990 The use of EIT techniques to measure interface pressure *Proc. 12th Ann. Int. Conf. IEEE Engineering in Medicine and Biology Society (Philadelphia, PA, 1–4 Nov.)* pp 2307–8
[27] Jeong Y J, Kim Y E, Kim K J, Woo E J and Oh T I 2020 Multilayered fabric pressure sensor for real-time piezo-impedance imaging of pressure distribution *IEEE Trans. Instrum. Meas.* **69** 565–72
[28] Yorkey T J, Webster J G and Tompkins W J 1987 Comparing reconstruction algorithms for electrical impedance tomography *IEEE Trans. Biomed. Eng.* **34** 843–52
[29] Basarab-Horwath I and Faraj M 1992 A prototype distributed pressure sensor utilizing electrical impedance tomography—initial results *Workshop on Tomographic Techniques for*

Process Design and Operation (ECAPT'92) (Manchester, Mar 26–29) (Computational Mechanics Publications Ltd) pp 277–83

[30] Fulton W S and Lipczynski R T 1993 Body-support pressure measurement using electrical impedance tomography *Proc. 15th Ann. Int. Conf. IEEE Engineering in Medicine and Biology Society (San Diego, CA, 31–31 Oct.)* pp 98–9

[31] Hou T C, Loh K J and Lynch J P 2007 Electrical impedance tomography of carbon nanotube composite materials Conf. on Sensors and Smart Structures Technologies for Civil, Mechanical and Aerospace Systems SPIE 6529 *(San Diego, CA, Mar 19–22)*

[32] Hou T C, Loh K J and Lynch J P 2007 Spatial conductivity mapping of carbon nanotube composite thin films by electrical impedance tomography for sensing applications *Nanotechnology* **18** 9

[33] Nagakubo A, Alirezaei H and Kuniyoshi Y 2007 A tactile distribution sensor based on inverse problem theory *J. Robot. Soc. Jap* **25** 960–9

[34] Nagakubo A, Alirezaei H and Kuniyoshi Y 2007 A deformable and deformation sensitive tactile distribution sensor *IEEE Int. Conf. Robot. Biomimetics (ROBIO) (Sanya, China, Dec. 15–18)* pp 1301–8

[35] Alirezaei H, Nagakubo A and Kuniyoshi Y 2007 A highly stretchable tactile distribution sensor for smooth surfaced humanoids *Humanoids '07: 7th IEEE-RAS Int. Conf. Humanoid Robots (Pittsburgh, PA, Nov. 29—Dec. 1)* pp 167–73

[36] Kato Y, Mukai T, Hayakawa T and Shibata T 2007 Tactile sensor without wire and sensing element in the tactile region based on EIT method *IEEE Sensors (Atlanta, GA, Oct. 28–31)* pp 792–5

[37] Kato Y and Mukai T 2008 Tactile sensor without wire and sensing element in the tactile region using new rbber material *Sensors, Focus on Tactile, Force and Stress Sensors* ed J G Rocha and S Lanceros-Mendez (Vienna: InTech) pp 399–408

[38] Alirezaei H, Nagakubo A and Kuniyoshi Y 2009 A tactile distribution sensor which enables stable measurement under high and dynamic stretch *IEEE Symp. 3D User Interfaces (Lafayette, LA, 14–15 March)* pp 87–93

[39] Tawil D S, Rye D and Velonaki M 2011 Improved EIT drive patterns for a robotics sensitive skin *Australasian Conf. Robotics and Automation (ACRA) (Sydney, Australia, Dec. 2–4)* p 112s111

[40] Yoshikai T, Fukushima H, Hayashi M and Inaba M 2009 Development of soft stretchable knit sensor for humanoids' whole-body tactile sensibility *9th IEEE-RAS Int. Conf. on Humanoid Robots (Paris, 7–10 Dec.)* pp 624–31

[41] Tawil D S, Rye D and Velonaki M 2011 Improved image reconstruction for an EIT-based sensitive skin with multiple internal electrodes *IEEE Trans. Robot.* **27** 425–35

[42] Tawil D S, Rye D and Velonaki M 2011 Touch modality interpretation for an EIT-based sensitive skin *2011 IEEE Int. Conf Robotics and Automation (ICRA) (Shanghai, 9–13 May)* pp 3770–6

[43] Elsanadedy A, Mamatjan Y, Ahmadi M and Adler A 2012 Characterisation of conductive polymer for EIT based sensor *Int. Conf. Electrical and Computer Systems (Ottawa, Aug 16–18)* p 117

[44] Tawil D S, Rye D and Velonaki M 2012 Interpretation of the modality of touch on an artificial arm covered with an EIT-based sensitive skin *Int. J. Robot. Res.* **31** 1627–41

[45] Tawil D S 2012 Artificial skin and the interpretation of touch in human–robot interaction *PhD Thesis* School of Aerospace, Mechanical and Mechatronic Engineering, University of Sydney, Australia

[46] Yao A and Soleimani M 2012 A pressure mapping imaging device based on electrical impedance tomography of conductive fabrics *Sensor Rev.* **32** 310–7

[47] Pugach G, Khomenko V, Melnyk A, Pitti A, Henaff P and Gaussier P 2013 Electronic hardware design of a low cost tactile sensor device for physical human–robot interactions *Electronics and Nanotechnology (ELNANO) (Kiev, Ukraine, 16–19 April)* (IEEE) pp 445–9

[48] Yao A, Yang C L, Seo J K and Soleimani M 2013 EIT-based fabric pressure sensing *Comput. Math. Method. Medicine* **2013** 405325

[49] Silvera-Tawil D, Rye D and Velonaki M 2014 Interpretation of social touch on an artificial arm covered with an EIT-based sensitive skin *Int. J. Soc. Robot.* **6** 489–505

[50] Tallman T and Wang K-W 2015 The influence of filler volume fraction on sensitivity to distributed strain in carbon nanofiber/polyurethane nanocomposites *25th Canadian Congress of Applied Mechanics (CANCAM) (London, ON, May 31–Jun 4)*

[51] Tallman T N, Gungor S, Wang K W and Bakis C E 2015 Tactile imaging and distributed strain sensing in highly flexible carbon nanofiber/polyurethane nanocomposites *Carbon* **95** 485–93

[52] Visentin F and Suzuki K 2015 Deformable sensors for soft robot by electrical impedance tomography *IEEE Int. Conf. Robotics and Biomimetics (ROBIO) (Zhuhai, China, 6–9 Dec.)* pp 1006–11

[53] Yang C L, Mohammed A, Mohamadou Y, Oh T I and Soleimani M 2015 Complex conductivity reconstruction in multiple frequency electrical impedance tomography for fabric-based pressure sensor *Sensor Rev.* **35** 85–97

[54] Russo S, Meziani S-N, Gulrez T, Carbonaro N and Tognetti A 2016 Towards the development of an EIT-based stretchable sensor for multi-touch industrial human-computer interaction dystems *Cross-Cultural Design* ed P-L P Rau (Berlin: Springer International Publishing) pp 563–73

[55] Tallman T N and Wang K W 2016 Damage and strain identification in multifunctional materials via electrical impedance tomography with constrained sine wave solutions *Struct. Health Monit.* **15** 235–44

[56] Visentin F, Fiorini P and Suzuki K 2016 A deformable smart skin for continuous sensing based on electrical impedance tomography *Sensors* **16** ARTN 1928

[57] Wang L, Gupta S, Loh K J and Koo H S 2016 Distributed pressure sensing using carbon nanotube fabrics *IEEE Sens.* J **16** 4663–4

[58] Jeong Y J, Oh T I, Woo E J and Kim K J 2017 Integration of piezo-capacitive and piezo-electric nanoweb based pressure sensors for imaging of static and dynamic pressure distribution *39th Ann. Int. Conf. IEEE Engineering in Medicine and Biology Society (EMBC) (Jeju, Korea, 11–15 July)* pp 21–4

[59] Lee H, Kwon D, Cho H, Park I and Kim J 2017 Soft nanocomposite based multi-point, multi-directional strain mapping sensor using anisotropic electrical impedance tomography *Sci. Rep.* **7** 39837

[60] Lee H, Park K, Kim Y and Kim J 2017 Durable and repairable soft tactile skin for physical human robot interaction *ACM/IEEE Int. Conf. Human–Robot Interaction (HRI) (Vienna, March 6–9)* (ACM) pp 183–4

[61] Russo S, Nefti-Meziani S, Carbonaro N and Tognetti A 2017 A quantitative evaluation of drive pattern selection for optimizing EIT-based stretchable sensors *Sensors* **17** ARTN 1999

[62] Russo S, Nefti-Meziani S, Carbonaro N and Tognetti A 2017 Development of a high-speed current injection and voltage measurement system for electrical impedance tomography-based stretchable sensors *Technologies* **5** 48

[63] Tallman T N, Gungor S, Koo G M and Bakis C E 2017 On the inverse determination of displacements, strains, and stresses in a carbon nanofiber/polyurethane nanocomposite from conductivity data obtained via electrical impedance tomography *J. Intell. Material Syst. Struct* **28** 2617–29

[64] Yoon S H, Huo K, Zhang Y, Chen G, Paredes L, Chidambaram S and Ramani K 2017 iSoft: a customizable soft sensor with real-time continuous contact and stretching sensing *Proc. 30th Ann. ACM Symp. User Interface Software and Technology* (Québec City, QC: Association for Computing Machinery) pp 665–78

[65] Zhang Y, Laput G and Harrison C 2017 Electrick: low-cost touch sensing using electric field tomography *Proc. 2017 CH, Conf. Human Factors in Computing Systems* (Denver, CO: Association for Computing Machinery) pp 1–14

[66] Chen Y, Yu M, Bruck H A and Smela E 2018 Compliant multi-layer tactile sensing for enhanced identification of human touch *Smart Mater. Struct.* **27** 125009

[67] Chen Y 2018 Tactile sensing with compliant structures for human–robot interaction *PhD Thesis* Department of Mechanical Engineering, University of Maryland

[68] Lee Y, Choi B, Yoon J, Kim Y, Park J, Kim H J, Kim D H, Kim D M, Kim S and Choi S J 2018 Highly transparent tactile sensor based on a percolated carbon nanotube network *AIP Adv.* **8** 6

[69] Oh J, Yang J C, Kim J-O, Park H, Kwon S Y, Lee S, Sim J Y, Oh H W, Kim J and Park S 2018 Pressure insensitive strain sensor with facile solution-based process for tactile sensing applications *ACS Nano* **12** 7546–53

[70] Yoon S H, Paredes L, Huo K and Ramani K 2018 MultiSoft: soft sensor enabling real-time multimodal sensing with contact localization and deformation classification *Proc. ACM Interact. Mob. Wearable Ubiquitous Technol* 2 Article 145

[71] Dai H B and Thostenson E T 2019 Large-area carbon nanotube-based flexible composites for ultra-wide range pressure sensing and spatial pressure mapping *ACS Appl. Mater. Interfaces* **11** 48370–80

[72] Duan X, Taurand S and Soleimani M 2019 Artificial skin through super-sensing method and electrical impedance data from conductive fabric with aid of deep learning *Sci. Rep.* **9** Number seag8831

[73] Russo S, Carbonaro N and Tognetti A 2019 EIT-based tactile sensing patches for rehabilitation and human machine interaction *Wearable Robotics: Challenges and Trends of the series Biosystems and Biorobotics* ed M C Carrozza, S Micera and J L Pons (Cham: Springer International Publishing) vol 22 pp 13–7

[74] Wang Y, Ju F, Cao Y, Yun Y, Wang Y, Bai D and Chen B 2019 An aero-engine inspection continuum robot with tactile sensor based on EIT for exploration and navigation in unknown environment *2019 IEEE/ASME Int. Conf. Advanced Intelligent Mechatronics (AIM) (Hong Kong, 8–12 July)* pp 1157–62

[75] Abdelwahed M, Pitti A, Romain O and Ouezdou F B 2020 Use of multi-frequency electrical impedance tomography as tactile sensor for material discrimination *5th Int. Conf. Advanced Robotics and Mechatronics (ICARM) (Shenzhen, China, 18–21 Dec.)* pp 588–94

[76] Duan X 2020 Electrical impedance tomography: methods and applications *PhD Thesis* Department of Electronic and Electrical Engineering, University of Bath, Bath, UK

[77] Sun L, Jiang S, Xiao Y and Zhang W 2020 Realization of flexible pressure sensor based on conductive polymer composite via using electrical impedance tomography *Smart Mater. Struct.* **29** 055004

[78] Yoshimoto S, Kuroda Y and Oshiro O 2020 Tomographic approach for universal tactile imaging with electromechanically coupled conductors *IEEE Trans. Ind. Electron.* **67** 627–36

[79] Zhao T, Wu C and Soleimani M 2020 Ionic liquid based distributed touch sensor using electrical impedance tomography *IOP Sci. Notes* **1** 025005

[80] Chen Y and Liu H 2021 Location-dependent performance of large-area piezoresistive tactile sensors based on electrical impedance tomography *IEEE Sens.* J **21** 21622–30

[81] Huuhtanen T, Lankinen A and Jung A 2021 Target tracking on sensing surface with electrical impedance tomography *28th European Signal Processing Conf. (EUSIPCO) (Amsterdam, 18–21 Jan)* pp 1817–21

[82] Li S J, Lin Y A and Loh K J 2021 Pressure mapping using a nanocomposite smartfoam and electrical impedance tomography *Conf. on Nano-, Bio-, Info-Tech Sensors and Wearable Systems* SPIE 11590*(Mar 22–26)*

[83] Zhao H and Yang W 2021 Flexible tactile sensing based on electrical resistance tomography and wavelet image fusion *2021 IEEE Int. Conf. Imaging Systems and Techniques (IST) (Kaohsiung, Taiwan, 24–26 Aug.)* pp 1–6

[84] Avery J, Runciman M, Fiani C, Sanchez E M, Akhond S, Liu Z, Aristovich K and Mylonas G 2022 Lumen shape reconstruction using a soft robotic balloon catheter and electical impedance tomography arXiv:2207.12536

[85] Chen H, Yang X, Wang P, Geng J, Ma G and Wang X 2022 A large-area flexible tactile sensor for multi-touch and force detection using electrical impedance tomography *IEEE Sens.* J **22** 7119–29

[86] Ellingham R and Giffney T 2022 Carbon black silicone composite piezoresistive electrical impedance tomography strain sensor device *Conf. on Electroactive Polymer Actuators and Devices (EAPAD) XXIV, SPIE Smart Structures and Nondestructive Evaluation Conf.* SPIE 12042 *(Long Beach, CA, Mar 06–09)*

[87] Smela E 2022 EIT for tactile sensing: considering artefacts in hyperparameter selection *Eng. Res. Express* **4** 035057

[88] Smela E 2022 EIT for tactile sensing: considerations regarding the injection-measurement pattern *Eng. Res. Express* **4** 045041

[89] Soleimani M and Friedrich M 2022 E-skin using fringing field electrical impedance tomography with an ionic liquid domain *Sensors* **22** 5040

[90] Wu H, Zheng B, Wang H and Ye J 2022 New flexible tactile sensor based on electrical impedance tomography *Micromachines* **13** 185

[91] Husain Z, Madjid N A and Liatsis P 2021 Tactile sensing using machine learning-driven electrical impedance tomography *IEEE Sens.* J **21** 11628–42

[92] Pugach G, Melnyk A, Tolochko O, Pitti A and Gaussier P 2016 Touch-based admittance control of a robotic arm using neural learning of an artificial skin *IEEE/RSJ Int. Conf. Intelligent Robots and Systems (IROS) (Daejeon, Korea, 9–14 Oct.)* pp 3374–80

[93] Sauerbrunn E, Chen Y, Didion J, Yu M, Smela E and Bruck H A 2015 Thermal imaging using polymer nanocomposite temperature sensors, EIT *Phys. Stat. Sol.* A **212** 2239–45

[94] Wissman J *et al* 2013 New compliant strain gauges for self-sensing dynamic deformation of flapping wings on miniature air vehicles *Smart Mater. Struct.* **22** 085031

[95] Bragaglia M, Paleari L, Lamastra F R, Puglia D, Fabbrocino F and Nanni F 2021 Graphene nanoplatelet, multiwall carbon nanotube, and hybrid multiwall carbon nanotube–graphene nanoplatelet epoxy nanocomposites as strain sensing coatings *J. Reinf. Plast. and Compos* **40** 1–12

[96] Chen Y, Yu M, Bruck H A and Smela E 2018 Characterization of a compliant multi-layer system for tactile sensing with enhanced sensitivity and range *Smart Mater. Struct.* **27** 065005

[97] Dahiya R S, Metta G, Valle M and Sandini G 2010 Tactile sensing—from humans to humanoids *IEEE Trans. Robot.* **26** 1–20

[98] Guardo R, Boulay C and Bertrand M 1991 A neural network approach to image reconstruction in electrical impedance tomography *Proc. Ann. Int. Conf. IEEE Engineering in Medicine and Biology Society* 13 *(Orlando, FL, 31 Oct.–3 Nov.)* pp 14–5

[99] Adler A and Guardo R 1994 A neural network image reconstruction technique for electrical impedance tomography *IEEE Trans. Med. Imag* **13** 594–600

[100] Biasi N, Gargano A, Arcarisi L, Carbonaro N and Tognetti A 2022 Physics-based simulation and machine learning for the practical implementation of EIT-based tactile sensors *IEEE Sens.* J **22** 4186–96

[101] Pugach G, Pitti A and Gaussier P 2015 Neural learning of the topographic tactile sensory information of an artificial skin through a self-organizing map *Adv. Robotics* **29** 1393–409

[102] Li J and Lee K M 2022 A novel method for soft contact sensing based on electrical impedance sensitivity images *IEEE Sens.* J **22** 9296–305

[103] Low K 2021 Electrical impedance tomography for wearable sensors: a deep convolutional neural network approach *MASc Thesis* Electrical Engineering, University of British Columbia

[104] Husain Z and Liatsis P 2019 A neural network-based local decomposition approach for image reconstruction in electrical impedance tomography *IEEE Int. Conf. Imaging Systems and Techniques (IST) (Abu Dhabi, UAE)*

[105] Park H, Lee H, Park K, Mo S and Kim J 2019 Deep neural network approach in electrical impedance tomography-based real-time soft tactile sensor *IEEE/RSJ Int. Conf. Intelligent Robots and Systems (IROS) (Macau, China)* pp 7447–52

[106] Biasi N, Carbonaro N, Arcarisi L and Tognetti A 2020 Combining physics-based simulation and machine learning for EIT-based tactile sensing *IEEE Sensors (Rotterdam, Netherlands)*

[107] Russo S, Assaf R and Nefti-Meziani S 2017 Towards a practical implementation of EIT-based sensors using artificial neural networks *2017 IEEE Sensors (Glasgow, UK, 29 Oct.-1 Nov.)* pp 1–3

[108] Russo S, Assaf R, Carbonaro N and Tognetti A 2019 Touch position detection in electrical tomography tactile sensors through quadratic classifier *IEEE Sens.* J **19** 474–83

[109] Park H, Park K, Mo S and Kim J 2021 Deep neural network based electrical impedance tomographic sensing methodology for large-area robotic tactile sensing *IEEE Trans. Robot.* **37** 1570–83

[110] Liu K, Qin Z, Wu Y, Chen B, Li F, Pan H and Yao J 2022 Fabrication of a tactile sensor for artificial skin based on electrical impedance tomography *Biosens. Bioelectron.* **10** 100116

[111] Quqa S, Shu Y N, Li S J and Loh K J 2022 Pressure mapping using nanocomposite-enhanced foam and machine learning *Front. Mater.* **9** 12

Chapter 3

Simulation conditions and performance metrics

Elisabeth Smela, with contributions by Ayush Nankani

This chapter describes the simulation methods employed in this work and it provides the definitions for the performance measures, or metrics, that were used to evaluate simulation results. Key metrics that have been established for electrical impedance tomography (EIT) are introduced, as are the important considerations for tactile imaging. Definitions are provided, along with how the metrics are calculated in the open-sourced code EIDORS. A table showing the important characteristics that must be determined of tactile contacts is given, together with the metrics associated with determining those characteristics; these differ somewhat from the metrics of interest for medical imaging.

3.1 Simulation methods

EIDORS (version 3.10, MATLAB version R2018b) [1–3] was used to solve both the forward and inverse problems, employing difference electrical impedance tomography (EIT) and a 2D model. (Our Matlab codes are available upon request.) In the forward problem, voltages at the electrodes are calculated from a given current injection and conductivity distribution, and in the reverse problem the conductivity distribution within the area is estimated from boundary voltages. Difference EIT compares voltages due to conductivity changes on the sensor with those from a uniform initial conductivity [4, 5].

3.1.1 Synthetic data

Synthetic data were generated using 'bipolar' injection and measurement configurations, so called because each use two electrodes. The configurations are denoted by the electrode position differences, known as the offset, and the combination of injection and measurement (I–M) patterns is denoted by the pair of differences (figure 3.1). For example, in a 16-electrode system pseudo-polar injection combined with adjacent measurement is denoted I–M = 7–1, while adjacent injection and

doi:10.1088/978-0-7503-5402-8ch3

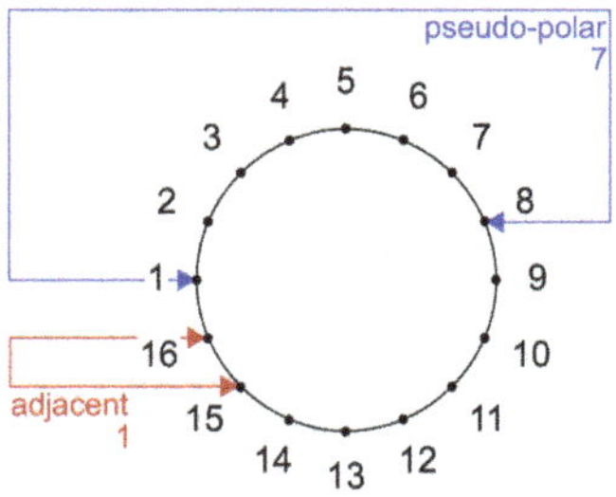

Figure 3.1. (a) Schematic showing two current injection or voltage measurement configurations: adjacent (1) and pseudo-polar (7), where the notation indicates the differences in position numbers of the two electrodes.

adjacent measurement is denoted 1–1, as shown in figure 3.1. (A detailed description of the EIT measurement process is given in section 4.2.)

3.1.2 Sensor model

A circular sensor with 16 electrodes equally spaced around a circular 2D sensor with a radius $r_S = 1$ was simulated. The units for EIDORS are MKS, so for a current in amps, distances in meters, and measurements in volts, conductivity is in Siemens/meter (S m^{-1}). (For further discussion of units in EIDORS 2D simulations, see section 3.1.4.) Based on our experimental conditions [6], a current of $I = 1 \times 10^{-3}$ (corresponding to 1 mA) or 3×10^{-3} was injected into one electrode and another electrode was made ground, depending on the injection pattern.

Simulation data were generated using 'bipolar' configurations that inject current between one pair of electrodes and measure voltages between a different pair of electrodes. The combination of current injection and voltage measurement (I–M) patterns is denoted by the position differences between each. For example in a 16-electrode system, when the injection electrode is eight positions away from ground (on directly opposite sides of the sensor) and the measurement electrodes are next to each other (adjacent) the I–M pattern is denoted 8–1. The base case pattern was I–M = 7–1 (pseudo-polar-adjacent).

The conductivity of the sensor was fixed at a uniform $\sigma_0 = 0.01$ (S m^{-1}). The constant background conductivity of the sensor was specified in the sensor model; without that, the output conductivity is incorrectly scaled by a constant. The baseline conductivity distribution σ_0 is an EIDORS parameter, as mentioned above. Using the default of '1' for a sensor with a uniform, isotropic conductivity will yield images that are proportionally correct in the conductivity change. To obtain quantitatively correct amplitudes, the baseline conductivity σ_0 must be specified; this gives the reconstruction the correct scaling. If the sensor baseline conductivity is non-uniform or anisotropic, it is essential to specify it to avoid a poor or even completely incorrect reconstruction. A mistaken assumption of a homogeneous background conductivity may result in substantial errors, as has been shown for medical imaging [7, 8] and for tactile sensors that have spatially-varying conductivity [9].

3.1.3 Targets

Targets consisted of a constant-amplitude contrast, with a step decrease of $\Delta\sigma$ from a constant baseline sensor conductivity σ_0 to the target conductivity σ_T. Unless otherwise specified, the target was circular with a radius $r_T = 0.2$ within which the conductivity was typically $0.9\sigma_0$, giving a change in conductivity $\Delta\sigma = -1$ mS m^{-1}, for a contrast of $(\sigma_T - \sigma_0)/\sigma_0 = -10\%$. In some cases σ_T was $0.6\sigma_0$, giving a change in conductivity $\Delta\sigma_T = -0.004$ for a contrast $(\sigma_0 - \sigma_T)/\sigma_0$ of -40%. It should be noted that such sharp edges would not be encountered in most experimental situations, such as touch by a finger or contact with a sensing skin over a cushioned surface: the transition from low to high would be more gradual. A negative $\Delta\sigma_T$ corresponds to using a tactile sensor whose resistance increases with strain (positive gauge factor), such as conductive-particle filled composites. Sensors such as conductive fabrics may have resistance decreases with strain [10]. In some cases triangular targets were employed. For a triangular-shaped target, the length along the x direction was $2r_T$ and its height in y was $1.4r_T$, giving a total area that was of 90% of that of a circular target of radius r_T.

3.1.4 Units for 2D EIDORS

Users of EIDORS for tactile imaging frequently wonder about the units in 2D simulations, which do not correspond to physically realizable systems. 3D EIDORS and ANSYS simulations do employ units, so simulations run in these were compared to those from 2D EIDORS using the same area dimensions and nominal properties. The sensor in all three cases was a circular region of radius 1 (m in the ANSYS simulations, unspecified unit in the other two), thickness 1 (m, unspecified), and conductivity 0.01 (S m^{-1}, unspecified). The configuration I–M = 1–1 was used with 16 electrodes having thickness 1 (m, unspecified) and width 0.1 (m, unspecified), and the injected current was 0.003 (Amps, unspecified). A circular target with radius 0.2 (m, unspecified) was located at the center (0,0), and it had a conductivity of 0.006 (S m^{-1}, unspecified). The values of the output voltages matched in all three cases, as did the EIT images. Thus, these SI units can be assumed in EIDORS 2D simulations.

3.1.5 The forward problem

A two-dimensional (2D) forward model was solved in EIDORS to generate voltages at the boundary due to the target conductivity change. Meshes were generated in EIDORS with *distmesh* using the function *mk_common_model.* The chosen mesh was *j2d4c*, which is the finest one for a circular area.

3.1.6 The inverse problem

Voltage measurements $\mathbf{V}_{touch}$ and $\mathbf{V}_{ref}$ obtained from the forward problem were used as inputs for the inverse problem. Voltages involving the driving electrodes were set to zero.

The algorithm used in this work was the one-step Gauss–Newton algorithm, commonly employed for tactile imaging because of its speed, which is essential for tactile imaging [11]. The Laplace prior was used unless otherwise noted. The nodal solver (*nodal_solve*), which solves for mesh nodes rather than mesh elements, was employed because it gave slightly more aesthetically pleasing images, but results were identical with both methods. The second-finest mesh *h2d4c* was chosen with a minimal noise to avoid an inverse crime [12, 13], except when the $\mathbf{V}^{\mathrm{T}}\boldsymbol{\sigma}$ were found, which requires using the same mesh and thus employed *j2d4c* for the inverse (which constitutes an inverse crime).

3.1.7 Noise

Normally distributed zero-mean noise was added to the synthetic forward voltage measurements; no noise was added to the injected current. The simulations typically had low noise, $N = 10^{-12}$. The noise, which had a standard deviation σ_{n}, was added to every element of the boundary voltage vectors $\mathbf{V}_{\mathrm{touch}}$ and $\mathbf{V}_{\mathrm{ref}}$ that came from the forward problem. Because the variances of independent random variables sum, the noise in the difference signal $\boldsymbol{\Delta}$ was $\sqrt{2\sigma_n}$. Note that in other work noise may have been added only to $\mathbf{V}_{\mathrm{touch}}$, with $\mathbf{V}_{\mathrm{ref}}$ coming from averaging many frames [14]. Because noise was added to both reference and measurement frames $\mathbf{V}_{\mathrm{ref}}$ and $\mathbf{V}_{\mathrm{touch}}$, these simulations have 40% greater noise than comparable simulations that add noise only to $\mathbf{V}_{\mathrm{touch}}$.

The noise level, or standard deviation of the voltage, was independent of the amplitude of the voltage and independent of electrode position, reflecting an experimental situation in which noise sources are independent of the input, for example when noise is primarily due to the data acquisition system [15]. This independence may not be the case in a given experiment: current may generate significant noise in the sensed medium [16]. It has been noted that most EIT systems have noise that is the same over the measurement channels [17], whereas others have found that noise can vary considerably among channels [5]. Simulated noise behavior may therefore not be representative of the noise in a particular system.

3.2 Metrics

Performance can be quantified by figures of merit, or metrics. In this chapter the key metrics for tactile imaging are defined, which are used in subsequent chapters to quantify system performance.

3.2.1 Key metrics

Metrics have been broadly categorized as measures of accuracy, distinguishability, and detectability [18]. Accuracy assesses whether a target is correctly represented and includes amplitude, resolution, and position and shape errors. Distinguishability addresses the reliability of identifying two targets, which is also determined by resolution. These are the key measures for tactile imaging. Detectability addresses the minimum size and conductivity contrast required for a target to be identified. Detectability is of considerable importance to medical imaging, but for tactile imaging the sensitivity of the sensor can in principle be increased through the materials or structure, and the challenge may instead be handling a large signal dynamic range [19]. Other differences between the requirements on EIT for medical imaging and tactile imaging were discussed in section 2.3.

The Graz consensus reconstruction algorithm for EIT (GREIT) defined key metrics for medical applications [20]. In order of importance they were amplitude uniformity, position error, ringing, resolution uniformity, shape deformation, and resolution. In EIDORS 3.10 [2, 18], five metrics are calculated: image amplitude, resolution, position error, shape deformation, and ringing. These five can be combined into one [21]. The following metrics were previously recommended for tactile imaging [11]: resolution, shape deformation, position error, and amplitude.

For tactile imaging, as opposed to pressure sensing, it is essential to know how many touches there are and approximately where, how hard (light, medium, strong), and what size (finger versus fist). *A priori*, none of these is predictable. The most important measures of performance and associated figures of merit for the reconstruction may therefore be: (a) absence of artefacts caused by noise (noise susceptibility is investigated in chapter 6 and chapter 7), (b) amplitude and (c) amplitude uniformity across the sensor, and (d) distinguishability of nearby contacts (resolution). For understanding the intensity of the contact, (e) preservation of the volume of the reconstructed feature is desirable. Depending on the application, (f) position error and (g) shape error may also be of interest. For applications involving human touch, it is typically unnecessary to resolve edge sharpness or to determine the exact shape of the touching object since fingers deform during the contact. Metrics related to the sensor, such as sensitivity, hysteresis, isotropy, and temperature dependence, are critical in experiments, but because they are indirectly related to EIT they are not treated here.

3.2.2 Definitions

Largely following [2], for completeness several of the standard metrics are illustrated in figure 3.2, which shows a circular sensor of radius r_S. Although the target cross-section is represented as an upward step in figure 3.2(b), it is typical for piezoresistive sensors to have a negative conductivity change, corresponding to an increase in resistance, which is what the simulations in this book cover. *In this work we have thus inverted the EIT images so that reductions in conductivity are represented as positive.* As in most prior work, the 'target' conductivity change imposed on the sensor was of constant amplitude $\Delta\sigma_T$ within an area A_T defined by a linear dimension r_T. In figure 3.2(a) this conductivity change is exemplified by a circular target of radius r_T, where the target size is specified as a fraction of r_S. In most cases in this book, $r_T = 0.2$, or 20% of the sensor radius. Figure 3.2(a) shows an example reconstruction, the color corresponding to the amplitude, from white indicating zero to dark red indicating large; negative values due to ringing, which would be representated as blue, are omitted. In addition to the peak due to the target, a false postive peak, or artefact, due to noise is shown for illustration.

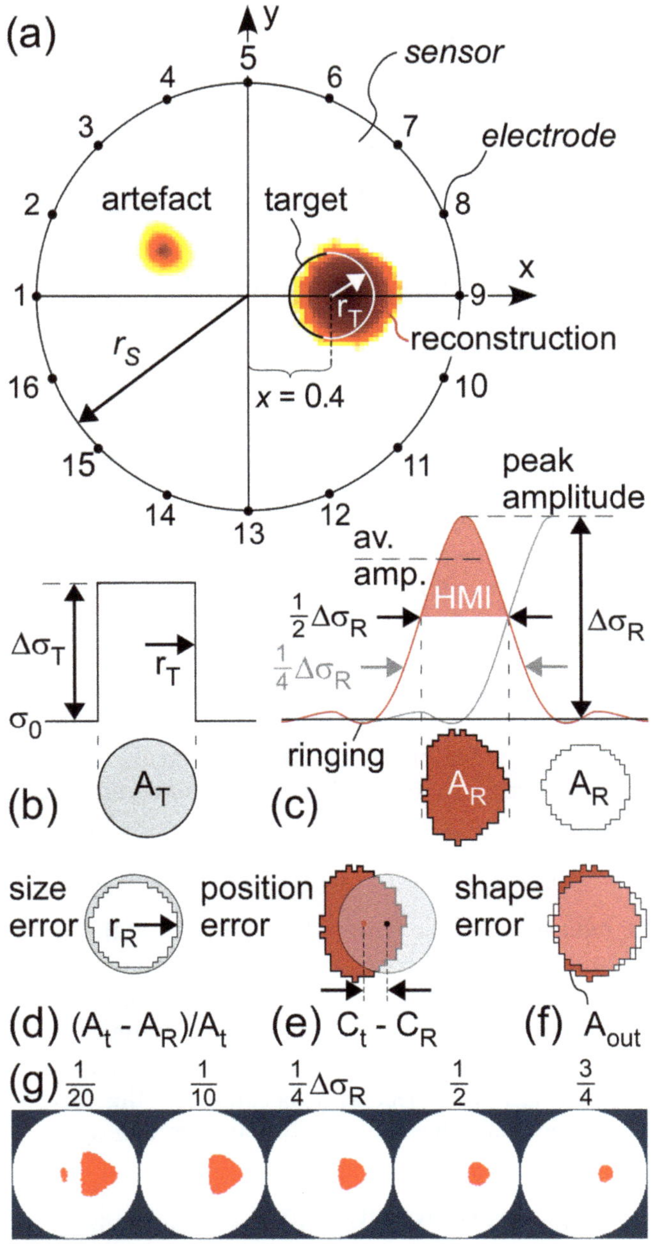

Figure 3.2. The metrics used to evaluate the EIT reconstructions. (a) A circular sensor with 16 electrodes at the boundary illustrating a target stimulus (circle) at $x = 0.4$ with radius $r_T = 0.2$, area A_T, and (b) constant amplitude $\Delta\sigma_T$, as well as the EIT reconstruction (red). Also shown is an example of a noise-induced artefact. (c) Cross-section of the reconstructed image of the target, which has a peak amplitude $\Delta\sigma_R$ and area A_R, defined as the region having values greater than some threshold, here $\Delta\sigma_R/2$; the commonly used $\Delta\sigma_R/4$ threshold is also indicated. Also shown is the equivalently-sized circular area and the average amplitude. The radius of A_R, r_R, is defined as the resolution. Although (b) and (c) indicate a positive amplitude, in this work $\Delta\sigma$ decreases, corresponding to an increase in resistance. The (d) size, (e) position, and (f) shape errors. (g) For a triangular target, threshold images showing the area of the reconstruction having an amplitude greater than the indicated fractions f of the peak maximum $\Delta\sigma_R$, known as elements belonging to the fMI or f max image. The '½' image is the half max set shown in (c).

Although metrics have been defined in numerous prior works, definitions have varied, so for clarity and completeness we here define the metrics used in this book.

3.2.3 Amplitude

The amplitude $\Delta\sigma_R$ of the reconstructed feature is the maximum value in the image, obtained in this work by averaging the 10 largest image points (either nodes or elements).

$$\text{Peak Amplitude} = \Delta\sigma_R = \max(\Delta\sigma)\big|_{\text{image}} \tag{3.1}$$

The peak amplitude varies in the presence of noise. There are thus other ways of reporting amplitude. EIDORS 3.10 reports the *image* amplitude, which is the sum over all the values in the image, which yields a 'volume' rather than an amplitude. An amplitude response metric has also been employed as the ratio of the elements above a threshold to the product of the target area and the relative conductivity change [21]. In this work, the average amplitude was used instead of the image amplitude, calculated as the average of those elements with values greater than $\Delta\sigma_R/2$ in all features (including artefacts):

$$\text{Average Amplitude} = \Delta\sigma_{R,\text{av}} = \text{E}(\Delta\sigma_i)|_{\Delta\sigma_i > \Delta\sigma/2} \tag{3.2}$$

where E refers to the expected value. (In an image with multiple features, this average can be found separately for each feature from MeanIntensity using regionprops in Matlab; for a single feature it gives the same result.) This average is, unlike the peak amplitude $\Delta\sigma_R$, sensitive to the chosen threshold, and for $\Delta\sigma_R/2$ the average is smaller than $\Delta\sigma_T$. An average amplitude error can be derived from the above as:

$$\text{Amplitude Error} = (\Delta\sigma_{R,\text{av}} - \Delta\sigma_T)/\Delta\sigma_T \tag{3.3}$$

A negative value indicates that the feature has a smaller amplitude than the target. A similar metric could be defined based on the peak amplitude, instead.

An amplitude uniformity metric can be defined, using either the peak or the average, as the ratio between the minimum and maximum amplitudes when the target position is moved along a line from the center to the periphery. (For a circular sensor only radial variation is necessary because, in the absence of electrode artefacts, reconstructions have been shown to have circular symmetry [9, 22, 23].) Using the peak:

$$\text{Amplitude Uniformity} = (\Delta\sigma_{R,\min}/\Delta\sigma_{R,\max})|_x \tag{3.4}$$

where x is the distance from the center. Spatial uniformity becomes more important when imaging multiple touches so that one touch does not mask others.

3.2.4 Resolution

The reconstructed feature is smooth, unlike the target, as indicated by the cross-section in figure 3.2(c). It has an area A_R; this area is often referred to in the literature as the region of interest (ROI). Here A_R was taken as the area occupied by half amplitude set, or the area with elements in the image having an amplitude greater than or equal to $\Delta\sigma_R/2$ (an area version of the full width at half maximum (FWHM) of a spectrum peak).

$$\text{ROI} = A_R = \sum_{\text{elements}} \text{element area}\Big|_{\Delta\sigma_i > \Delta\sigma/f} \tag{3.5}$$

This definition includes the areas of all image features, including artefacts, that have a conductivity change greater than the threshold. (Feature and target areas can be found using the Area item of regionprops in Matlab.) A different threshold can be set for the amplitude used in metrics calculations. For example, the set of elements in the area associated with $\Delta\sigma_R/4$, the area at quarter maximum, is the default employed by EIDORS (see *calc_hm_set.m*). Using $\Delta\sigma_R/4$, the area of the target and the reconstruction are approximately equal for the smallest hyperparameters, while using $\Delta\sigma_R/2$ results in A_R being somewhat smaller than A_T. For higher noise conditions it may be of interest to use $3\Delta\sigma_R/4$. It has been argued that the ½ max image (HMI) set is the best choice [21]. Figure 3.2(g) shows binary images of the points above various thresholds. Elements within A_R belong to the $1/f$ max amplitude in the image set (fMI), where f is the threshold.

The resolution of the reconstructed features determines the ability to distinguish adjacent touches. Peak widths are used in numerous fields to define resolution or resolvability: two peaks of equal size separated by a distance d = FWHM can be readily resolved, having a dip between them of roughly half their heights (figure 3.2(c)), while peaks separated by FWHM/2 can just be resolved, having a small dip between them. In EIT resolution is usually defined as the square root of the normalized area, or the radius of the feature if the sensor radius is 1:

$$\begin{aligned} \text{Resolution} &= \sqrt{A_R/A_s} = r_R/r_s \\ &= r_R \text{ if } r_S = 1 \\ &= \text{FWHM for circular features using } \Delta\sigma_R/2 \text{ as the threshold} \end{aligned} \tag{3.6}$$

By this definition smaller numbers are preferable since they show finer resolution. EIDORS 3.10 calculates resolution using a threshold of $\Delta\sigma_R/4$ by default; this threshold can be changed in *eval_GREIT_fig_merit.m.*

Resolution has been defined in multiple other ways in the literature [24]. For example, in some work [21, 22] resolution is given as the relative area A_R/A_S, or fraction of elements in the half amplitude set, rather than a radius. In others, it is the reciprocal of the FWHM of the point spread function (PSF) [25], where the PSF is refers to the area resulting from a single-point target. Depending on the definition, a higher or lower value of resolution is desired.

Using a point target in equation (3.6) gives the *blur radius* [25] in analogy with the use of this term in optical imaging systems, which is a measure of the PSF. The blur radius depends on target position and the extent of regularization, as do the other metrics.

$$R_{\text{blur}}(x, \lambda) = \left(r_{\text{point}}/r_{\text{S}}\right)\Big|_{x,\lambda} \tag{3.7}$$

The resolution uniformity can be defined analogously to the one for amplitude uniformity:

$$\text{Resolution Uniformity} = (r_{\text{R,min}}/r_{\text{R,max}})|_{x} \tag{3.8}$$

Since resolution may differ along x and y, depending on the target and particularly near the perimeter, the maximum dimensions of the feature can be found separately along x and y directions:

$$\begin{aligned} \text{x-resolution} &= \text{FWHM}_x \\ \text{y-resolution} &= \text{FWHM}_y \end{aligned} \tag{3.9}$$

(These values can be found from the BoundingBox property of regionprops in Matlab.) In some cases resolution uniformity may be more important than fine resolution, since non-uniformity can result in distortion of the shape and position of targets [20].

Size error is another way of looking at resolution, but it is based on area. It can be taken as the normalized difference between the reconstructed feature area A_{R} and the original target area A_{T} (figure 3.2(d)).

$$\text{Size Error} = (A_{\text{R}} - A_{\text{T}})/A_{\text{T}} \tag{3.10}$$

Positive size error indicates that the size of reconstructed target is greater than the size of the original target. For $r_{\text{T}}= 0.2$ and target positions $x > 0.8$ along the x-axis, the target area extends beyond the sensing area, reducing the size of both the original target and the feature.

3.2.5 Energy

The 'volume' of the feature, also referred to as its energy [12], takes into account both its area and amplitude. Here it was found as the sum of the elements in the half amplitude set:

$$\text{Volume} = \text{Energy} = \sum_{\text{elements}} \Delta\sigma_i|_{\Delta\sigma_i > \Delta\sigma/2} \tag{3.11}$$

Note that this sum will also include elements in artefacts. Volume is related to the EIDORS image amplitude metric, but instead of summing over the entire image, this sum is restricted to the HMI.

3.2.6 Position

Position error is defined as the distance between the weighted center C_{T} of the original target and the center C_{R} of the reconstructed feature (figure 3.2(e)).

$$\text{Position Error} = C_{\text{R}} - C_{\text{T}} \tag{3.12}$$

This error is computed by EIDORS as the difference in the center of mass distances from the origin. A negative position error indicates that the center of the reconstructed feature is closer to the center of the sensor than the target. Since the sensor radius $r_S = 1$ using *mk_common_model*, this distance is a value between 0 and 1. The position error can be affected by shape errors.

3.2.7 Shape

Shape error (figure 3.2(f)), also called shape deformation, refers to the extent of spatial distortion of the feature, such as stretching toward the perimeter. For a circular target, it is found by creating a circle with an equivalent area A_R and radius r_R (figure 3.2(c)) around the position C_R and then finding the area of the reconstructed feature lying outside of that (figure 3.2(e)), normalized by A_R.

$$\text{Shape Error} = A_{OUT}/A_R \tag{3.13}$$

For positions $x > 0.8$, the shape of the original target within the sensing area was no longer circular, so this metric was not used for those positions. Likewise, the metric was not used for triangular targets.

For non-circular targets, circularity can be considered as an alternative metric. It has a value of 1 for a circle, and it decreases with decreasing numbers of sides of the shape. For an equilateral triangle with 45° angles, circularity = 0.54. (Circularity can be obtained in Matlab from regionprops.) Circularity is calculated as:

$$\text{Circularity} = 4\pi A_R/\text{perimeter}_R^2 \tag{3.14}$$

3.2.8 Artefacts, or non-target features

Artefacts are features in the reconstructed image that do not correspond to targets, typically caused by noise, electrode motion or strain at electrodes, or reconstruction errors. Since contact can in principle be made anywhere on the sensor, and since the size and strength of contacts may vary by an order of magnitude, artefacts can be difficult to distinguish from real contacts. It has been found that image degradation in tactile imaging is caused mainly by artefacts [26]. One can define:

$$\text{Artefacts} = \text{number of features with } \Delta\sigma > \Delta\sigma_R/f - \text{number of targets} \tag{3.15}$$

(This metric can be found using the Matlab function regionprops on thresholded images.) Unlike resolution the identification of artefacts isolates the effects of noise since it does not reflect broadening due to increases in λ.

An efficient metric for noise susceptibility is the noise threshold, N_{th} at a particular hyperparameter. It is a measure of the onset of (in)stability. N_{th} is the highest value of noise N at which no artefacts are observed in five trials.

$$N_{th} = \max(\text{N})|_\lambda \in \text{Artefacts} = 0 \text{ in 5 trials} \tag{3.16}$$

Ringing error is generally not of high importance in tactile imaging, since conductivity changes with the opposite sign of those induced by a touch are not physically meaningful and the amplitude of same-sign conductivity changes surrounding that is small. Negative values can be disregarded or masked, for example by displaying the reconstructed feature using a threshold [26, 27] as in figure 3.2(g). However, ringing can lead to distortions in the image, as shown below, and are one indication of the stability of the reconstruction. Ringing is calculated within EIDORS as the sum of the negative values in the image divided by the sum of the values in the half amplitude set (or quarter maximum set):

$$\text{Ringing} = \frac{\sum\limits_{\text{pixels}} \Delta\sigma_i \,|_{\Delta\sigma_i < 0}}{\text{volume}} \tag{3.17}$$

3.2.9 Critical metrics for tactile imaging

Table 3.1 summarizes the most critical characteristics of tactile contacts and the associated metrics required for capturing each of them. All depend on the absence of artefacts, which translates to a required minimum hyperparameter for a given system at a given noise, explored in chapter 6. The performance measures also depend on the uniformity of the distortions caused by regularization: non-uniformity masks the presence of contacts near the center, misrepresents the relative sizes of contacts, distorts the shape of the features, misleads about the strength and intensity of the touch, and contributes to position error (as shown in chapter 5). Since non-uniformity can result in masking when there are multiple simultaneous touches, particularly of touches having different strength, uniformity is a significant metric for tactile imaging. Correct determination of the number, size, and shape of contacts further depends on having sufficiently fine resolution. To detect low-strength contacts, where strength means either pressure or displacement, depending on the sensor, loss of amplitude of the reconstruction must be minimized. To correctly represent high-strength contacts requires good performance of the algorithm when changes in conductivity are high, when the linearity assumption begins to fail. Because EIT performance is severely degraded by regularization, the elimination of noise to allow the use of a small hyperparameter must be a primary emphasis of an experimental set-up.

Table 3.1. Characteristics of tactile contacts and the key associated metrics.

<table>
<tr><th>Number</th><th>Area</th><th>Shape</th><th>Strength</th><th>Intensity</th><th>Location</th></tr>
<tr><td colspan="6">Absence of artefacts</td></tr>
<tr><td colspan="6">Uniformity of amplitude and volume over the sensor</td></tr>
<tr><td colspan="3">Resolution</td><td>Amplitude</td><td>Volume</td><td>Position Error</td></tr>
<tr><td>Ringing</td><td>Size Error</td><td>Shape Error</td><td>Ringing</td><td></td><td></td></tr>
</table>

References

[1] Vauhkonen M, Lionheart W R, Heikkinen L M, Vauhkonen P J and Kaipio J P 2001 A MATLAB package for the EIDORS project to reconstruct two-dimensional EIT images *Physiol. Meas.* **22** 107–11

[2] Adler A and Lionheart W R B 2006 Uses and abuses of EIDORS: an extensible software base for EIT *Physiol. Meas.* **27** S25–42

[3] Adler A 2019 *EIDORS: Electrical Impedance Tomography and Diffuse Optical Tomography Reconstruction Software* http://eidors3d.sourceforge.net/

[4] Adler A and Boyl A 2020 Electrical impedance tomography *Wiley Encyclopedia of Electrical and Electronics Engineering* ed J G Webster (New York: Wiley)

[5] Grychtol B, Elke G, Meybohm P, Weiler N, Frerichs I and Adler A 2014 Functional validation and comparison framework for EIT lung imaging *PLoS One* **9**

[6] Chen Y, Yu M, Bruck H A and Smela E 2018 Compliant multi-layer tactile sensing for enhanced identification of human touch *Smart Mater. Struct.* **27** 125009

[7] Grychtol B and Adler A 2013 Uniform background assumption produces misleading lung EIT images *Physiol. Meas.* **34** 579–93

[8] Grychtol B and Adler A 2014 Choice of reconstructed tissue properties affects interpretation of lung EIT images *Physiol. Meas.* **35** 1035–50

[9] Chen Y 2018 Tactile sensing with compliant structures for human-robot interaction *PhD Thesis* Department of Mechanical Engineering, University of Maryland

[10] Russo S, Nefti-Meziani S, Carbonaro N and Tognetti A 2017 A quantitative evaluation of drive pattern selection for optimizing EIT-based stretchable sensors *Sensors* **17** *AR*TN 1999

[11] Silvera-Tawil D, Rye D, Soleimani M and Velonaki M 2015 Electrical impedance tomography for artificial sensitive robotic skin: a review *IEEE Sensors J.* **15** 2001–16

[12] Graham B M and Adler A 2006 Objective selection of hyperparameter for EIT *Physiol. Meas.* **27** S65–79

[13] Mueller J L and Siltanen S 2012 Chapter 2: Naïve reconstructions and inverse crimes *Linear and Nonlinear Inverse Problems with Practical Applications* (Philadelphia, PA: SIAM) pp 7–34

[14] Gaggero P O 2011 Miniaturization and distinguishability limits of electrical impedance tomography for biomedical application *PhD Thesis* Nanomedecine Division, Centre Suisse d'Electronique et de Microtechnique (CSEM), University of Neuchâtel, Landquart, Switzerland

[15] Shi X T, Dong X Z, Shuai W J, You F S, Fu F and Liu R G 2006 Pseudo-polar drive patterns for brain electrical impedance tomography *Physiol. Meas.* **27** 1071–80

[16] Bera T K and Nagaraju J 2012 Studying the resistivity imaging of chicken tissue phantoms with different current patterns in Electrical Impedance Tomography (EIT) *Measurement* **45** 663–82

[17] Adler A, Gaggero P O and Maimaitijiang Y 2011 Adjacent stimulation and measurement patterns considered harmful *Physiol. Meas.* **32** 731–44

[18] Yasin M, Bohm S, Gaggero P O and Adler A 2011 Evaluation of EIT system performance *Physiol. Meas.* **32** 851

[19] Chen Y, Yu M, Bruck H A and Smela E 2018 Characterization of a compliant multi-layer system for tactile sensing with enhanced sensitivity and range *Smart Mater. Struct.* **27** 065005

[20] Adler A *et al* 2009 GREIT: a unified approach to 2D linear EIT reconstruction of lung images *Physiol. Meas.* **30** S35–55

[21] Naushad A, Rashid A and Mazhar S 2014 Year Analysing the performance of EIT images using the point spread function *Int. Conf. Emerging Technologies (ICET) (Islamabad, 8–9 Dec)* pp 36–41

[22] Tawil D S, Rye D and Velonaki M 2009 Improved EIT drive patterns for a robotics sensitive skin *Australasian Conf. Robotics and Automation (ACRA) (Sydney, Dec. 2–4)* pap112s111

[23] Tawil D S 2012 Artificial skin and the interpretation of touch in human-robot interaction *PhD Thesis* School of Aerospace, Mechanical and Mechatronic Engineering, University of Sydney, Australia

[24] Wheeler J L, Wang W and Tang M X 2002 A comparison of methods for measurement of spatial resolution in two-dimensional circular EIT images *Physiol. Meas.* **23** 169–76

[25] Adler A and Guardo R 1996 Electrical impedance tomography: regularized imaging and contrast detection *IEEE Trans. Med. Imag.* **15** 170–9

[26] Elsanadedy A 2012 Application of electrical impedance tomography to robotic tactile sensing *MS Thesis* Mechanical Engineering, Carleton University, Ottawa, Ontario, Canada

[27] Duan X, Taurand S and Soleimani M 2019 Artificial skin through super-sensing method and electrical impedance data from conductive fabric with aid of deep learning *Sci Rep.* **9** seag8831

Chapter 4

In layperson's terms, how does electrical impedance tomography work?

Elisabeth Smela, with contributions by Ayush Nankani

This chapter explains the basics of electrical impedance tomography (EIT) for sensor experimentalists who are new to the field, focusing on piezoresistive sensing. It closely examines how EIT works starting from the data collection process and going through the inverse problem to produce an image, with reference to the computations made in the open-source EIDORS software. Using figures and examples, key concepts are explained, including singular value decomposition (SVD), the prior, regularization, and Picard coefficients. The scaling relationships among current, conductivity, and the hyperparameter are presented. The implications for handling noise and image quality are then discussed.

4.1 Overview

Section 2.2.2 gave a high-level overview of the EIT process; figure 2.2 is repeated here as figure 4.1. This chapter goes in depth through each step of EIT imaging: data collection (section 4.2), representation of the data (section 4.3), parameters and mechanics of the inverse problem (sections 4.4 and 4.5), and practical ramifications for imaging (section 4.6).

4.2 The measurements

4.2.1 Data collection

Figure 4.2(a) shows a typical tactile imaging measurement configuration at one snapshot in the sequence of measurements. A circular sensor is shown for illustration, although other shapes have been employed. The sensors can be considered two-dimensional. Usually 16 electrodes are employed [1–5] and roughly 200 measurements are made per image, systematically switching the positions of the injection, measurement, and ground electrodes. In EIT, the cost of the small number of electrodes placed solely at the perimeter is an increased complexity of the data acquisition electronics as well as of the subsequent signal processing. Figure 4.2(a)

doi:10.1088/978-0-7503-5402-8ch4

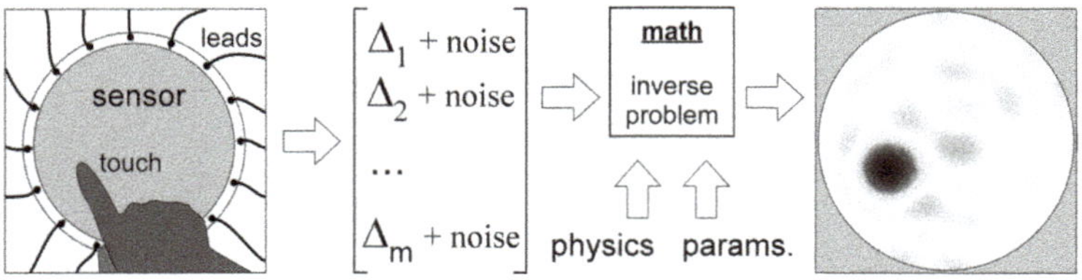

Figure 4.1. The EIT process (left to right) from the experiment to the output difference data, the physical system and model choices, algorithm, and final reconstruction.

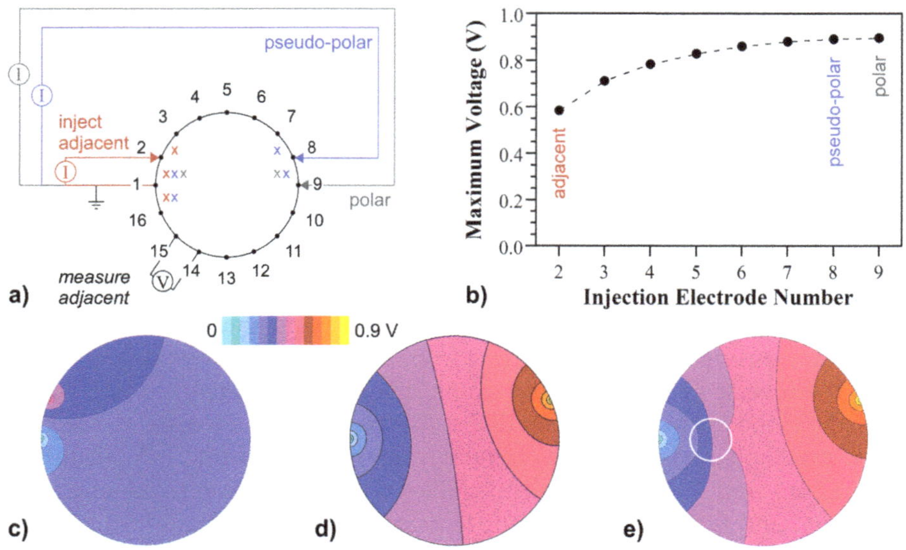

Figure 4.2. (a) Schematic showing three commonly used current injection patterns: adjacent, pseudo-polar, and polar for a circular sensor. An adjacent measurement pattern is also indicated. The x symbols indicate pairs of electrodes between which voltages are not recorded (colors correspond to those of the injection pattern labels). (b) The calculated DC voltage drop between the injection electrodes, which is the maximum value seen anywhere in the sensor, as a function of the position of the current injection electrode, with ground at electrode 1. (Conditions: 2D sensor, constant $I = 3$ mA injection current, uniform baseline conductivity $\sigma_0 = 10$ mS; see units discussion in section 3.1.4.) Simulated equipotential lines for (c) the adjacent and (d) the pseudo-polar injection patterns for a sensor of uniform baseline conductivity (the reference state). Note that the maximum values at the electrodes differ between the two patterns, as expected from (b). (The color bar indicates the voltages, from yellow at 0.9 V to blue at 0 V, with intervals of 0.07 V.) (e) Distorted equipotential lines for the pseudo-polar injection pattern when the sensor has a lower conductivity within the circular area indicated by the white line.

shows a *bipolar* or single current source injection system, also referred to as pair drive, which is the one most commonly employed in tactile imaging. It also shows a bipolar voltage measurement configuration. Software-controlled switches define the injection and measurement electrodes by changing connections throughout the sequence of measurements.

To obtain one element of $\mathbf{V}_{\text{touch}}$ or $\mathbf{V}_{\text{ref}}$, a current is injected at one electrode. It flows throughout the entire conductive sensor to ground, and voltages are measured between other electrode pairs. Various voltage measurement patterns have been used, but the dominant one has been the 'adjacent' pattern [5, 6] (also called neighboring), as shown in figure 4.2(a), in which voltage differences between neighboring electrodes are obtained. In practice the voltages are often recorded between each electrode and ground, and the differences between the electrodes are calculated in software.

Various electrode pairs can also be used to inject the current [1, 6]. In the adjacent injection pattern the current-injecting, or driving, electrodes are again immediate neighbors, such as electrodes 1 and 2, whereas in the 'polar' pattern (also called opposite) they are on opposite sides of the sensor (i.e. electrodes 1 and 9). Other, non-bipolar injection patterns, such as trigonometric [7], optimal (multiple current source) [8], and diagonal [9], have also been proposed, but the hardware complexity required for implementation [4, 10, 11], which may require multiple current sources, means that they are rarely used in practice [12, 13], so we do not treat them here.

To name the electrode pairs, we refer to the gaps or offsets between them, and the injection–measurement (I–M) pattern is named with the injection electrode pair followed by the measurement pair. Therefore the adjacent–adjacent I–M pattern is, for 16-electrode systems, called 1–1 and the polar-adjacent pattern is 8–1. Another commonly used pattern, pseudo-polar-adjacent, is 7–1. If polar injection is used with polar measurement, it is called 8–8. The latter configuration has a high symmetry since rotation by 90°, 180°, and 270° produces identical results for a uniform initial sensor conductivity. One disadvantage of this naming convention is that the names change if a different number of electrodes is used. For example, with 32 electrodes, 8–8 becomes 16–16. In this book, all the I–M pattern designations refer to a 16-electrode system unless otherwise noted.

For each pair of injection electrodes, voltages are measured between multiple other pairs. For adjacent current injection combined with adjacent measurement (1–1), when the injection pair is at positions 1, 2, the measurement pairs are first 3,4 then 4,5, etc, ending at 15,16. (In practice, the voltages may be measured simultaneously rather than sequentially [14].) Voltages are not measured (or they are recorded and discarded) between injecting electrodes and their immediate neighbors, as indicated in figure 4.2(a), to avoid contact resistance errors [12], so 13 voltage differences are obtained for the adjacent measurement pattern and 12 for most others, except for 8–8, for which 14 are collected. The injection electrodes are then rotated to the next position (e.g. for adjacent from 1.2 to 2.3, while for polar from 1.9 to 2.10), and voltages are once again obtained between the other electrodes. The process continues around the perimeter for a total of m measurements. For the 1–1 pattern this sequence leads to a total of $m = 16 \times 13 = 208$ voltage measurements and for most other patterns, 192 measurements. This set of measurements is known as a 'frame'. Due to various symmetries, however, the number of independent measurements is only on the order of 100, further discussed below. The number of measurements in the frame increases approximately with the square of the number of electrodes: for 7–1, 32 electrodes requires 896 measurements.

4.2.2 Potential drops

In tactile imaging, constant DC current, rather than AC excitation, is typically used and the sensors can be considered two-dimensional. Figure 4.2(b) shows the voltage drop for a planar sensor between the injecting electrode and ground as a function of injecting electrode offset position; electrode 1 is kept at ground [15]. For a constant injection current, the voltage between the injecting electrodes is higher the further apart they are, since $V = IR$ and R increases with distance. These simulation results agree with calculations of the resistance between points on a resistive circular area [16]. Since voltage differences between any other two points on the perimeter are fractions of this largest voltage difference, measured voltages will be highest overall for the polar injection pattern.

As mentioned above, to obtain an image of a conductivity change, such as due to a touch on a tactile sensor, the conductivity within the sensing area is compared to a reference image, which for tactile imaging is typically one obtained without a touch. Simulated equipotential lines are shown in figure 4.2(c) for I–M = 1–1 (adjacent–adjacent) and in figure 4.2(d) for 7–1 (pseudo-polar–adjacent) for a circular sensing area with uniform background conductivity. These are the reference images. Consistent with figure 4.2(b), the voltage drop between the current injecting electrodes is larger for pseudo-polar injection, as shown by the color scale. These figures also illustrate the greater voltage gradient (field strength) in the center of the sensor for pseudo-polar than for adjacent injection [17], since in the latter the current flows primarily at the periphery of the sensor. Figure 4.2(e) shows the equipotential lines for pseudo-polar injection for a sensor with a circular region of lower conductivity (higher resistance) than the background, indicated by the white line, which could be the result of a touch. The equipotential lines are distorted from those in figure 4.2(d) by the change in conductivity $\Delta\sigma$: more voltage is now dropped over that region of locally higher resistance and there are thus small changes in the perimeter voltages. EIT algorithms 'reconstruct' the conductivity changes that led to the voltage changes. Figure 4.2 is key for understanding why some injection patterns have been preferred in the literature: the further apart the injection electrodes, the greater the voltage drops between all other electrodes, and the larger the field gradients at the location of the perturbation, the larger the relative voltage changes.

4.2.3 Voltage data

Figure 4.3(a) shows the 208 voltages in the arrays $\mathbf{V}_{\mathrm{ref}}$ and $\mathbf{V}_{\mathrm{touch}}$ for simulations of the I–M = 1–1 pattern without and with a conductivity change near the perimeter, respectively, from a sensor with 16 electrodes. The voltages in the reference state are high when the measurement electrode is near the injection electrode, which occurs cyclically as the measurement pair position performs its rotation for each injection position in the frame. (For example, referring to figures 4.2(a) and (c), the voltage difference between the pair of measurement electrodes is highest when the injection electrode pair is 1,2 and measurement electrode pair is 3,4 or 15,16 and again when the injection electrode pair is 2,3 and measurement electrode pair is 4,5 or 16,1.) For 1–1, there are 13 points in each voltage measurement sub-cycle. The voltage

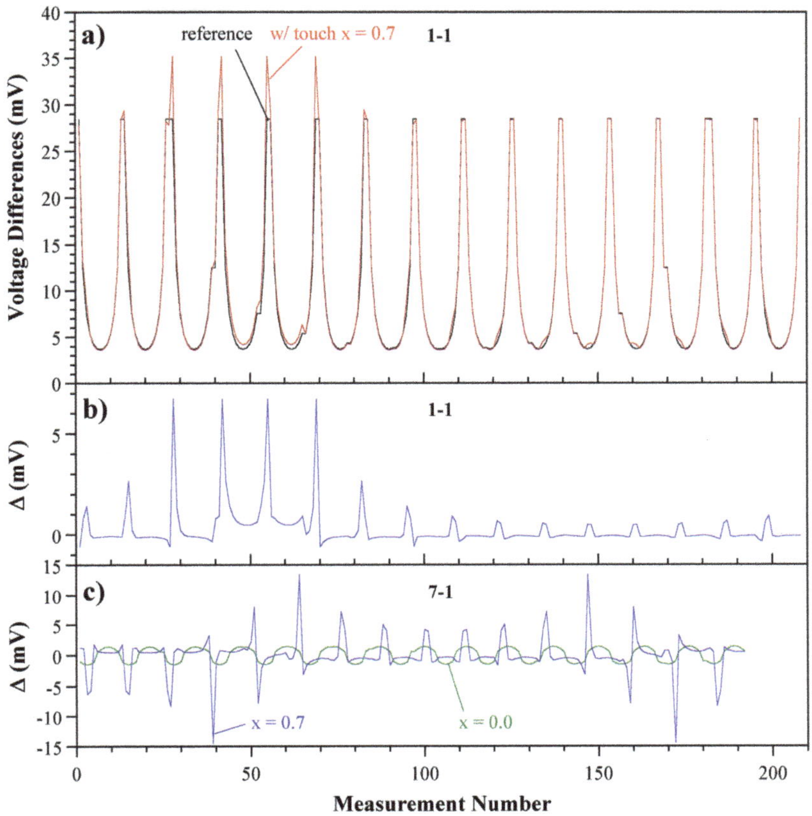

Figure 4.3. (a) For a 16-electrode system, boundary potential measurement frames $\mathbf{V}_{\text{touch}}$ and $\mathbf{V}_{\text{ref}}$ resulting from the 1–1 I–M pattern with (red) and without (black) a touch near the perimeter (at $x = 0.7$, $y = 0.0$, circular target, radius of conductivity change $r_T = 0.2$). (b) The difference $\Delta = \mathbf{V}_{\text{touch}} - \mathbf{V}_{\text{ref}}$ associated with (a). (c) For I–M = 7–1, Δ for a target at $x = 0.7$ (blue) and for a target at $x = 0.0$ (green). The vertical scales in these plots differ. (Simulation conditions: $I = 3 \times 10^{-3}$, $\sigma_0 = 10^{-2}$ $\Delta\sigma = -4 \times 10^{-3}$; no noise; see units discussion in section 3.1.4.)

difference decreases with distance from the injection pair, resulting in a series of 16 *U*-shaped features. (If the injection electrode pair is 1,2 the voltage differences between adjacent electrodes is smallest when the measurement electrode pair is 9,10.) For I–M = 7–1 and 7–7, on the other hand, there are regions where the voltage differences are negative (figure 4.4), because, referring to figure 4.2(d), the orientation of the measurement pair with respect to ground switches in half of the sub-cycle.

In figure 4.3(b) $\mathbf{V}_{\text{ref}}$ is subtracted from $\mathbf{V}_{\text{touch}}$, giving the difference array, $\mathbf{\Delta} = \mathbf{V}_{\text{touch}} - \mathbf{V}_{\text{ref}}$, which is the information used by the EIT algorithms (figure 4.1). (The values in $\mathbf{V}_{\text{touch}}$ and $\mathbf{V}_{\text{ref}}$ are voltage differences between pairs of measurement electrodes, while the values in $\mathbf{\Delta}$ are differences in those same pairs *at different times*.) Note that in some places the differences are positive while in others they are negative; all contain information about the touch and contribute to the EIT image. The m values Δ_i in $\mathbf{\Delta}$ are small, with many of them near zero (note the difference in

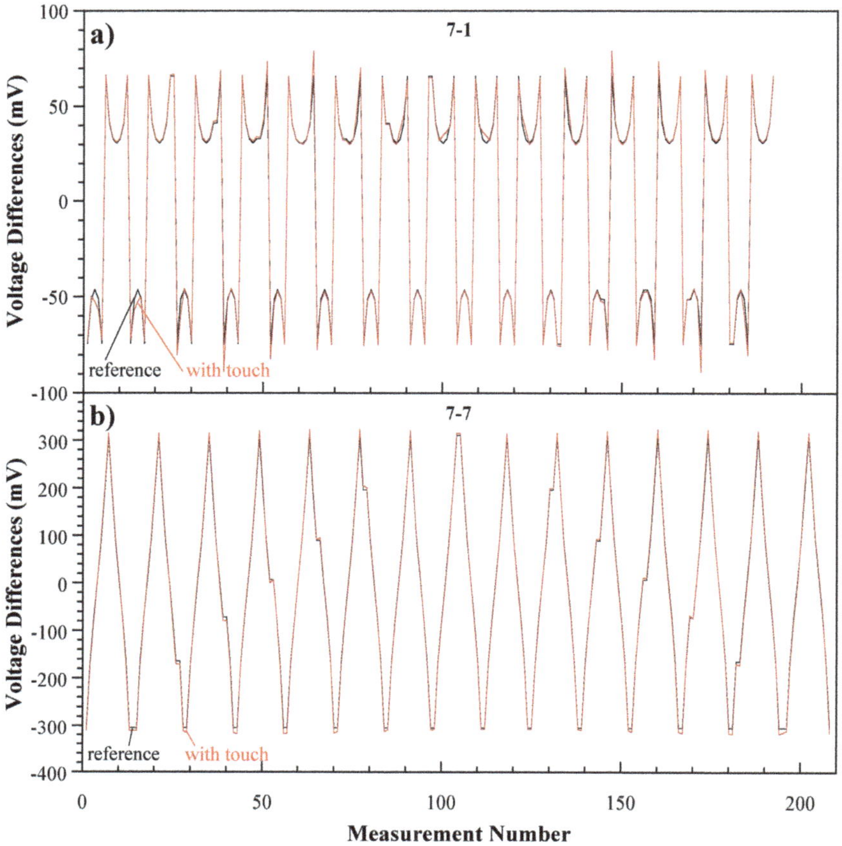

Figure 4.4. Using the same simulation conditions as in figure 4.3, $\mathbf{V}_{touch}$ (red) and $\mathbf{V}_{ref}$ (black) resulting from the (a) 7–1 and (b) 7–7 I–M pattern for a circular target at $x = 0.7$. Note differences in vertical scales of these plots.

y-axis scales between figures 4.3(a) and (b)). In this simulation the target was near the perimeter, closer to some of the electrodes, so the differences Δ_i are largest there. The Δ_i increase proportionally with the size of the stimulus, i.e. the strength of the touch.

Figure 4.3(c) shows $\mathbf{\Delta}$ for the 7–1 pattern under identical conditions. The Δ_i are larger than in figure 4.3(b) (again note the difference in y-axis scales), as expected from figure 4.2(e). Also note that, as expected from figures 4.2(c) and (d), the maxima are more uniform across the vector instead of more focused at a few positions. Figure 4.3(c) also illustrates that $\mathbf{\Delta}$ changes with the location of the target. The Δ_i for a target at $x = 0$ were smaller and showed periodicity.

The simulated data in figure 4.3 were noise-free. Experimentally, noise may be contributed by both $\mathbf{V}_{touch}$ and $\mathbf{V}_{ref}$, and if these are in turn obtained from the difference of two measurements between an electrode and ground, then there are noise contributions in both of those measurements. In practice each voltage is typically obtained by averaging multiple readings on each electrode to reduce noise, although this increases the data collection time. Often V_{ref} is obtained by averaging a large number of frames, making it essentially noise-free. The standard deviation of the noise may be 1–300 μV [18]. At minimum the noise between an electrode and ground is at the level of the least significant bit of the analog-to-digital converter (ADC).

4.3 The forward problem, using the sensitivity matrix approach

Given a known conductivity distribution in a region Ω (the sensor area), one can obtain the potentials at the perimeter; this is called the 'forward' problem [19]. For DC current injection, typically used in tactile imaging, to simulate the experimental situation the continuum version of Ohm's law is used,

$$\mathbf{j} = \sigma \mathbf{E} \tag{4.1}$$

where $\boldsymbol{j}$ is the current density, σ the conductivity, and $\boldsymbol{E}$ the electric field, together with the conservation of current [20] and the continuum version of Kirchhoff's law,

$$\nabla \cdot \sigma \nabla \phi = 0 = \nabla \cdot \mathbf{j} \tag{4.2}$$

where ϕ is the electric potential. Equation (4.2) is known as the Laplace equation [60]. (At DC or low frequency AC, magnetic fields do not need to be considered.)

4.3.1 The Jacobian or sensitivity matrix

If the sensor area Ω is divided into spatial sub-regions Ω_k (figure 4.5(a)), the voltage V_i between the measurement electrodes is the sum of contributions from all the Ω_{k}. The contribution to a change in V_i due to a change in the conductivity $\Delta\sigma_k$ of Ω_k depends on the amount of current flowing through Ω_k, the distance of Ω_k to that electrode, and the field lines ($\boldsymbol{E} = -\nabla\phi$) at Ω_k associated with the injection and measurement electrodes [19]. Specifically, the sensitivity to $\Delta\sigma_k$, or the amount that each element Ω_k contributes to the measured signal [17], is highest where the injection and measurement fields are parallel: it depends on their dot product, where the field due to the measurement electrodes is taken as if they had been used for driving [21–23]. The value of the dot product is the same upon reversing the injecting and measuring electrodes by the reciprocity theorem or lead theorem [23]. Expressing the above mathematically:

$$J_{i,\,k} = \nabla\, \varphi_{i,\,k} \cdot \nabla\, \varphi_{I,\,k} \tag{4.3}$$

where $\nabla\, \varphi_{i,\,k}$ is the potential gradient that would arise at element k if current were injected into the voltage-measuring electrode pair and $\nabla\, \varphi_{I,\,k}$ is the potential gradient arising from the current-injecting electrode pair.

In finite element modeling (FEM) the regions Ω_k are mesh elements. The matrix $\mathbf{J}$ of terms

$$J_{i,\,k} = \left.\frac{\partial V_i}{\partial \sigma_k}\right|_{\sigma_0} \tag{4.4}$$

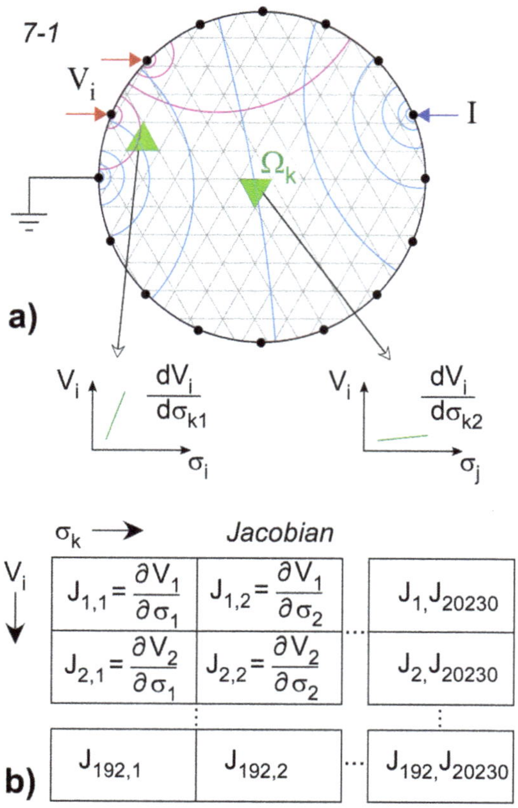

Figure 4.5. (a) The contribution of each mesh element Ω_k to the voltage difference V_i between a pair of electrodes depends on the dot product of the injection and measurement fields there, the current flowing through it, and its distance from the electrodes. In this figure, the 7–1 configuration is shown for illustration. Two mesh elements at different locations 1 and 2 are indicated in green as examples. V_i indicates a particular combination of driving and measuring electrodes. (b) Example elements of the Jacobian, or the sensitivity matrix for an injection-measurement pattern having 192 measurements in the frame. Rows correspond to the injection-measurement positions in the measurement frame. Each row of J is an image showing the sensitivity at all locations on the mesh for that measurement.

which depends on the sensor conductivity $\boldsymbol{\sigma}_0$, is called the Jacobian or sensitivity matrix (figure 4.5(b)), where i goes from 1 to the m, the length of $\boldsymbol{\Delta}$ (the frame size), and k goes from 1 to n, the number of mesh elements. In general the Jacobian of a matrix **F** is a matrix whose (i,k)th entry is $\partial F_i/\partial x_k$. In EIT, the Jacobian relates changes in voltages at each electrode to changes in conductivity at each mesh element for every drive-measurement pair in the particular I–M pattern. *This transformation matrix is a linearized mapping between the boundary voltages and the internal conductivity, assuming small variations for which the derivative (slope) is sufficient to describe the dependence.* (**J** is $m \times n$. For the I–M pattern 7–1 in a 16-electrode system, $m = 16 \times 12 = 192$. Using the EIDORS 2-D mesh model j2d4c, the number of mesh elements $n = 20{,}230$; so **J** is $192 \times 20{,}230$.) The linear approximation can be used with voltage difference data because the changes in voltages are small. On the other hand, for a 'static' image reconstruction of a medium's absolute conductivity from a single set of data, the reconstruction problem is highly nonlinear [24].

We can write

$$\mathbf{J}\sigma = \Delta \tag{4.5}$$

where $\boldsymbol{\sigma}$ is a vector of the conductivity changes $\Delta\sigma_k$ of the mesh elements and $\boldsymbol{\Delta}$ is the vector of voltage differences (figures 4.3(b) and (c)). The vector $\boldsymbol{\sigma}$ encodes an image. In EIT forward problem simulations, $\boldsymbol{\sigma}$ is the difference between the baseline conductivity reference image and the image with the target (figure 2.3). The assumption in equation (4.4) should be emphasized: inverse solution methods often assume that the conductivity changes $\Delta\sigma_k$ in $\boldsymbol{\sigma}$ are small in order to linearize the problem. However, in tactile imaging this assumption may easily be violated. For example, near the edge of the sensor large-area or multiple high-contrast contacts result in incorrect reconstructions.

The Jacobian is found from the reference baseline conductivity and from the I–M pattern: it comes from the reference forward model (e.g. figures 4.2(c) and (d)). *It contains no information about the target or the noise.*

The sensitivity of individual injection and measurement electrode combinations in the data frame to different locations on the sensor can be visualized [61, 62], as shown in figure 4.6; each row of J is one such image (normalized by mesh element size). The first seven rows (i.e. $J_{1,:} - J_{7,:}$, figure 4.5) out of the total m are shown for the adjacent (1–1) and pseudo-polar (7–1) patterns, with red indicating regions of high positive sensitivity (positive slope in equation (4.4)) and blue high negative sensitivity. (The other rows can be inferred by symmetry.) The adjacent pattern has high sensitivity at the perimeter, highest when the injection and measurement electrode pairs are close together (e.g. $J_{1,:}$) as discussed above, and low sensitivity at the center, whereas the pseudo-polar pattern sensitivity is just as high or higher at

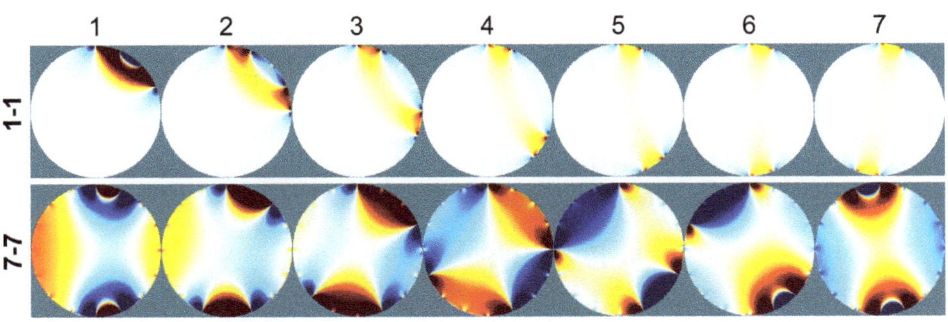

Figure 4.6. Visualization of some of the rows of the Jacobian **J**, or sensitivity matrix, for two patterns, I–M = 1–1 (top) and 7–7 (bottom), for a 16-electrode system and a circular sensor with uniform conductivity. The images correspond to the first current injection position and the first seven voltage measurement positions; the rest of the measurement positions are mirror images and the rest of the injection positions are rotations of the first. Red indicates high positive sensitivity, blue high negative sensitivity, and white no sensitivity. (The same color scale was used for all 14 images.)

the perimeter but extends into the center for some combinations, particularly $J_{1,:}$ and $J_{7,:}$. (Other patterns are shown in appendix C.) Note that many values of the Jacobian are close to zero (represented as white in the images), which poses a challenge for the inverse problem, as discussed below.

4.3.2 Singular value decomposition

To go from voltages at the perimeter to a conductivity distribution over the region, i.e. to take the measured data and create a conductivity image, is called the inverse problem, discussed in section 4.4. This involves inverting the Jacobian to find $\boldsymbol{\sigma} = \mathbf{J}^{-1}\boldsymbol{\Delta}$.

One way this inversion can be done, and which allows valuable insight into the reconstructions, is by factoring $\mathbf{J}$ into three matrices by performing a singular value decomposition (SVD) [20, 25, 26]:

$$\mathbf{J} = \mathbf{UST}^{\mathrm{T}} \tag{4.6}$$

where $\mathbf{S}$ is a diagonal matrix of so-called singular values $s_i = \mathbf{S}_{ii}$, ordered from highest to lowest (see section 4.3.4). The columns of $\mathbf{U}$, $\mathbf{u}_{\mathrm{j}}$, and the columns of $\mathbf{V}$, $\mathbf{v}_{\mathrm{k}}$, are the left and the right singular vectors of $\mathbf{J}$. The superscript T indicates the transpose, since the values are real. (For a lucid discussion of SVD in the context of image processing and 'eigenfaces' see [27], and for SVD discussed theoretically see [28].) The number of nonzero values in $\mathbf{S}$, and also the number of nonzero columns in $\mathbf{V}$, is given by the rank r of $\mathbf{J}$, or the number of linearly independent columns. By the reciprocity theorem and because of various symmetries, depending on I–M, r is less than m (the matrices are rank deficient). (For I–M = 7–1, $r = 104$ while for I–M = 8–8, $r = 28$.)

What SVD does is re-express $\mathbf{J}$, the linearized relationship between voltage changes and conductivity changes, in terms of two orthonormal bases: the $\mathbf{u}_{\mathrm{j}}$ are the basis vectors for the voltage measurements for a particular I–M pattern ('eigen-Δ', so to speak, discussed in section 4.3.5) and the $\mathbf{v}_{\mathrm{k}}$ are the basis vectors, or eigen-images, for the conductivity changes (section 4.3.3). $\mathbf{S}$, like $\mathbf{J}$, is size $m \times n$, $\mathbf{U}$ is $m \times m$, and $\mathbf{V}$ is $n \times n$. (For I–M = 7–1, $\mathbf{S}$ is 192 × 20,230 with 104 nonzero diagonal values and all other entries zero, or, due to numerical rounding errors, near zero. Note: for 7–1 the command *svd* in Matlab returns $\mathbf{U}$ as 192 × 192, but it returns $\mathbf{S}$ as a sparse 192 × 1 matrix and $\mathbf{V}$ as only 20,230 × 192.) Because the $\mathbf{u}_{\mathrm{j}}$ and $\mathbf{v}_{\mathrm{k}}$ are orthonormal bases we can write:

$$\mathbf{J} = \mathrm{s}_1\mathbf{u}_1\mathbf{v}_1^{\mathrm{T}} + \mathrm{s}_2\mathbf{u}_2\mathbf{v}_2^{\mathrm{T}} + \cdots + \mathrm{s}_r\mathbf{u}_r\mathbf{v}_r^{\mathrm{T}} \tag{4.7}$$

where each of the r terms $\mathrm{s}_i\mathbf{u}_i\mathbf{v}_i^{\mathrm{T}}$ is also $m \times n$. (For 7–1, each $\mathrm{s}_i\mathbf{u}_i\mathbf{v}_i^{\mathrm{T}}$ consists of 104 image vectors.) From here forward we use the same subscript i for all three components to highlight that they are matched in this way.

$\mathbf{U}$ and $\mathbf{V}$ are spectral bases [29]. Just as a Fourier expansion of sines and cosines can be used to represent any voltage signal, sums of $\mathbf{u}_i$ can represent any measurement signal and sums of $\mathbf{v}_i$ any spatial conductivity change, and the singular values s_i

are analogous to the coefficients of a Fourier expansion and show the overall importance of the *i*th component to **J**, in descending order. Recapitulating, the $\mathbf{u}_i$ form the basis for $\boldsymbol{\Delta}$ (the perimeter voltage frames can be created by combining these orthogonal vectors) and the $\mathbf{v}_i$ form the basis for $\boldsymbol{\sigma}$ (the conductivity image can be created from these orthogonal basis functions). The terms with the largest s_i are those that contribute most of the information to the conductivity image for a given I–M pattern.

Matrix inversion is an important application of SVD. The inverse (or pseudo-inverse or Moore–Penrose generalized inverse or minimum 2-norm least squares inverse) is found by:

$$\mathbf{J}^{-1} = \mathbf{V}\mathbf{S}^{-1}\mathbf{U}^{\mathrm{T}} \tag{4.8}$$

where $\mathbf{S}^{-1}$ is formed simply by taking the reciprocals of the nonzero diagonal elements, $1/s_i$, and transposing.

If the sensitivity matrix has values near zero, for example because little current passes through an element Ω_k, as is the case for the 1–1 pattern near the center of the sensor (figure 4.6), then the inversion will be unstable because of division by such small values [19]. This instability makes the inverse problem 'ill-posed'.

4.3.3 The image modes or eigen-images, $\mathbf{v}_i$

The eigen-images resemble standing waves or mode shapes of the head of a drum (figure 4.7). As explained in [30], these can be visualized by treating the vectors as image data in EIDORS. Figure 4.7(a) shows, for a 16-electrode system, examples of $\mathbf{v}_i$ that have circular symmetry with the index i increasing left to right; note how the spatial frequency increases with i. Note that the amplitudes of the $\mathbf{v}_i$ do not depend on current or sensor conductivity—that information is contained in the singular values, not the basis functions. Figure 4.7(b) shows examples of $\mathbf{v}_i$ with four lobes, two positive and two negative, and figure 4.7(c) illustrates a peripheral pattern as the index and angular frequencies increase. The first eight $\mathbf{v}_i$ (i = 1–8) for I–M = 1–1 and 7–1 are shown in figures 4.7(d) and (e), respectively. (All the $\mathbf{v}_i$ for these two I–M are shown appendix B). By comparing figures 4.7(d) and (e), it can be seen that the relative importance of the particular $\mathbf{v}_i$ differ for 1–1 and 7–1, as indicated by their order, and that while 1–1 and 7–1 share some of the mode shapes, some that are found in one are not found in the other.

To obtain an image with fine resolution, a large number of $\mathbf{v}_i$ is needed, just as in a Fourier expansion a large number of terms is needed to recreate the corner of a step function from sine waves. (For an illustration of how low-frequency modes form the main features of the target and high-frequency components reveal its details, see [21].) To separate adjacent targets (figure 2.1) or to recreate pointed features, a full, or nearly full, complement of $\mathbf{v}_i$ is required. Importantly, a large number of $\mathbf{v}_i$ is also needed to image features at the center of the sensor [25, 31]: note in figure 4.7 how *the higher i modes have fine structure at the image center*, whereas the lower i modes do not.

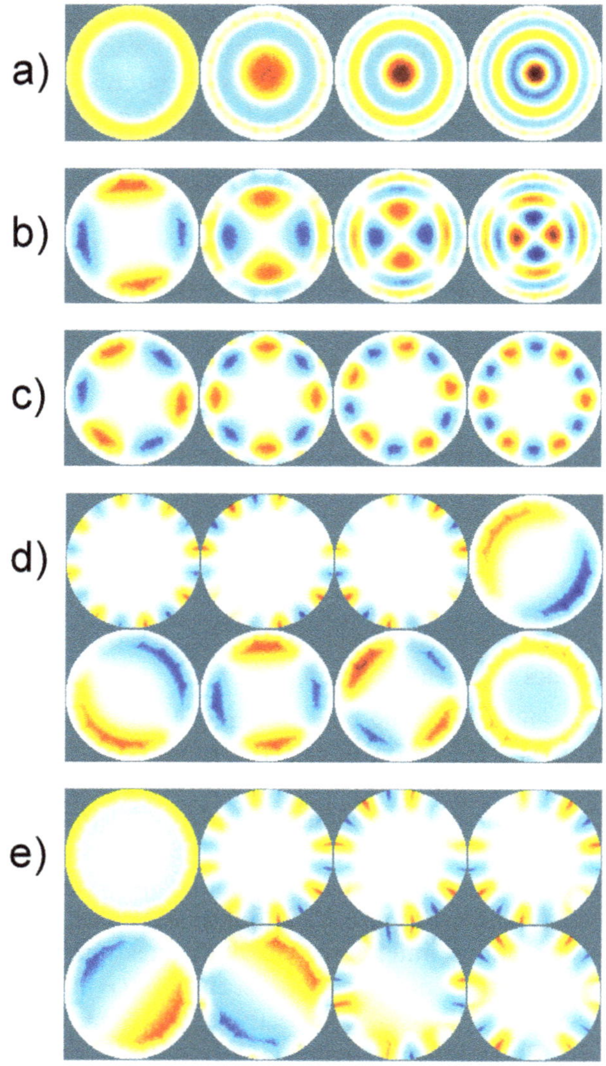

Figure 4.7. Examples of the $\mathbf{v}_i$, or eigen-images or modes, for a 16-electrode system. Red colors indicate positive amplitude, blue negative, and white zero; the same color scale was used for all the images. With increasing i from left to right, $\mathbf{v}_i$ with (a) circular symmetry and (b) four lobe symmetry. (c) Examples of $\mathbf{v}_i$ having a single peripheral ring of lobes, increasing in spatial frequency. The first eight $\mathbf{v}_i$ for two I–M patterns, (d) 1–1 and (e) 7–1.

Both 1–1 and 7–1 have a total of 104 $\mathbf{v}_i$ (the rank of $\mathbf{J}$) in 16-electrode systems; for eight electrodes the equivalent patterns 1–1 and 3–1 have only 20, and for 32 electrodes the equivalent patterns 1–1 and 15–1 have 430. Other I–M patterns have fewer $\mathbf{v}_i$ due to symmetries. For example 8–8 has the highest symmetry in the 16-electrode system and has only 28 modes. Thus, 1–1 confers greater resolution than 8–8 under low noise conditions.

Combinations of the $\mathbf{v}_i$ can produce images that little resemble the individual $\mathbf{v}_i$, as shown in the reconstructions of figure 2.1. The process of combining eigen-images is

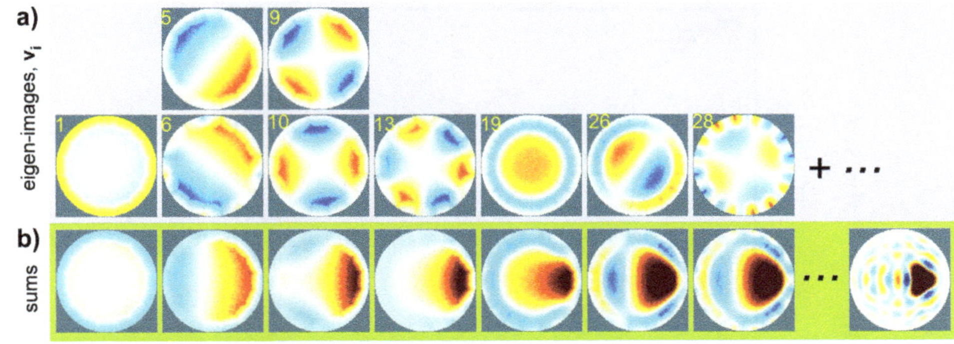

Figure 4.8. Example of how an EIT image is created from a sum of $\mathbf{v}_i$ for a triangular target at $x = 0.5$. (a) The $\mathbf{v}_i$ that contribute most significantly to this target, up to $i = 28$. Yellow numbers indicate the index i. (b) The weighted sums as the $\mathbf{v}_i$ above each image in the bottom row are added. (Same color scales.) The final image is on the lower right.

illustrated in figure 4.8 for a triangular target. The top two rows show the $\mathbf{v}_i$ that make the most significant contributions for this target, up to $i = 28$. The images in the bottom row show the weighted running sums as the $\mathbf{v}_i$ are added, moving left to right, with the final EIT image on the right. Note that the weight for $\mathbf{v}_1$ is negative, so height is added to the center of the sensor and subtracted from the perimeter; the 'energy' is focused in the center of the sensor. Weights are further discussed in section 4.6.2. Adding the next two $\mathbf{v}_i$ with significant weights, $\mathbf{v}_5$ and $\mathbf{v}_6$, adds height to the right side, and so forth.

4.3.4 The singular values, s_i

A plot of the singular values s_i for 7–1 and 8–8 are shown in figure 4.9. The s_i are usually plotted on a log scale (the y-axis on the right). (Sometimes plots of s_i/s_1 are used instead.) Note the large range of values. The ratio of the largest to the smallest s_i is the condition number, and the large ratio makes $\mathbf{S}$ *ill-conditioned* for inversion, as will be discussed below. Also note the sudden fall-off by many decades for 7–1 above $i = 104$ and the fall-off for 8–8 above $i = 28$, which are the ranks of $\mathbf{S}$ for these two patterns. The tiny values for $i > r$ are not zero due to numerical rounding errors in the FEM.

The singular values depend on the I–M pattern and number of electrodes, and they scale with the current and conductivity, but they do not depend on target or on noise characteristics since $\mathbf{J}$ is based on the reference conductivity distribution. As discussed further below, the singular values are critical to understanding the effects of noise and regularization. *Signal and image components* (which are linked) *with smaller singular values are more affected by noise and are preferentially removed by regularization.*

4.3.5 The voltage difference modes or eigen-Δs, $\mathbf{u}_i$

As discussed above, the $\mathbf{u}_i$ form an orthonormal basis for $\boldsymbol{\Delta}$: sums of the modes $\mathbf{u}_i$ can create any voltage difference vector $\boldsymbol{\Delta}$ (figures 4.3(b) and (c)), just as the eigen-

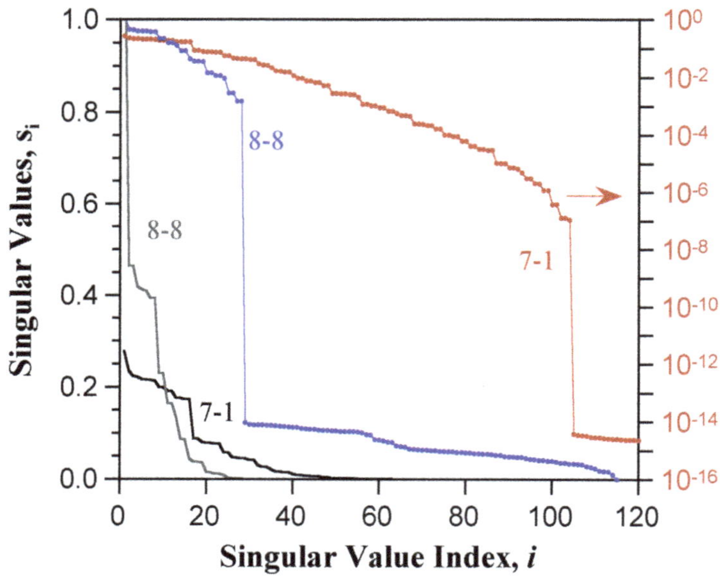

Figure 4.9. Singular values s_i from I–M = 7–1 and 8–8 shown on both linear (left, gray and black lines) and log scales (right, color points on lines) up to index i = 120 (16 electrodes, $I = 1 \times 10^{-3}$, $\sigma_0 = 0.01$).

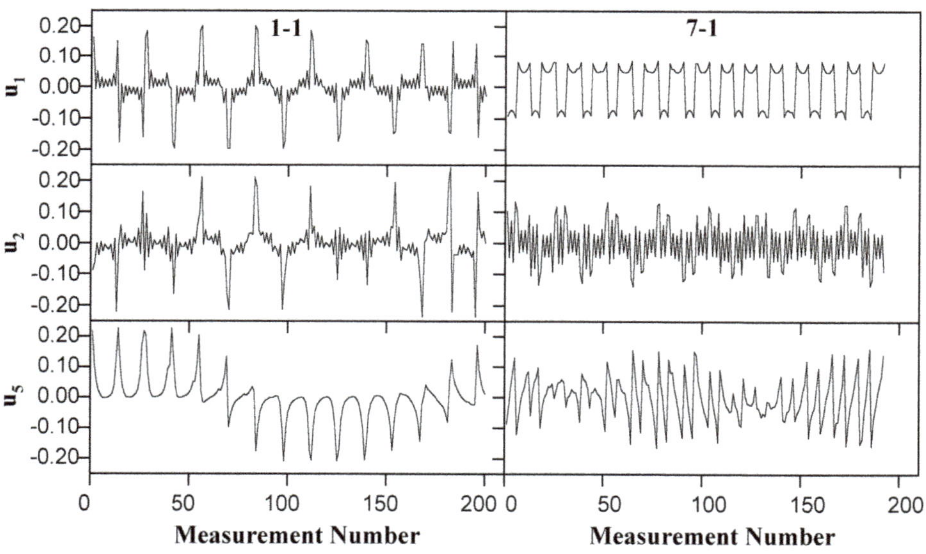

Figure 4.10. The first two and the fifth $\mathbf{u}_i$ for (left) 1–1 and (right) 7–1 (16 electrodes).

images are summed to form the final EIT image (figure 4.8). A plot of $\mathbf{u}_1$, $\mathbf{u}_2$, and $\mathbf{u}_5$ for 1–1 and 7–1 are plotted in figure 4.10, illustrating that the $\mathbf{u}_i$ also differ for various I–M patterns. For example, $\mathbf{u}_1$ for 7–1 is not found anywhere in the set of modes for 1–1. The amplitudes of the $\mathbf{u}_i$ do not depend on current or sensor conductivity.

Examples of the component matrices contributing to **J** are included in appendix D.1. The first 10 entries of $s_5\mathbf{u}_5\mathbf{v}_5$ for I–M = 7–1 are shown.

4.4 The inverse problem for reconstruction

As mentioned above, the goal of EIT is to invert **J** to reconstruct the conductivity changes over the sensor area Ω from the measured voltage differences **Δ** measured at the perimeter. The inverse problem can be stated as:

$$\sigma = \mathbf{J}^{-1}\Delta. \tag{4.9}$$

However, we are looking for more detail in **σ** than we have meaningful information from **Δ** [22]. The number of unknowns (the number of mesh elements in **σ**) is much larger than the number of independent equations (given by the rank of **J**), and because of the large condition number of **S**, this problem is *ill-conditioned* and thus *ill-posed* [19, 32]. (Note: these two terms are often used interchangeably in the literature. The problem is also called under-determined.) *This means that small changes in* **Δ** *due to noise can result in large changes in* **σ** [33]. Because of noise, the problem to be inverted is actually this one [30]:

$$\mathbf{J}\sigma + \mathbf{n} = \Delta \tag{4.10}$$

where **n** is the noise on each measurement and is assumed to be additive. Since the inverse problem is ill-posed, the solution in the presence of noise is not unique, and it requires so-called *regularization* to obtain an accurate approximate reconstruction. (Alternatively stated, noise is amplified, resulting in meaningless solutions, as shown in section 6.1.3.3.2.) The regularized equation that is solved is:

$$\boldsymbol{\sigma} = \mathbf{J}_{\mathbf{reg}}^{-1}\,\Delta \tag{4.11}$$

4.4.1 Regularization

Regularization approaches were reviewed in [22], and the advantages of various methods have receive much consideration [34–39]. We focus on Tikhonov regularization, a so-called penalty method, and in particular on the approach in [40]. Numerous prior treatments have already provided mathematical justifications and derivations, so the following discussion focuses first on the general idea in plain English, and then on the implementation mechanics.

Regularization essentially entails using known information about the physical reality of the conductivity and how it changes as a constraint on the solution. It involves balancing the measured data with that prior information (figure 4.11), employing a *hyperparameter* λ to act as a dial that controls the amount of regularization. The raw data may contain a lot of high frequency components, while the assumption about the physical reality may be that the conductivity changes are smooth, with conductivities not being greatly different in immediately neighboring elements Ω_k. Also, it can be assumed that the conductivity of the medium is everywhere real, positive, and nonzero [33]. The baseline conductivity is typically known.

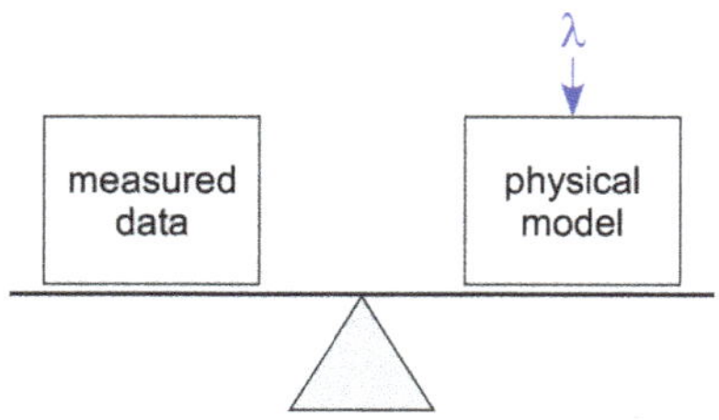

Figure 4.11. The concept of regularization. The difference between an image solution that is a good fit to the noisy measured data is balanced with an image that is a good fit to a sensor model with known information and assumptions about the conductivity. For tactile imaging the baseline conductivity is a uniform σ_0.

Regularization penalizes particular image features, as determined by a 'prior', discussed below, to eliminate destabilizing large variations and make the inverse problem better posed [20]. If high spatial frequency components are penalized, for example by down-weighting components of the solution for which $s_i < \lambda$ [21, 41], the image is smoothed. Of course, the greater the smoothing, the lower the resolution. On the other hand, if λ is too small the inversion becomes numerically unstable or the image becomes dominated by noise.

The terms L1 and L2 norm are frequently encountered in discussions of penalizing high frequency contributions. In regularization based on the L1 norm, distances are calculated as the sum of the absolute values of terms $||x|| = \sum|x_i|$. These approaches are also known as *total variation* [22]. Regularization using an L2 norm (also known as a *Euclidian norm*), as is used in Tikhonov regularization, calculates distances instead as Euclidean lengths $||x|| = \sqrt{\sum x_i^2}$.

4.4.2 Algorithms for the inverse problem, Gauss–Newton one-step method

Much has been written about algorithms that can be used for the inverse problem (see for example [36, 42–44]). They have been grouped in various ways (use of L1 vs L2 norm, projection methods versus penalty methods, etc), but for tactile imaging the most important distinction is whether they are one-step or iterative. Higher accuracy and finer resolution can be achieved using iterative methods, but they take more time and computational power, and speed is essential for tactile imaging [4, 45]. Iterative methods are required for using the L1 norm [46]. Importantly, one-step methods can pre-calculate the regularized inverse of the sensitivity matrix [23, 47], so they require one matrix multiplication instead of matrix inversions [40]. In order to provide real-time imaging that allows immediate responses to tactile cues, we therefore limit the discussion here to the Gauss–Newton (GN) one-step method [35, 40], which uses an L2 norm, because of its speed [37, 48].

In the GN one-step inversion, the regularized inverse, equation (4.11), is obtained by finding $\mathbf{J}_{\text{reg}}^{-1}$ this way:

$$\mathbf{J}_{\text{reg}}^{-1} = (\mathbf{J}^{\mathrm{T}}\,\mathbf{W}\,\mathbf{J} + \lambda^2\,\mathbf{R}^{\mathrm{T}}\,\mathbf{R})^{-1}\,\mathbf{J}^{\mathrm{T}}\mathbf{W} \tag{4.12}$$

(For images based on element nodes, this step is performed in the Matlab file *nodal_solve.m*, and for elements, in *inv_solve_diff_GN_one_step.m*.) Before examining the components of equation (4.12), it should be noted that it is an example of *generalized Tikhonov regularization*, which solves the problem of an ill-posed inverse, in this case the near-singular matrix $\mathbf{J}^T\mathbf{J}$ (meaning that the ratio of the largest to smallest singular values, s_1/s_r is large) by adding positive elements, given by the regularization term $\lambda^2\mathbf{R}^T\mathbf{R}$. Equation (4.12) is further discussed in appendix D.3.

In equation (4.12), **W** is a weight matrix (calculated in *calc_meas_icov.m*), which is the identity matrix ($m \times m$) by default if no measurement covariances are specified. For uncorrelated noise, **W** is a diagonal matrix with the noise variance at each measurement [46].

The important **R** is the regularization matrix, and $\mathbf{R}^T\mathbf{R}$ ($n \times n$) (obtained in *calc_RtR_prior.m*) acts as a 'filter', chosen to give preference to solutions that are considered to be desirable. For example, with the *Tikhonov prior*, $\mathbf{R}^T\mathbf{R} = \mathbf{I}$. (If $\mathbf{W} = \mathbf{I}$ and $\mathbf{R}^T\mathbf{R} = \mathbf{I}$, then the method is called zeroth order Tikhonov regularization; for difference imaging assuming identical channels $\mathbf{W} = \mathbf{I}$ [35]). Note that the Tikhonov prior should not be confused with Tikhonov regularization, with which it is used. The *NOSER prior* instead scales the identity matrix by the sensitivity [46] (table 4.1, table D.1) (specifically, the diagonal elements of $\mathbf{R}^T\mathbf{R}$ are $(\mathbf{J}^T\mathbf{J})^p$ where p = 0 to 1, typically 0.5 [35]). The EIDORS default is the *Laplace prior* (implemented in *prior_laplace.m*), which is a second order high pass filter (defined for a general mesh as a factor of 3 for the element and −1 for each adjacent element); it adds matrix elements not only to the diagonal but also to places off the diagonal. The Laplace prior was compared to others in [39] and found to better preserve feature edges, while the performance of various priors with the GN algorithm was discussed in [37]. It is important to specify the prior if this type of approach to finding the inverse is used: the effect of different priors on EIT images is shown below, in section 4.5. $\mathbf{R}^T\mathbf{R}$

Table 4.1. The first five row and column entries of $\mathbf{R}^T\mathbf{R}$ for two priors. (2D circular sensor, constant conductivity).

NOSER	1	2	3	4	5
1	0.0068	0	0	0	0
2	0	0.0068	0	0	0
3	0	0	0.0105	0	0
4	0	0	0	0.0100	0
5	0	0	0	0	0.0010
Laplace	**1**	**2**	**3**	**4**	**5**
1	6	0	−2	0	0
2	0	6	−2	0	0
3	−2	−2	6	−2	0
4	0	0	−2	6	0
5	0	0	0	0	4

is unchanged with forward model parameters such as current, conductivity, and I–M pattern.

In equation (4.12), $\lambda^2\mathbf{R}^T\mathbf{R}$ begins to noticeably contribute to the sum in the denominator, and thus to affect the image, when it is greater than $\mathbf{J}^T\mathbf{W}\mathbf{J}$ (= $\mathbf{J}^T\mathbf{J}$, $n \times n$, when $\mathbf{W} = \mathbf{I}$), which *does* depend on forward model parameters. Examples of matrix values are shown in appendix D.2 for a relatively large hyperparameter, i.e. $\lambda^2\mathbf{R}^T\mathbf{R} > \mathbf{J}^T\mathbf{W}\mathbf{J}(1,1)$, showing how this term affects the denominator.

In the truncated SVD (TSVD) method of approximating the inverse, the ill-conditioned problem $\boldsymbol{\sigma} = \mathbf{J}^{-1}\boldsymbol{\Delta}$ is handled differently. $\mathbf{J}$ can be approximated by using only terms with the highest singular values. Instead of using the full expansion of $\mathbf{J}$ into r terms of $s_i\mathbf{u}_i\mathbf{v}_i^T$ as in equation (4.7), in TSVD the expansion is truncated at j terms, where $j < r$ [41]. This truncation removes small-value diagonal terms in the matrix, corresponding to high frequency components.

4.4.3 The effect of the hyperparameter on images

The optimal choice of hyperparameter has received much attention, as reviewed in [49, 50]. The effects of the hyperparameter are covered in depth in chapter 5, but are introduced here.

Figure 4.12 shows example reconstructions for a ring-shaped target at different positions between $x = 0$ and 0.8 for increasing λ. Greater regularization results in greater smoothing, while features broaden and fall, or 'defocus'. By $\lambda = 1$, almost all information about the contact has been lost. For a small hyperparameter, amplitudes and resolutions do not change appreciably with the target's position

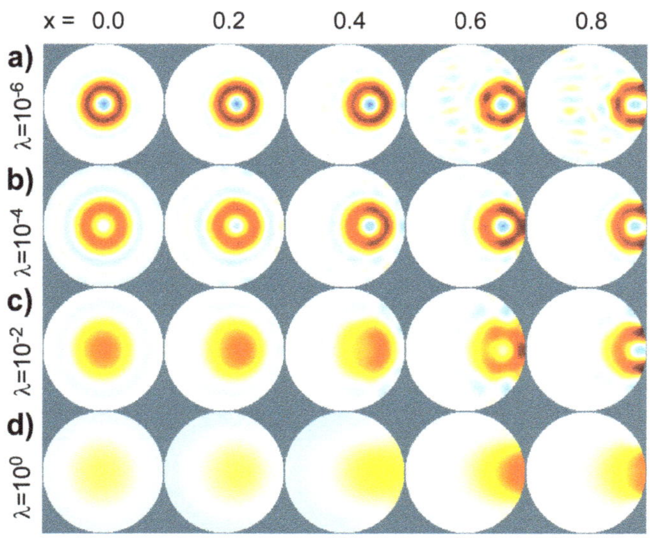

Figure 4.12. Effect of the hyperparameter λ on noise-free reconstructions of a ring-shaped target of outer radius $r_{T,o} = 0.4$ and inner radius $r_{T,i} = 0.2$ at different x-positions as λ increases from top to bottom: (a) $\lambda = 10^{-6}$, (b) $\lambda = 10^{-4}$, (c) $\lambda = 10^{-2}$, and (d) $\lambda = 10^{0}$ (16 electrodes, I–M = 7–1, $I = 1 \times 10^{-3}$, $\sigma_0 = 0.01$, $\sigma_T = 0.9\sigma_0$, $N = 10^{-12}$, $\lambda_s = 10^{-7}$ to 10^{-1}).

(figure 4.12(a)). For larger λ, however, the reconstructed feature *does* depend on position, being more 'defocused', at the center of the sensor (figure 4.12(c)). The images thus misrepresent the relative sizes and strengths of targets. This spatial dependence is detrimental for interpreting tactile contacts, since they are represented very differently at different sensor locations. Furthermore, when imaging multiple contacts, a touch at the center can be masked, or hidden, by touches at the edges. In addition, non-uniformity leads to distorted feature shapes and position errors. Spatial non-uniformity increases with λ. Since sensitivity to changes in conductivity, $\partial V_i/\partial \sigma_k = J_{i,\,k}$ are smaller at the center of the sensor than at the edge, the $\mathbf{J}^T\mathbf{W}\mathbf{J}$ terms are smaller there, and the prior information $\lambda^2\mathbf{R}^T\mathbf{R}$ makes a relatively larger contribution to the sum. Thus, to retain image information, the smallest possible λ must be used, and this, in turn, necessitates the smallest levels of noise.

It should also be noted in figure 4.12 that at small hyperparameters, most pronouncedly at the periphery of the sensor, the ring is not of uniform amplitude. Rather, there are several points at which the amplitude is higher, shown by the darker red. This variation arises because the image is created from a sum of eigen-functions, as shown in figure 4.7.

The sum of eigen-functions is clearly apparent when looking at cross-sections along $y = 0$, through the center of the target. Figure 4.13 shows cross-sections for a range of target sizes r_T, at two target positions and two hyperparameters. As the target radius increases beyond $r_T = 0.2$, it becomes too wide to represent with a single peak; the reconstruction then employs by two peaks along x; the center of the feature becomes a local minimum. The number of peaks increases stepwise with r_T. Below $r_T = 0.1$, the reconstructed peak decreases in amplitude but not significantly in width, since the eigen-functions have a fixed width. (Simplifying the display to show only values above a threshold eliminates the rippled representation, but this may hinder distinguishability of closely positioned touches.) Another thing to note is that the width of the eigen-functions increases with λ.

When the target is off center (figures 4.13(b) and (d)) the reconstructed feature becomes increasingly asymmetric, since the effects of the hyperparameter are spatially varying. Beyond a certain radius (in this example, at $r_T = 0.6$) the reconstruction can fail because the assumption of small conductivity changes used to linearize the problem no longer holds. Yet such stimuli might occur during tactile imaging.

4.4.4 Effects of conductivity, contrast, and current

The product $\mathbf{J}^T\mathbf{W}\mathbf{J}$ in equation (4.12) depends on the sensor conductivity, the injection current, and the I–M pattern. Since $\mathbf{J}$ (equation (4.4)) has units of $V\Omega m$ = Am S^{-2} (current distance/conductance^2), then $\mathbf{J}^T\mathbf{W}\mathbf{J}$ has units of A^2m^2/S^4. This term therefore increases as the square of the current and decreases as the 4th power of the conductivity.

Thus, to have the same level of influence on the sum in equation (4.12), λ must be increased or decreased commensurately with changes in current and conductivity (table 4.2). The higher the current, the larger $\lambda^2\mathbf{R}^T\mathbf{R}$ must be to challenge $\mathbf{J}^T\mathbf{W}\mathbf{J}$. For each 10× increase in current, the size of λ must be increased by 10× for it to have

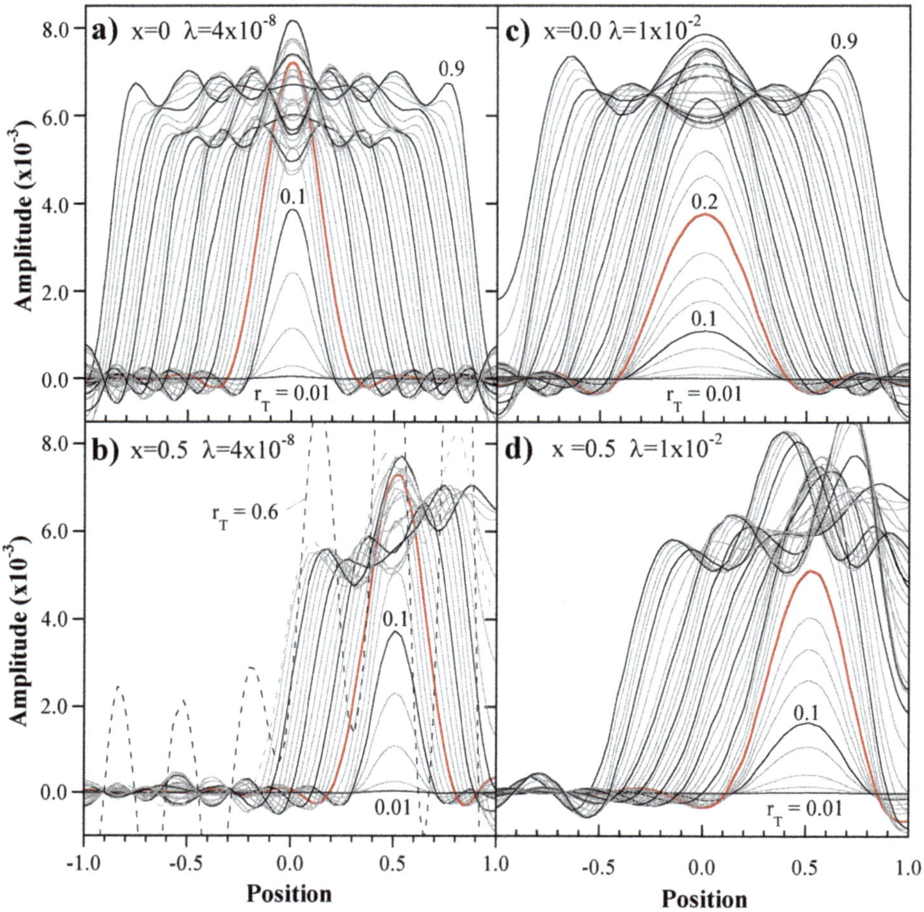

Figure 4.13. Cross-sections taken along the x-axis of reconstructed EIT images of a circular target with different radii for the ADJ–ADJ pattern (I–M = 1–1). (a) At the smallest hyperparameter $\lambda = 4 \times 10^{-8}$ ($\lambda_s = 1.3 \times 10^{-9}$) a target at the center of the sensor, $x = 0$. Black lines show $r_T = 0.01$ and r_T at multiples of 0.1, the red line shows $r_T = 0.2$, and gray lines show intermediate target radii, while dashed lines show problematic reconstructions. (b) The same λ as (a) with the target at $x = 0.5$. (c) The same $x = 0$ as (a) but with a larger hyperparameter, $\lambda = 1 \times 10^{-2}$ ($\lambda_s = 3.3 \times 10^{-4}$). (d) The same $\lambda = 1 \times 10^{-2}$ as (c) but with the target at $x = 0.5$. (16 electrodes, $I = 3 \times 10^{-3}$, $\sigma_0 = 10^{-2}$, $\sigma_T = 0.6\sigma_0$, noise-free)

Table 4.2. Scaling λ to maintain the same level of regularization, provided that variations in conductivity are small enough for the linear approximation made in the solution to hold.

Vary	Direction, amount	Fix	For same effective regularization, change numerical value of λ
I	↑ 10	σ_0, $\Delta\sigma$	↑ 10
$\Delta\sigma$	↑ 10	σ_0, I	—
σ_0	↑ 10	$\Delta\sigma$, I	↓ 10^{-2}

the same relative strength. In other words, the numerical value for λ entered into the simulation goes up, but the image resolution will be the same. This effect is illustrated by the cross-sections in figure 4.14 (blue versus black curves). Alternatively stated, using a higher current at the same hyperparameter results in finer resolution (see also appendix E.1). On the other hand, the higher the sensor conductivity, the smaller λ must be set to have the same influence. This relationship goes as the inverse square: for each 10× increase in conductivity, the size of λ must be decreased by 100× for it to have the same relative strength, as shown in figure 4.14 (red versus black curves). (See also appendix E.2.) Note that changing the contrast $\Delta\sigma_T$ does not change the effective strength of λ, although it does improve noise immunity by increasing the SNR.

We therefore introduce a scaled hyperparameter λ_s that allows comparison across experimental conditions:

$$\lambda_s = \lambda\sigma_0^2/I \tag{4.13}$$

Thus, we can consider the values of the unscaled λ to be per (S/cm)^2/A. The λ_s in figure 4.14 are all the same: $\lambda_s = 10^{-3}$. Another scaling that has been used is to give λ in terms of $\mathbf{J}^T\mathbf{J}$ [31].

Increasing the current at a given σ_0 results in a larger signal $\mathbf{\Delta}$ since $V = IR$. A larger $\mathbf{\Delta}$ is beneficial in the presence of a fixed noise level. Increasing I is not usually possible in medical imaging, since the current injected into the patient must be limited for safety [47, 51]. In tactile imaging, on the other hand, it is feasible to

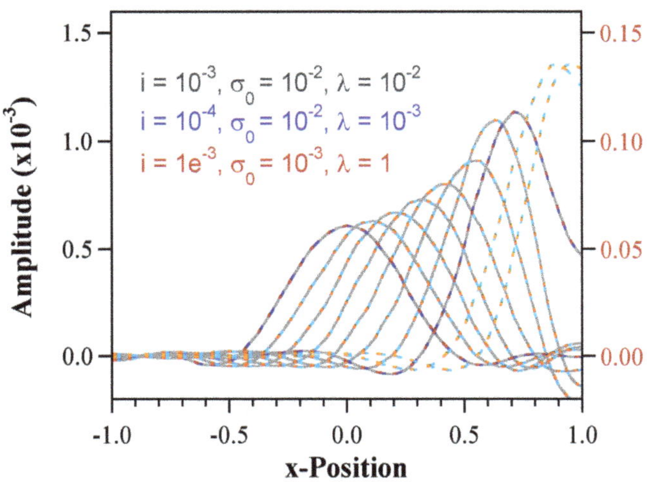

Figure 4.14. Cross-sections along the center line of the image, at $y = 0$ (along the x-axis), through a circular target at various x-positions. The base case curves with current $I = 1 \times 10^{-3}$, conductivity $\sigma_0 = 10^{-2}$, and hyperparameter $\lambda = 10^{-2}$are shown in black and gray. The curves for a 10× reduction in I and a 10× reduction in λ are shown in dashed blue at two positions of the target, at the center and near the edge. The curves for a 10× reduction in σ_0 and a 100× increase in λ are shown in dashed red and employ the secondary y-axis, on which values are reduced by a factor of 10. Dotted gray lines indicate peaks at positions where the target was so close to the edge of the sensor that it touched it or extended partially outside the sensor area. For all three sets of curves $\lambda_s = 10^{-3}$ (16 electrodes, I–M = 7–1, $r_T = 0.2$, $\sigma_T = 0.9\sigma_0$ (−10% target contrast), $N = 10^{-12}$).

increase I, but while the issue is not one of safety, the power consumption ($P = I^2R$) increases, which is a problem. In addition, increasing I may result in additional noise on the signal, or may result in heating that alters the sensor's conductivity [52].

In a piezoresistive material formed by mixing conductive particles into an insulating host, σ_0 is determined by the 'loading', or fraction of particles. For the experimentalist wondering whether σ_0 should be high or low, decreasing σ_0 (increasing resistivity) generates a larger signal $\mathbf{\Delta}$ for a fixed injection current, and thus improves susceptibility to noise, but at the cost of greater power consumption.

A higher conductivity change or contrast $\Delta\sigma$ can be achieved with a larger gauge factor (GF), or sensor sensitivity: $\mathrm{GF} = (\Delta R/R_0)/\varepsilon$, where ΔR is the change in resistance and ε is the strain. (Stronger touches also result in greater $\Delta\sigma$, but that is not controlled by sensor design.)

Increasing the target contrast $\Delta\sigma$ increases the peak amplitude, the relationship being linear. Unlike for changes to σ_0, there is no change in resolution for a fixed λ. The gauge factor should therefore be as high as possible, an intuitively obvious conclusion. A caveat applies, however: since the inverse is approximated by solving a linear system of equations, changes in resistance are recommended to be limited to approximately 20% [19].

4.5 Regularization method—the prior

The question of the most appropriate type of regularization to employ has received much consideration [34–39, 43, 44]. As summarized in [22], two main types of techniques have been widely used: 'projection methods', such as TSVD, and 'penalty methods', such as Tikhonov regularization. For the latter, the regularization matrix **R**, known as the prior, was introduced in section 4.4.2.

Four priors are available for use with the GN one-step algorithm, which employs Tikhonov regularization, in EIDORS: Laplace, Tikhonov (not to be confused with Tikhonov regularization generally), NOSER (Newton's one-step error reconstructor), and Gaussian_HPF (high pass filter). These have been compared in prior studies with differing conclusions. For example, Laplace, Tikhonov, and NOSER were evaluated experimentally in [39], and the shape of the feature found to be more accurate using Laplace. Simulated EIT images and cross-sections using all four priors found that the Laplace prior had the smallest amplitude error and that NOSER failed to reconstruct in the presence of noise [37]. On the other hand, it was concluded in [53] that the Gaussian HPF prior showed the best compromise between resolution and position error. NOSER, Laplace, and Tikhonov were compared, along with Markov random field (MRF), experimentally and in simulation, showing that NOSER showed poor noise performance, Laplace was the slowest, and Tikhonov resulted in artefacts [54]. The assumption in the Tikhonov prior of independent targets was said not to work well [47]. The NOSER prior was found not to reproduce conductivity changes accurately [55]. The Laplace prior has been characterized as edge-preserving [39].

The work in this book utilized the Laplace prior. To shed light on the use of this regularization method as the EIDORS default, this section compares Laplace with two of the other priors, Tikhonov and NOSER, and also with a completely different regularization approach, TSVD. There are other regularization methods that are more complex to implement, which are not examined here.

For TSVD, regularization is accomplished by simply truncating the number of terms (e.g. the number of $\mathbf{v}_i$) used in the reconstruction [26, 41]. Unlike the gradual diminution of the eigen-image amplitudes seen in figure 5.3, higher index terms are simply not included in solving the inverse problem. The number of eliminated terms is given by the number of singular values s_i that are greater than $\lambda/100$. For example, using $\lambda = 1$ in TSVD only the first 50 terms are retained using the simulation conditions employed below.

The three priors are implemented in EIDORS (in *calc_RtR_prior.m*) via the regularization matrix $\mathbf{R}^T\mathbf{R}$ (section 4.4). The Tikhonov prior, called zeroth order [37], is the identity matrix (when shown using elements rather than nodes). The NOSER prior instead scales $\mathbf{R}$ by the sensitivity $\mathbf{J}$ [46], so $\mathbf{R}^T\mathbf{R} = \mathbf{J}^T\mathbf{J}$. Thus, for NOSER, $\mathbf{R}^T\mathbf{R}$ is a diagonal matrix with values that vary in amplitude. The Laplace prior incorporates a spatial filter to penalize non-smooth image elements, which reduces 'speckle' in the image [47]. It has been called a second order high pass filter, defined as having, for a 2D sensed area, a value of 3 on each element and −1 on each adjacent element. Using the simulation conditions below, $\mathbf{R}^T\mathbf{R}$ had values of 6 along the main diagonal, along with 4 and −2 at occasional off-diagonal locations.

The hyperparameter does not have equivalent strength across different regularization methods [35], so image metrics at nominally the same λ are not directly comparable. Figure 4.15 shows the reconstructed feature's peak amplitude, normalized to its value at $\lambda = 10^{-6}$, as a function of λ for the different regularization methods. Indeed, the extent of regularization at a given value of λ was greater for some than others. For example, with the Tikhonov prior the peak height was reduced more for the same nominal value of λ than with the Laplace prior, while for TSVD it was reduced less. The four curves also had different shapes, with the one for NOSER crossing over two of the others. Also shown in the figure are results with the Laplacian prior obtained solving the inverse problem using elements instead of nodes; the results were identical.

Using the information in figure 4.15, hyperparameters for each regularization method were chosen so that the peak amplitudes were roughly comparable: 10^{-1} for Laplace and NOSER, 10^{-2} for Tikhonov, and 10^{0} for TSVD, with a large amount of regularization chosen to accentuate the differences in the methods. EIT images and cross-sections are shown in figure 4.16 for varying target position x. One clear difference among the approaches was the well-known tendency of the Laplace prior to stretch the feature toward the perimeter; the Tikhonov prior and TSVD method kept the feature more rounded as it approached the edge. However, at $x = 0.9$, that rounding resulting in feature distortion, and the Laplace prior instead more accurately represented the target position. TSVD resulted in greater ringing, and the contributions of the small number of eigen-images were more visually evident (e.g. see figure 5.3). Another difference, even more apparent in the cross-sections, was that the Tikhonov and TSVD images had rougher profiles, compared to the smoother shapes obtained with Laplace and NOSER. The 'speckle' patterns resulting from Tikhonov have previously been noted [47].

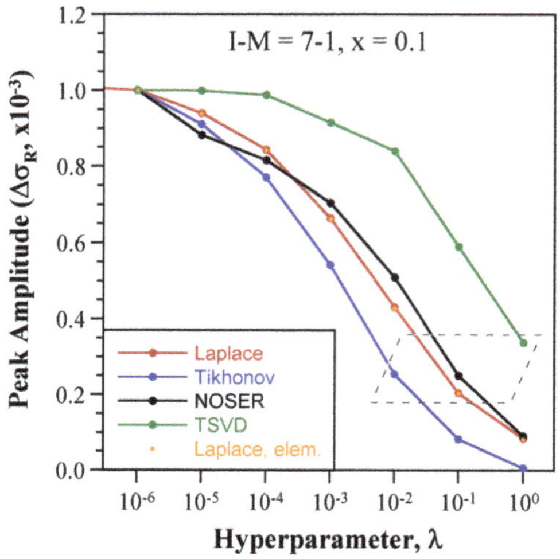

Figure 4.15. Normalized peak amplitude as a function of hyperparameter for a circular target at $x = 0.1$. The four regularization approaches are compared using nodal solve, and elemental solve is also shown for the Laplace prior. The dashed gray box indicates which values of λ were used for each method in subsequent plots (16 electrodes, I–M = 7–1, $r_T = 0.2$, $I = 10^{-3}$, $\sigma_0 = 10^{-2}$, $\sigma_T = 0.9\sigma_0$, $N = 10^{-12}$).

The four approaches were quantitatively compared at varying target positions using four performance metrics, as shown in figure 4.17. Looking at peak amplitude (figure 4.17(a)), the dependence on x differed among the four methods. For example, the TSVD spatial dependence was not smooth, reflecting the abrupt elimination of eigen-images rather than weighted changes in their contributions. (The complete sets of curves for each method at all λ are shown in appendix D.4.) The curves for the Laplace and Tikhonov priors were most nonlinear moving from the center to the perimeter. The Laplace prior resulted in the most smooth and uniform curve.

Turning to resolution (figure 4.17(b)), and keeping in mind that the levels of regularization differ somewhat among the four methods so that the magnitudes are not directly comparable, the Laplace prior produced the most linear dependence on position. TSVD and Tikhonov had the most irregular position dependence of resolution, even before the flattening that occurred for all four near the perimeter. As mentioned previously, the spatial uniformity of resolution is considered to be even more important than fine resolution, since non-uniformity will result in distortion of the shape and position of larger targets [56].

The volume or 'energy' of the feature (figure 4.17(c)) was again most uniform for the Laplace prior, although the three priors were similar up to $x = 0.4$. In contrast, TSVD showed the feature as being significantly larger in the center, whereas the volume for the NOSER prior decreased markedly near the perimeter. Thus, the change in conductivity was most misrepresented by NOSER and TSVD. For the Laplace prior, even though the energy defocused toward the center it was preserved. Lastly, the Laplace prior produced the smallest position errors (figure 4.17(d)). It should be noted that given the differences in behavior resulting from the choice of regularization method, the method should be reported in publications.

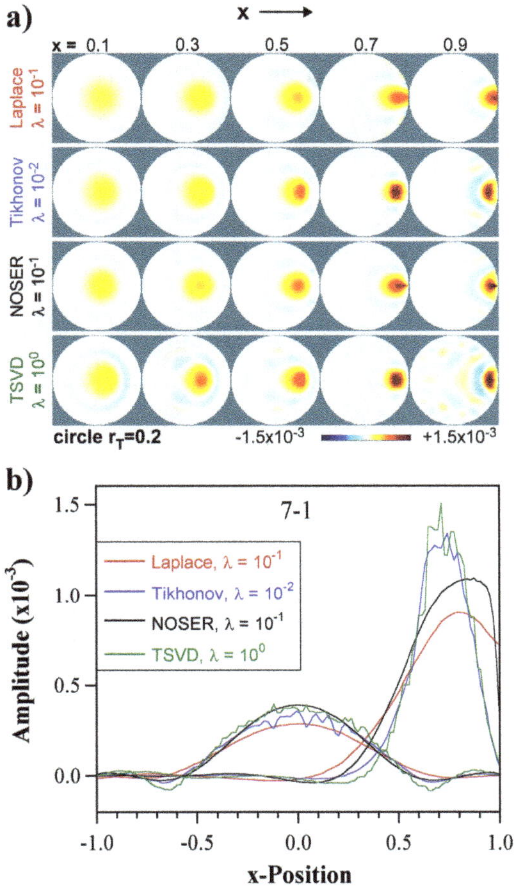

Figure 4.16. The Laplace prior compared to three other approaches at comparable levels of regularization for I–M = 7–1 at $\lambda = 0.1$. (a) EIT images at different x-positions and (b) cross-sections at $x = 0.0$ and 0.7 (16 electrodes, $r_T = 0.2$, $I = 10^{-3}$, $\sigma_0 = 10^{-2}$, $\sigma_T = 0.9\sigma_0$, $N = 10^{-12}$, $\lambda_s = 10^{-2}$).

Regarding the choice of a regularization method, it is clear why the Laplace prior is so frequently employed. It has greater uniformity, smoother spatial dependence, smaller position error, and higher fidelity to total peak energy, in addition to aesthetically pleasing images. The remainder of this book employs the Laplace prior for regularization.

Among the regularization approaches, an advantage of the Laplace prior is the preservation of feature volume over much of the sensor area and over a large range of λ, which conserves the overall intensity or 'touch energy' of the contact. If the volume of the reconstructed feature is constant, then as the hyperparameter broadens the peak height drops commensurately; the two are predictably linked. Other advantages of the Laplace prior include smooth, monotonic changes in metrics with target position and small position error.

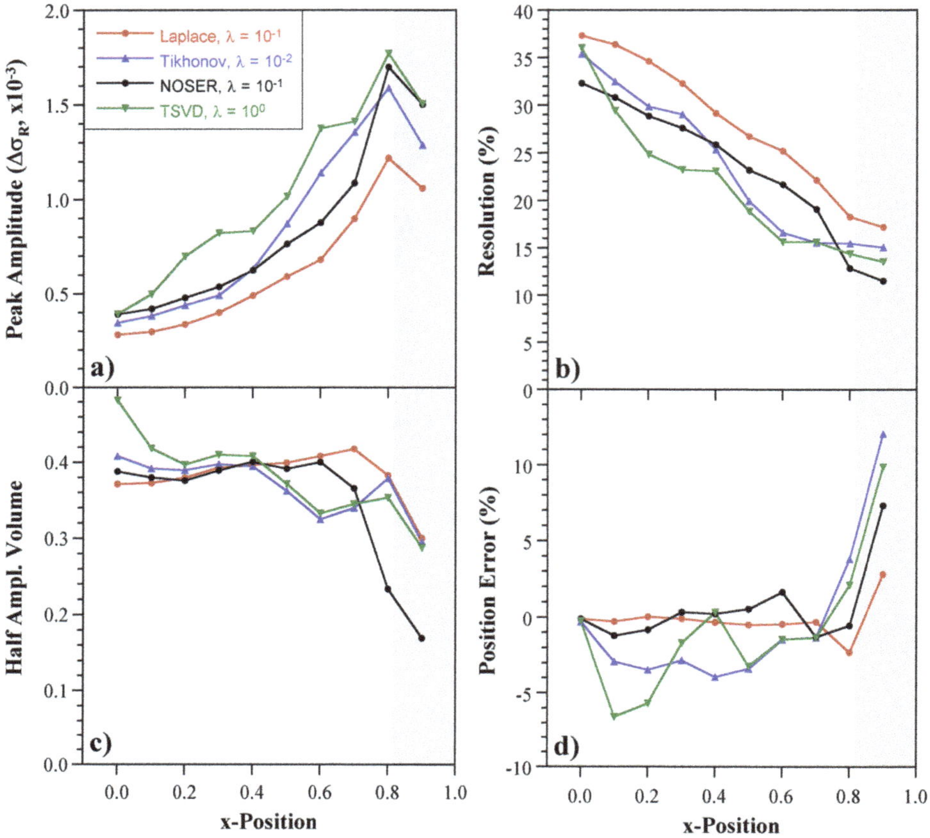

Figure 4.17. For levels of regularization for the three other approaches comparable to that of the Laplace prior at $\lambda = 0.1$ (given in figure 4.15), (a) peak amplitude (b) resolution, (c) volume, and (d) position error as a function of target position (16 electrodes, 7–1, $r_T = 0.2$, $I = 10^{-3}$, $\sigma_0 = 10^{-2}$, $\sigma_T = 0.9\sigma_0$, $N = 10^{-12}$, $\lambda_s = 10^{-2}$).

4.6 Practical implications: experimental configurations and parameter selection

The challenge of the EIT inverse problem, as shown above, is noise, and imaging decisions revolve around the strength and type of regularization to handle it. In this chapter we introduce two spectra or fingerprints, $|\mathbf{U}^T\mathbf{\Delta}|$ and $|\mathbf{V}^T\boldsymbol{\sigma}|$, that elucidate the roles of noise and regularization. The first, $|\mathbf{U}^T\mathbf{\Delta}|$, is a measure of the signal strength for understanding the signal-to-noise ratio (SNR) in EIT, and the second, $|\mathbf{V}^T\boldsymbol{\sigma}|$, clearly illustrates the process of regularization. The two spectra are closely related, but the former contains only forward problem information while the latter also contains inverse problem information. Here we also begin to discuss the role of the injection–measurement (I–M) pattern (a discussion continued in sections 5.3 and 7.2) as elucidated by $|\mathbf{V}^T\boldsymbol{\sigma}|$ spectra.

4.6.1 Noise and $|\mathbf{U}^T\mathbf{\Delta}|$

In EIT, even tiny amounts of noise more than a thousand times smaller than the measured voltage differences Δ_i can overwhelm an image because of the ill-posed nature of the inverse problem. (This topic is taken up in detail in chapter 6.) The effects of noise are illustrated in figure 4.18. In general, as noise N increases the image becomes distorted, begins to show artefacts, and then breaks up completely. Artefacts are features that appear in the reconstruction that are not associated with the target. Given the importance of identifying the correct number, locations, and strengths of touches, which may be highly variable, the onset of artifacts is unacceptable. At the lowest noise level (figure 4.18(a)), the chosen hyperparameter $\lambda = 10^{-2}$ was large enough to correctly show a single target; the triangular shape, however, was lost at this combination of λ and noise. As the noise increased (figure 4.18(d)) it became increasingly unclear what the original target was, and finally (figure 4.18(f)) the noise dominated the image. This image deterioration is what necessitates the use of increasing levels of regularization with noise.

To guide experimental decisions such as how many data points to record at each electrode to reduce noise by averaging, versus spending that time instead on employing a larger number of electrodes to try to increase resolution, one needs to understand SNR in the context of EIT. There are several conceptualizations of 'signal' that can be compared with noise. It has been stated that the smallest values in $\mathbf{\Delta}$ determine the quality of the image since they are the most changed by noise [10] and large voltages can be measured more precisely than small ones [57]. *This assertion turns out not to be the case*, as can be shown by simulations that apply noise selectively to the largest or smallest Δ_i (see chapter 6), and for reasons that become evident below. Alternatively, the average amplitude of $\mathbf{\Delta}$ has been used as a measure of signal strength, which works well, but only for a given system and target. For

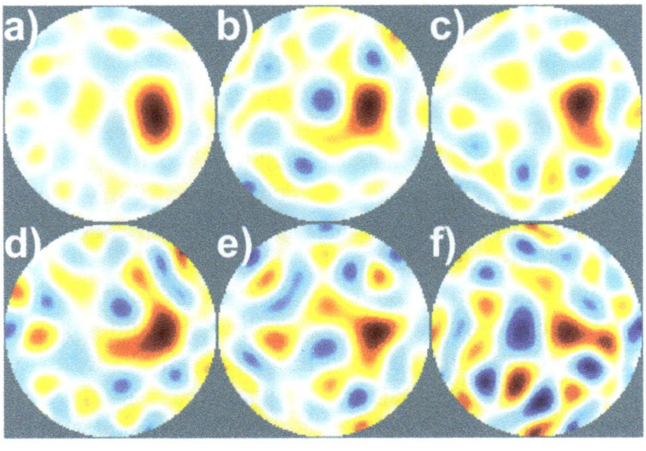

Figure 4.18. Effect of increasing noise at $\lambda = 10^{-2}$. Representative images of a triangular target at $x = 0.5$ for (a) $N = 6 \times 10^{-5}$ (b) $N = 7 \times 10^{-5}$, (c) $N = 8 \times 10^{-5}$, (d) $N = 9 \times 10^{-5}$, (e) $N = 10 \times 10^{-5}$, and (f) $N = 20 \times 10^{-5}$ V (16 electrodes, I–M = 7–1, $r_T = 0.2$, $I = 3 \times 10^{-3}$, $\sigma_0 = 0.01$ $\sigma_T = 0.6\sigma_0$, noise-free).

example, it has been suggested that I–M patterns having a larger average **Δ** should be more immune to noise [5, 10, 30], *but that is also not necessarily the case.*

It is instructive to examine $|\mathbf{U}^T\mathbf{\Delta}|$ spectra [20, 26, 58] to appreciate how small levels of noise can destabilize an image. The use of $|\mathbf{U}^T\mathbf{\Delta}|$ also has the advantage of allowing comparison of different systems and targets. To judge the impact of a certain level of noise on a measurement, the signal basis vectors $\mathbf{u}_i$ are multiplied by the measured voltage differences **Δ** [20]. Recall that the $\mathbf{u}_i$ (figure 4.10) depend only on the system forward-problem parameters, such as the I–M pattern and number of electrodes. The $\mathbf{u}_i$ with the smallest indices i correspond to the largest singular values s_i (figure 4.9) and thus have the most importance in determining the reconstructed image. To understand this product, return to the Fourier expansion analogy: the coefficient b_n in the sum over n of $b_n\sin(n\pi x/L)$ is found for a particular $f(x)$ by integrating the product $f(x)\sin(n\pi x/L)$ over the interval –L to L. Likewise, the product $\mathbf{U}^T\mathbf{\Delta}$ (size $m \times 1$) gives the amplitudes of coefficients in the expansion of **Δ** into eigen-**Δ**s.

The absolute values $P_i = |\mathbf{u}_i^T\mathbf{\Delta}|$ are known as Picard coefficients. *The P_i have units of volts and can be directly compared to the noise.* (The P_i can be found by adapting the Matlab EIDORS code; our codes are available upon request.) Using the Picard coefficients for SNR dates back to employing SVD for solving inverse problems and regularizing ill-conditioned matrices [59].

Figure 4.19(a) shows the first 50 P_i without noise for two targets, circular and triangular, plotted in order of their singular value index i on a logarithmic axis. Differences in **Δ** for the two targets are translated into differences in P_i. Likewise, differences in I–M pattern would also be manifested in the P_i.

Figure 4.19(b) shows the first 130 P_i for the triangular target without noise and when two levels of noise were added, indicated by the dashed horizontal lines. Without noise the P_i decay with i and then drop abruptly above $i = r$. Terms with index greater than the rank of **J**, here beyond position 104, which are nominally zero but are actually small values near 10^{-17} V due to numerical noise, do not play a role in the reconstruction. Raising their values by 8 orders of magnitude by adding $N = 1 \times 10^{-9}$ V did not interfere with the creation of a good image. With noise, the P_i instead level off at the noise level. The index i at which the leveling begins is called the Picard threshold. Using the smallest hyperparameter that permitted reconstruction, $\lambda = 10^{-7}$, at $N = 3 \times 10^{-9}$ V the target was well represented, as shown by the EIT inset. At $N = 6 \times 10^{-9}$ V the images broke up and showed artefacts. Even though 6 nV might seem like a tiny amount of noise compared to values in **Δ**, which may be 10 mV (figure 4.3), it *is large compared to the amplitudes of the smaller* $\mathbf{u}_i$. The largest several $\mathbf{u}_i$ are, however, unaffected until the noise reaches mV levels.

Thus, noise creates inaccurate images because of the incorrect amplitudes of the affected $\mathbf{u}_i$. Recalling from equation (4.7) that the s_i, $\mathbf{u}_i$, and $\mathbf{v}_i$ at the singular value index i are linked, the corresponding eigen-images $\mathbf{v}_i$, which then also have corrupted amplitudes, are used in the reconstruction when they should be disregarded, as shown below. This is called 'over-fitting'. As noise increases, the number of eigen-images $\mathbf{v}_i$ that can be beneficially employed in the reconstruction decreases, being equal to the number of P_i above the noise level. The $\mathbf{v}_i$ corresponding to P_i in the noise plateau are excluded by increasing λ, the mechanism of which is shown in the

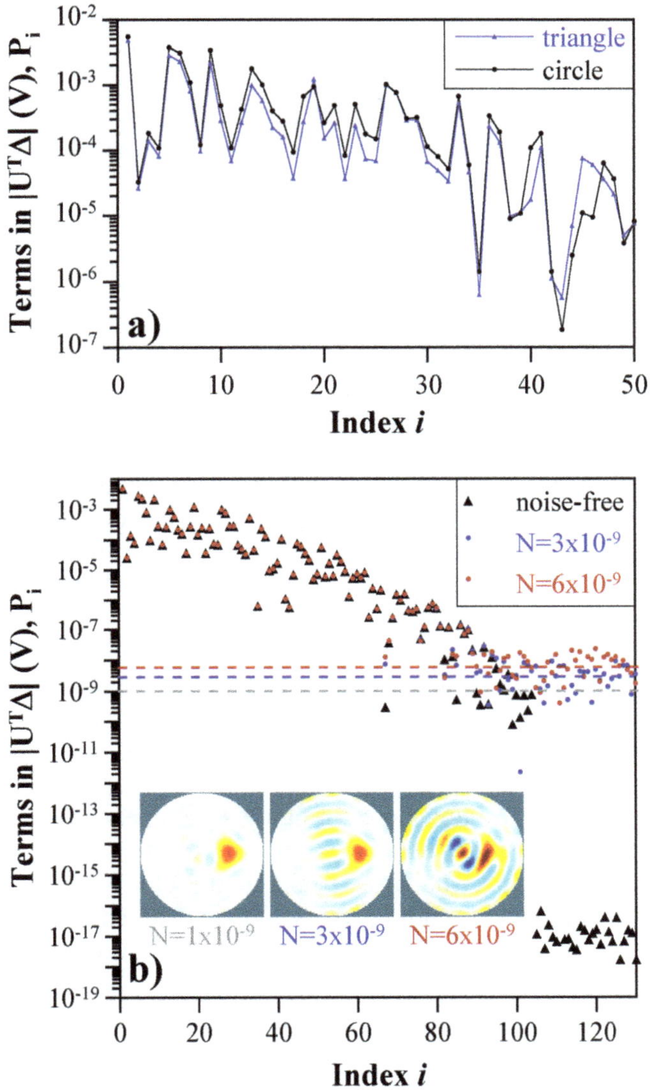

Figure 4.19. (a) The first 50 $|\mathbf{U}^{\mathrm{T}}\mathbf{\Delta}|$ terms, or Picard coefficients P_i, as a function of singular value index i for triangular and circular targets at $x = 0.5$, with negligible noise ($N = 10^{-12}$ V). (b) The first 130 $|\mathbf{U}^{\mathrm{T}}\mathbf{\Delta}|$ terms for the triangular target with negligible noise and with noise at two levels, $N = 3 \times 10^{-9}$ and $N = 6 \times 10^{-9}$. The corresponding EIT images made using $\lambda = 10^{-7}$ ($\lambda_s = 10^{-8}$) are included as insets (16 electrodes, I–M = 7–1, $r_{\mathrm{T}} = 0.2$, $I = 1 \times 10^{-3}$, $\sigma_0 = 10^{-2}$, $\sigma_{\mathrm{T}} = 0.6\sigma_0$).

next section. When using truncated SVD for regularization, the truncation is chosen to start at the index i at which the P_i begin to flatten due to noise [32]. In summary, the number of $\mathbf{u}_i$ that can be used to correctly represent the signal decreases with noise, and only the corresponding correct image components $\mathbf{v}_i$ should be retained.

Changing injection current, sensor conductivity, and contrast produces proportional up or down shifting of the $|\mathbf{U}^{\mathrm{T}}\mathbf{\Delta}|$ spectra because $\mathbf{\Delta}$ is linearly proportional to contrast and current and inversely proportional to conductivity (section 4.4.4). (The basis functions $\mathbf{u}_i$ are unaffected by these parameters.) Downward shifts make the system more susceptible to noise.

Noise has alternatively been compared to the singular values s_i. $|\mathbf{U}^T\mathbf{\Delta}|$ and $\mathbf{S}$ spectra have similar appearance (see appendices D.5 and D.6). However, the s_i pertain to $\mathbf{J}$ and therefore only characterize the measurement system, whereas the P_i also carry information about the current, the target, and other factors through the measured voltage differences $\mathbf{\Delta}$.

4.6.2 $|\mathbf{V}^T\boldsymbol{\sigma}|$ and regularization

While $|\mathbf{U}^T\mathbf{\Delta}|$ spectra are related to the input, or signal, side of the EIT process, there is an analogous spectrum on the output, or image, side, which is $|\mathbf{V}^T\boldsymbol{\sigma}|$. The two spectra strongly resemble each other, as would be expected from equation (4.7). *However,* $|\mathbf{V}^T\boldsymbol{\sigma}|$ *reflects the regularization used to obtain the inverse.* Given the profound effects of regularization on the quality of the image (figure 4.12), it is instructive to examine its effects on the various image components. (This topic is taken up in detail in chapter 5.) Taking the product of $\mathbf{V}$ and the image vector $\boldsymbol{\sigma}$ [20], provides the coefficients, or weights, C_i of the $\mathbf{v}_i$ that sum to form the particular EIT image: $C_i = |\mathbf{v}_i{}^T\boldsymbol{\sigma}|$. Thus $|\mathbf{V}^T\boldsymbol{\sigma}|$ shows the contributions of particular eigen-images $\mathbf{v}_i$ to the final reconstructed image, as was illustrated figure 4.8. (Note that to obtain the $|\mathbf{V}^T\boldsymbol{\sigma}|$, the same mesh must be used for the forward and inverse problems, constituting an inverse crime.)

As a side note, the product $\mathbf{S}\mathbf{V}^T\boldsymbol{\sigma}$ can also be found. At small λ, $C_i = P_i/s_i$ [26] since $\mathbf{J}\boldsymbol{\sigma} = \mathbf{U}\mathbf{S}\mathbf{V}^T\boldsymbol{\sigma} = \mathbf{\Delta}$.

Examples of $|\mathbf{V}^T\boldsymbol{\sigma}|$ spectra are shown in figure 4.20 (linear axis) at $\lambda = 10^{-6}$ with increasing noise levels, as well as at $\lambda = 10^{-5}$ at the top noise level. The most significant coefficients C_i are shown as peaks in the plot. (Again, C_i for i above $r = 104$ are due to numerical rounding errors and are near zero.) The corresponding EIT images are shown above the plot, and the contributions of eigen-image $\mathbf{v}_{101}$ are shown in the inset.

Below index $i = 80$, the four spectra were identical. With negligible noise (black line), the larger C_i were of comparable amplitude up to $i = 104$, and the EIT image was a good approximation to the target. With increasing noise, the spectra began to show increasing, unpredictable contributions from the high-index $\mathbf{v}_i$, due to the corruption of the corresponding $\mathbf{u}_i$ (figure 4.19(b)): the $\mathbf{v}_i$ that are sensitive to noise is determined by the amplitude of the corresponding P_i. For example, the amplitude of $\mathbf{v}_{101}$ was virtually zero at $N = 10^{-12}$ V and increased in intensity with N. At $N = 2 \times 10^{-8}$ V (green line) the EIT image developed ringing but still had no artifacts. At $N = 3 \times 10^{-8}$ V, with the incorrect Picard coefficients being even larger, the EIT image developed artifacts. At an even higher noise level, contributions of the high-frequency eigen-images dominated the final image, resulting in a solution that was no longer approximately correct. Raising λ to 10^{-5}, the amplitudes of terms above $i = 87$ were dampened, effectively eliminating those eigen-images from the sum and thereby removing artefacts from the image.

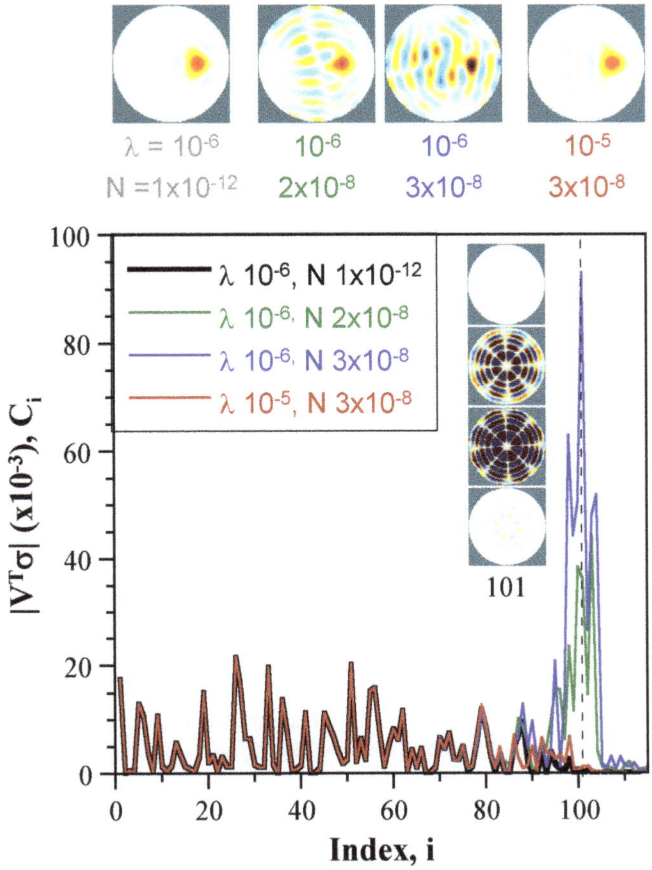

Figure 4.20. The effects of increasing noise and λ on the $\mathbf{V}^{\mathrm{T}}\boldsymbol{\sigma}$ spectrum of a triangular target at $x = 0.5$. The corresponding EIT images are included at the top. Also shown are the $\mathbf{v}_{101}$ for each case, ordered top to bottom in the same way as the legend (16 electrodes, I–M = 7–1, $r_{\mathrm{T}} = 0.2$, $I = 1 \times 10^{-3}\sigma_0 = 10^{-2}$, $\sigma_{\mathrm{T}} = 0.6\sigma_0$, Laplace prior).

As discussed above, regularization results in smoothing because above a certain i, image information, carried by the $\mathbf{v}_i$, is removed. (As phrased in [29], regularization schemes are spectral filtering methods.) Raising λ increases the number of $\mathbf{v}_i$ that are diminished, and the damping effect of λ on the C_i moves from right to left as λ increases. The images are changed in different ways depending on the I–M pattern and the prior, and to different extents depending on target position. For very large hyperparameters, which for the simulation conditions used in this book means $\lambda = 1$, only a handful of low-frequency eigen-images remain and almost all information about the contacts with the sensor is lost (figure 4.12(d)).

Turning to examine the operation of the prior, noise-free $|\mathbf{V}^{\mathrm{T}}\boldsymbol{\sigma}|$ spectra for four regularization methods (section 4.4.1) at comparable levels of regularization, as used in figure 4.16, are illustrated in figure 4.21 for a target at $x = 0.1$. (These spectra have a small number of peaks because they are dominated by the circularly symmetric $\mathbf{v}_i$.) The

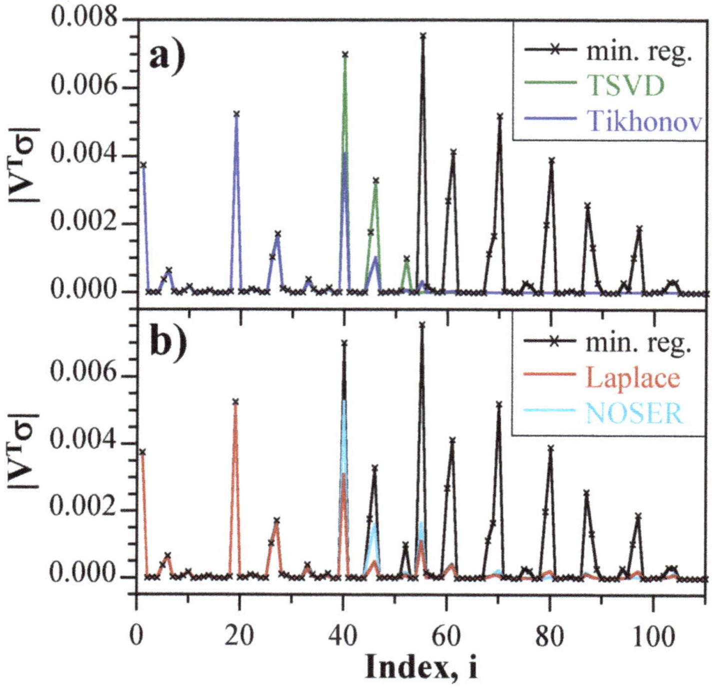

Figure 4.21. The $|\mathbf{V}^{\mathrm{T}}\boldsymbol{\sigma}|$ spectra for a target at $x = 0.1$ obtained using minimal regularization (black line) and (a) the Tikhonov prior ($\lambda = 10^{-2}$) and the TSVD method ($\lambda = 10^{0}$) and (b) and the Laplace and NOSER priors ($\lambda = 10^{-1}$) (16 electrodes, I–M = 7–1, $r_{\mathrm{T}} = 0.2$, $I = 10^{-3}$, $\sigma_0 = 10^{-2}$, $\sigma_{\mathrm{T}} = 0.9\sigma_0$, $N = 10^{-12}$).

un-regularized spectrum is shown in black. The TSVD method (figure 4.21(a), green) simply sets all the C_i above a particular index, here $i = 52$, to zero [41]; below that the terms were equal to those without regularization (the green and black lines in the figure overlap perfectly so that the back line is hidden). TSVD acts as a stepwise low-pass filter on i. The Tikhonov prior (blue) instead reduced the amplitudes gradually, the decrease being visually apparent starting from $i = 40$, where the blue line drops below the green one, and ending with near zero amplitudes at $i = 62$. It behaved as a ramped low-pass filter on i. The Laplace and NOSER priors (figure 4.21(b)), on the other hand, instead penalize different properties of the image damping C_i based on image criteria rather than i. Note how even at high i, some of the amplitudes did not go entirely to zero. Since the four filters have different effects on the C_i, the resulting EIT images better retain different types of information. ($|\mathbf{V}^{\mathrm{T}}\boldsymbol{\sigma}|$ spectra for a range of hyperparameters are shown in appendix D.7.)

4.6.3 Role of the injection–measurement pattern

$|\mathbf{V}^{\mathrm{T}}\boldsymbol{\sigma}|$ spectra also provide insight into differences in performance among I–M patterns, as shown in figure 4.22. At small λ, all full-rank I–M patterns provide virtually identical reconstructions, since a similar number of $\mathbf{v}_i$ are used; differences in performance only arise when regularizing. For a circular target at $x = 0.0$, EIT

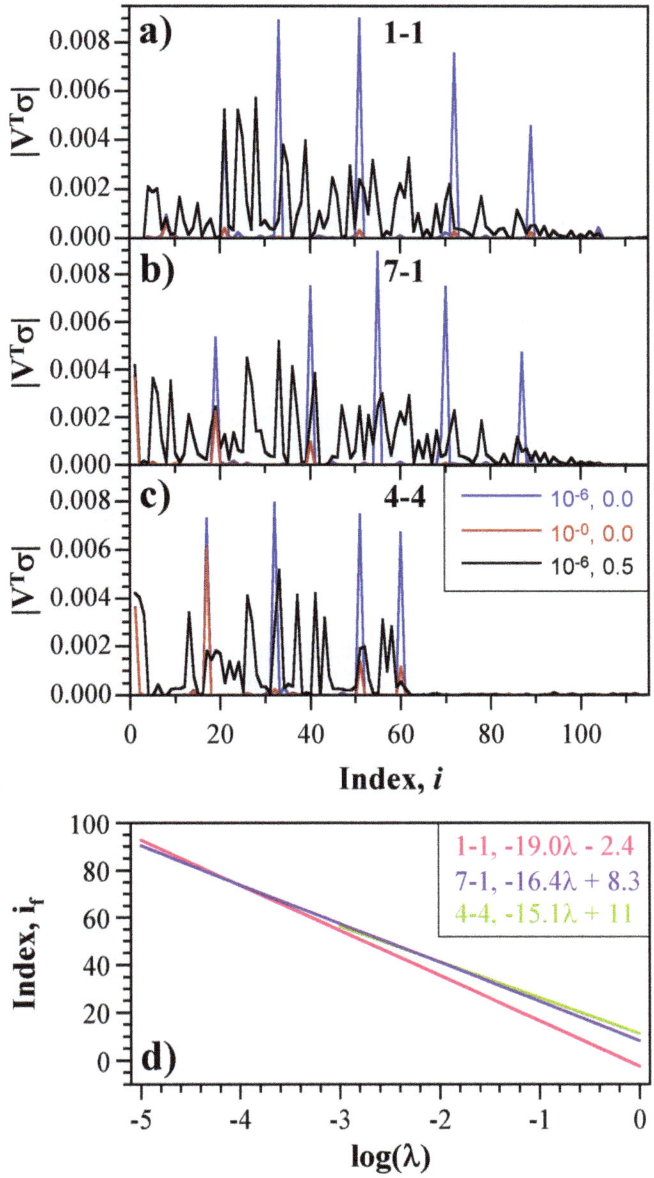

Figure 4.22. The absolute values of $\mathbf{V}^{\mathrm{T}}\boldsymbol{\sigma}$ for a circular target at $x = 0.0$ for $\lambda = 10^{-6}$ (blue) and $\lambda = 10^{0}$ (red) and at $x = 0.5$ for $\lambda = 10^{-6}$ (black) for I–M = (a) 1–1, (b) 7–1, and (c) 4–4. (d) Index i_{f} at which C_i are first damped as a function of λ (Laplace prior) (16 electrodes, $r_{\mathrm{T}} = 0.2$, $I = 10^{-3}$, $\sigma_0 = 10^{-2}$, $\sigma_{\mathrm{T}} = 0.9\sigma_0$, $N = 10^{-12}$).

images made using $\lambda = 10^{-6}$ (blue lines) with full-rank patterns (here 1–1 and 7–1, figures 4.22(a) and (b)) were constructed from six circularly symmetric $\mathbf{v}_i$. The indices i for these $\mathbf{v}_i$ varied with the I–M pattern. Again, more $\mathbf{v}_i$ were needed for a target at $x = 0.5$ (black lines). For lower rank patterns, such as 4–4 (figure 4.22(c)), the spectra terminate at smaller i, so the final EIT images are constructed from fewer

$\mathbf{v}_i$ and suffer from poorer resolution and diminished peak height. The spectra make clear the nature and origin of the deleterious effects of low rank due to symmetry. At $\lambda = 1$ (red lines, overlying the blue ones at small i) the C_i were diminished except at the smallest i. For I–M = 4–4, increasing λ had no effect on the image until λ was large enough to reach $i = 62$.

Looking more closely at the spectrum for I–M = 1–1, its reputation for poor performance compared to other full-rank patterns becomes clear: the $\mathbf{v}_i$ at $i = 1$ and 2 were insignificant for targets away from the perimeter, and the first peak for the target at $x = 0$ was located not at $i = 1$ but at $i = 8$ and was small. Because the lowest index patterns are the largest contributors to an image and the last to be affected by regularization, it is clear that targets at the center of the sensor using 1–1 would suffer more from regularization than with other patterns. This is how the lower sensitivity of 1–1 than 7–1 at the center of the sensor (figure 4.6) manifests itself in the SVD.

The singular value indices i_f can be found at which the larger C_i ($C_i > 2 \times 10^{-4}$) were first lowered by more than 5% from their values at $\lambda = 10^{-6}$, for hyperparameters between 10^{-5} and 10^{0}. The points can be well fit to the form $i = -a\log(\lambda) + b$ as shown in figure 4.22(d) for the circular target at $x = 0.5$ (black curves in figures 4.22(a)–(c)). The fit for 1–1 had a steeper slope than the others, showing a more rapid advance over i with λ; it also had a negative intercept, showing that even C_1 was affected at $\lambda = 1$: the effect of regularization was more severe for 1–1 than other I–M patterns. (The line for 4–4 did not begin until $\lambda = 10^{-3}$.)

To summarize, the I–M pattern affects performance in two ways. The first is symmetry, which plays a role primarily at small hyperparameters. Symmetry results in less information gathered despite an equal number of measurements, shown by a reduced rank r. Symmetry results in missing higher-order $\mathbf{v}_i$, leading to lower-quality reconstructions. (The highest-symmetry patterns also result in mirror image features, not shown here.) For full-rank patterns, at small hyperparameter it makes little difference which I–M is chosen. The second consideration applies at large hyperparameters: low sensitivity at the center of the sensor. This manifests itself in higher indices i of centrally-concentrated modes, so they are attenuated at relatively lower λ, and stronger dampening versus i for a given λ. The examination of the role of I–M pattern continues in sections 5.3, 6.2.1, and 7.2.

4.6.4 Discussion

A critical concept is that the EIT image can be considered to be a sum of eigen-images, with a resolution determined by the number of independent terms in that series whose amplitudes are greater than the noise. High symmetry measurement configurations such as polar have fewer independent terms, and thus inherently lower possible resolution.

To understand the action of the hyperparameter it can thus be helpful to look at $|\mathbf{V}^{\mathrm{T}}\boldsymbol{\sigma}|$ spectra, which are alternative views of the EIT image in the form of fingerprints that show the coefficients C_i of the eigen-images that sum to produce the EIT image. The spectra reveal how the coefficients change with the particular coupling of injection and measurement pairs at different locations on the surface and with target properties. The hyperparameter controls the number of eigen-images contributing to the reconstruction; more specifically, λ controls the amplitudes of those eigen-images, which are systematically reduced in favor of prior information as λ increases. The prior information is typically a uniform background conductivity for a tactile sensor. Therefore, the features broaden and fall.

Since the $|\mathbf{V}^T\boldsymbol{\sigma}|$ spectra reflect the action of the hyperparameter, through the final image $\boldsymbol{\sigma}$, they demonstrate explicitly how smoothing occurs and show the relative rate versus index i at which increases in λ affect the coefficients. The eigen-images corresponding to the highest index singular values, which are associated with the highest spatial frequency information, are removed first. With increasing λ, the number of eigen-images contributing to the EIT image drops as $\log\lambda$. The rule of thumb that regularization removes image components for which the singular values $s_i^2 < \lambda^2$ holds for a broad range of i but finally breaks down at large λ. For large hyperparameters, which for the simulation conditions used in this chapter means $\lambda = 1$, only a handful of low-frequency eigen-images remain. Thus almost all information about the contacts is lost, including the radius. The scheme governing the details of coefficient reduction is determined by the prior that is chosen. While regularization acts broadly as a low-pass filter, where the index i plays the role of frequency, the details depend on the image filtering strategy.

The I–M pattern and the target characteristics determine the original coefficients in the $|\mathbf{V}^T\boldsymbol{\sigma}|$ spectra. For the simulations in this chapter, the coefficients were unaffected below $\lambda = 10^{-6}$. The particulars of which coefficients are large, and thus which associated $\mathbf{v}_i$ make a substantial contribution to the final image, provide insight into the reconstructions. Some I–M patterns yield no appreciable peaks at low index for a given target, while others have a peak immediately at $i = 1$. The former are thus affected at a smaller hyperparameter than the latter. These differences reflect the underlying physics: the current flow through different locations on the sensor depending on the injection pattern. For the same reason the I–M pattern determines the rate at which the hyperparameter advances across the spectrum of eigen-image coefficients. The steepness of that slope and the particular eigen-images contributing to forming the reconstructed feature determine the image metrics.

4.7 Summary and conclusions

While it is possible for experimentalists to use EIT as a 'black box' because of the user-friendliness of EIDORS, it is helpful to understand what the algorithms are doing in order to obtain the most informative images possible under given conditions. This chapter illustrated the basic manipulations and concepts behind the techniques that have been frequently used in tactile imaging without assuming a previous high level of comfort with the mathematical methods.

EIT is attractive for tactile imaging because a relatively detailed image can be created from a comparatively small number of electrodes placed only at the sensor periphery by interrogating those electrodes in multiple combinations, using them at various times for current injection and voltage measurement, as specified by the I–M pattern. The resulting frame of measurements at given time is compared to one from a reference time, yielding a noisy set of small voltage differences $\mathbf{\Delta}$, with many values near zero.

The continuum version of Ohm's law returns the voltage difference between any two points on the periphery, given a current flowing between two other periphery points and a knowledge of the sensor conductivity. The relationship between a conductivity change at a particular interior location and a voltage change at particular perimeter location is approximated in a linearized sensitivity matrix, or Jacobian, $\mathbf{J}$, which depends on the I–M pattern. This mapping is the straightforward 'forward problem'. The 'inverse problem' involves inverting this mapping to find interior conductivity changes from measured perimeter voltage changes, which is more difficult because the matrix $\mathbf{J}$ is 'ill-conditioned' and highly sensitive to noise.

Visualizations of $\mathbf{J}$ show where on the sensor different I–M patterns have high and low sensitivities to conductivity changes. As a result of the perimeter placement of the electrodes, the terms in the sensitivity matrix $\mathbf{J}$ are larger at the perimeter than at the center. So, regardless of the I–M pattern, EIT is most sensitive to conductivity changes near the sensor edges, and regularization affects features in the center to a greater extent. This non-uniformity in the effects of regularization is highly detrimental to tactile images.

One technique for understanding the challenges and choices in EIT is singular value decomposition, which expresses $\mathbf{J}$ in terms of two orthonormal bases $\mathbf{U}$ and $\mathbf{V}$, the former for the measured voltage differences $\mathbf{\Delta}$ (eigen-Δs, $\mathbf{u}_i$) and the latter for the predicted conductivity changes $\boldsymbol{\sigma}$ (eigen-images, $\mathbf{v}_i$). EIT images can be constructed from a sum of the modes $\mathbf{v}_i$, with image fidelity depending on the number of terms in this series. Higher indices i correspond to higher spatial frequency image components. Increasing the number of electrodes increases the number of terms, thereby increasing resolution, whereas high symmetry in the current injection or voltage measurement electrode placements, such as on opposite sides of the sensor, results in fewer terms and thus inherently worse reconstruction performance. Likewise, the measured voltages can be represented as a sum of the $\mathbf{u}_i$. Even small amounts of noise can overwhelm the higher order terms of this series, which is why noise is so detrimental.

Among the reconstruction algorithms, the GN one-step has been the most attractive for tactile imaging because of its speed, even though it has lower resolution compared to iterative algorithms. It employs a regularized inverse of $\mathbf{J}$ that can be pre-calculated, subsequently only requiring matrix multiplication. An examination of this $\mathbf{J}_{\mathbf{reg}}^{-1}$ illustrated how the extent of regularization is controlled by the hyperparameter λ and the manner by the prior. Hyperparameter values must be adjusted if different values of current and sensor conductivity are employed. For a 10× decrease in injected current, a hyperparameter 10× smaller provides the same influence on the EIT image, whereas for a 10× decrease in sensor conductivity, a hyperparameter 100× larger has the same effect. Increases in contrast due to stronger touches or higher GF do not affect the required λ. While regularization stabilizes the reconstruction in the presence of noise, it broadens or defocuses the reconstructed features in a spatially-dependent manner, with the effects varying with the prior. The

Laplace prior, which is the one most commonly employed in tactile imaging, is advantageous from the perspective of uniformity across the sensor area. In particular, it best conserves feature volume, which is related to the strength of a tactile contact. To obtain images of reasonable resolution, to have sensitivity to small and to light touches, and to reduce non-uniformity over the sensor with its resulting distortions and masking, every effort must be made to reduce noise so that a smaller λ can be employed.

There are two sets of coefficients that are helpful to understanding the performance of an EIT system. The spectrum of Picard coefficients $P_i = |\mathbf{u}_i^{\mathbf{T}}\boldsymbol{\Delta}|$, which have units of V, allows comparison of the various signal components for a particular scenario to the noise amplitude N. Only signal components $\mathbf{u}_i$ with $P_i > N$ correspond to image components $\mathbf{v}_i$ that are meaningful. Those $\mathbf{v}_i$ associated with $P_i < N$ must be diminished by an appropriately set λ. The spectrum of coefficients $C_i = |\mathbf{v}_i^{\mathbf{T}}\boldsymbol{\sigma}|$ shows the importance of the various components to the image and how they are affected by regularization. The $\mathbf{v}_i$ with the largest i, which are associated with the highest spatial frequency information, are diminished by λ first. While regularization acts broadly as a low-pass filter on based on i, the details depend on the image filtering strategy, or prior, as well as on the I–M pattern. The rank of the I–M pattern determines the maximum number of $\mathbf{v}_i$, and thus image quality at small λ. The sensitivity of the pattern at the center of the sensor determines how strongly features are defocused there at large λ.

References

[1] Booth M J 2000 Design and development of a distributed planar pressure sensor utilising electrical impedance tomography *PhD Thesis* Sheffield Hallam University

[2] Alirezaei H, Nagakubo A and Kuniyoshi Y 2007 A highly stretchable tactile distribution sensor for smooth surfaced humanoids Humanoids'07: 7th IEEE-RAS Int. Conf. Humanoid Robots *(Pittsburgh, PA, Nov. 29–Dec. 1)* pp 167–73

[3] Nagakubo A, Alirezaei H and Kuniyoshi Y 2007 A deformable and deformation sensitive tactile distribution sensor IEEE Int. Conf. Robot. Biomimetics (ROBIO) *(Sanya, China, Dec. 15–18)* pp 1301–8

[4] Silvera-Tawil D, Rye D, Soleimani M and Velonaki M 2015 Electrical impedance tomography for artificial sensitive robotic skin: a review *IEEE Sens.* J **15** 2001–16

[5] Russo S, Nefti-Meziani S, Carbonaro N and Tognetti A 2017 A quantitative evaluation of drive pattern selection for optimizing EIT-based stretchable sensors *Sensors* **17** ARTN 1999

[6] Adler A, Gaggero P O and Maimaitijiang Y 2011 Adjacent stimulation and measurement patterns considered harmful *Physiol. Meas.* **32** 731–44

[7] Tawil D S, Rye D and Velonaki M 2012 Interpretation of the modality of touch on an artificial arm covered with an EIT-based sensitive skin *Int. J. Robot. Res.* **31** 1627–41

[8] Kaipio J P, Seppänen A, Voutilainen A and Haario H 2007 Optimal current patterns in dynamical electrical impedance tomography imaging *Inverse Prob.* **23** 1201–14

[9] Dickin F and Wang M 1996 Electrical resistance tomography for process applications *Meas. Sci. Technol.* **7** 247–60

[10] Shi X T, Dong X Z, Shuai W J, You F S, Fu F and Liu R G 2006 Pseudo-polar drive patterns for brain electrical impedance tomography *Physiol. Meas.* **27** 1071–80

[11] Bera T K and Nagaraju J 2012 Studying the resistivity imaging of chicken tissue phantoms with different current patterns in Electrical Impedance Tomography (EIT) *Measurement* **45** 663–82

[12] Visentin F, Fiorini P and Suzuki K 2016 A deformable smart skin for continuous sensing based on electrical impedance tomography *Sensors* **16** ARTN 1928

[13] Schuessler T F and Bates J H T 1998 Current patterns and electrode types for single-source electrical impedance tomography of the thorax *Ann. Biomed. Eng.* **26** 253–9

[14] Russo S, Nefti-Meziani S, Carbonaro N and Tognetti A 2017 Development of a high-speed current injection and voltage measurement system for electrical impedance tomography-based stretchable sensors *Technologies* **5** 48

[15] Nankani A 2019 EIT based piezoresistive tactile sensors: a simulation study *MS Thesis* Department of Mechanical Engineering, University of Maryland, Digital Repository at the University of Maryland (DRUM)

[16] McDonald K T 2000 *Physics Examples and Other Pedagogic Diversions: Resistance of a Disk* (Princeton University)

[17] Kauppinen P, Hyttinen J and Malmivuo J 2006 Sensitivity distribution visualizations of impedance tomography measurement strategies *Int. J. Bioelectromag* **8** 63–71

[18] Chen Y 2018 Tactile sensing with compliant structures for human-robot interaction *PhD Thesis* (Department of Mechanical Engineering, University of Maryland)

[19] Holder D S 2005 Introduction to biomedical electrical impedance tomography *Electrical Impedance Tomography: Methods, History and Applications, Series in Medical Physics and Biomedical Engineering* ed C G Orton, J H Nagel and J G Webster (Bristol: IOP Publishing) appendix B

[20] Lionheart W, Polydorides N and Borsic A 2005 The reconstruction problem *Electrical Impedance Tomography: Methods, History and Applications, Series in Medical Physics and Biomedical Engineering* ed C G Orton, J H Nagel and J G Webster (Bristol: IOP Publishing) ch 1

[21] Polydorides N and Lionheart W R B 2002 A Matlab toolkit for three-dimensional electrical impedance tomography: a contribution to the Electrical Impedance and Diffuse Optical Reconstruction Software project *Meas. Sci. Technol.* **13** 1871–83

[22] Tehrani J N, McEwan A, Jin C and van Schaik A 2012 L1 regularization method in electrical impedance tomography by using the L1-curve (Pareto frontier curve) *Appl. Math. Model.* **36** 1095–105

[23] Wang M, Wang Q and Karki B 2016 Arts of electrical impedance tomographic sensing *Philosoph. Trans.* A **374** 20150329

[24] Adler A and Guardo R 1994 A neural network image reconstruction technique for electrical impedance tomography *IEEE Trans. Med. Imag* **13** 594–600

[25] Zadehkoochak M, Blott B H, Hames T K and George R F 1991 Spectral expansion analysis in electrical-impedance tomography *J. Phys.* D **24** 1911–6

[26] Hansen P C 2010 *Discrete Inverse Problems: Insight and Algorithms, Fundamentals of Algorithms* (Philadelphia, PA: Society for Industrial and Applied Mathematics (SIAM))

[27] Bagheri R 2020 Understanding singular value decomposition and its application in data science *TDS Towards Data Science* https://towardsdatascience.com/understanding-singular-value-decomposition-and-its-application-in-data-science-388a54be95d#:~:text=In%20linear%20algebra%2C%20the%20Singular,important%20applications%20in%20data%20science

[28] Strang G 2018 6. Singular value decomposition (SVD) *MIT 18.065 Matrix Methods in Data Analysis, Signal Processing, and Machine Learning* https://www.youtube.com/watch?v=rYz83XPxiZo

[29] Hansen P C 2010 Computational aspects: regularization methods *Discrete Inverse Problems: Insight and Algorithms* ed N J Higham (Philadelphia, PA: Society for Industrial and Applied Mathematics (SIAM)) ch 4

[30] Gaggero P O 2011 Miniaturization and distinguishability limits of electrical impedance tomography for biomedical application *PhD Thesis* Nanomedecine Division, Centre Suisse d'Electronique et de Microtechnique (CSEM), University of Neuchâtel Landquart, Switzerland

[31] Tang M X, Wang W, Wheeler J, McCormick M and Dong X Z 2002 The number of electrodes and basis functions in EIT image reconstruction *Physiol. Meas.* **23** 129–40

[32] Hansen P C 2010 Fundamentals of algorithms *DIAS 006—Discrete Inverse Problems—Day 1, slides based on Discrete Inverse Problems: Insight and Algorithms* (Philadelphia, PA: Society for Industrial and Applied Mathematics (SIAM)) vol 2020

[33] Barber D C 2005 EIT: the view from Sheffield *Electrical Impedance Tomography: Methods, History and Applications of the Series Series in Medical Physics and Biomedical Engineering* ed C G Orton, J H Nagel and J G Webster (Bristol: Institute of Physics Publishing) ch 11

[34] Vauhkonen M, Vadasz D, Karjalainen P A, Somersalo E and Kaipio J P 1998 Tikhonov regularization and prior information in electrical impedance tomography *IEEE Trans. Med. Imag* **17** 285–93

[35] Adler A, Dai T and Lionheart W R B 2007 Temporal image reconstruction in electrical impedance tomography *Physiol. Meas.* **28** S1–S11

[36] Dai T 2008 Image reconstruction in EIT using advanced regularization frameworks *PhD Thesis* Department of Systems and Computer Engineering, Carleton University

[37] Islam M R and Kiber M A 2014 Electrical impedance tomography imaging using Gauss–Newton algorithm Int. Conf. Informatics, Electronics & Vision (ICIEV) *(Dhaka, Bangladesh, 23–24 May)* pp 1–4

[38] Ranade N V and Gharpure D C 2019 Enhancing sharp features by locally relaxing regularization for reconstructed images in electrical impedance tomography *J. Electr. Bioimp* **10** 2–13

[39] Sarode V, Patkar S and Cheeran A N 2013 Comparison of 2-D algorithms in EIT based image reconstruction *Int. J. Comput. Appl* **69** 6–11

[40] Adler A and Guardo R 1996 Electrical impedance tomography: regularized imaging and contrast detection *IEEE Trans. Med. Imag* **15** 170–9

[41] Hansen P C 1987 The truncated SVD as a method for regularization *BIT* **27** 534–53

[42] Lionheart W R B 2004 EIT reconstruction algorithms: pitfalls, challenges, and recent developments *Physiol. Meas.* **25** 125–42

[43] Grychtol B, Elke G, Meybohm P, Weiler N, Frerichs I and Adler A 2014 Functional validation and comparison framework for EIT lung imaging *PLoS One* **9**

[44] Hamilton S J, Lionheart R B and Adler A 2019 Comparing D-bar and common regularization-based methods for electrical impedance tomography *Physiol. Meas.* **40** ARTN 044004

[45] Elsanadedy A 2012 Application of Electrical Impedance Tomography to Robotic Tactile Sensing *MS Thesis* Mechanical Engineering, Carleton University, Ottawa

[46] Dai T and Adler A 2008 Electrical impedance tomography reconstruction using L1 norms for data and image terms 30th Annual Int. Conf. IEEE Eng. in Medicine and Biology Soc 1–8 2721–4

[47] Adler A and Boyle A 2017 Electrical impedance tomography: tissue properties to image measures *IEEE Trans. Biomed. Eng.* **64** 2494–504

[48] Widodo A and Endarko 2018 Experimental study of one step linear Gauss–Newton algorithm for improving the quality of image reconstruction in high-speed electrical impedance tomography (EIT) *J. Phys.: Conf. Ser.* **1120** 012067

[49] Graham B M and Adler A 2006 Objective selection of hyperparameter for EIT *Physiol. Meas.* **27** S65–79

[50] Braun F, Proença M, Solà J, Thiran J-P and Adler A 2017 A versatile noise performance metric for electrical impedance tomography algorithms *IEEE Trans. Biomed. Eng.* **64** 2321–30

[51] Saulnier G J 2005 EIT instrumentation *Electrical Impedance Tomography: Methods, History and Applications, Series in Medical Physics and Biomedical Engineering* ed C G Orton, J H Nagel and J G Webster (Bristol: IOP Publishing) ch 2

[52] Sauerbrunn E, Chen Y, Didion J, Yu M, Smela E and Bruck H A 2015 Thermal imaging using polymer nanocomposite temperature sensors *EIT Phys. Stat. Sol.* A **212** 2239–45

[53] Tawil D S 2012 Artificial skin and the interpretation of touch in human-robot interaction *PhD Thesis* School of Aerospace, Mechanical and Mechatronic Engineering, University of Sydney

[54] Zhou Z, Malone E, dos Santos G S, Li N, Xu H and Holder D 2015 Comparison of different quadratic regularization for electrical impedance tomography 6th Eur. Conf. Int. Fed. Medical and Biological Engineering (MBEC 2014) IFMBEvol 45 *(Dubrovnik, Sept. 7–11)*I Lacković and D Vasic pp 200–3

[55] Cheney M, lsaacson D, Newell J C, Simske S and Goble J 1991 NOSER: An algorithm for solving the inverse conductivity problem *Int. J. Imag. Syst. Technol.* **2** 66–75

[56] Adler A *et al* 2009 GREIT: a unified approach to 2D linear EIT reconstruction of lung images *Physiol. Meas.* **30** S35–55

[57] Zhang l, Wang H and Zhang L 2010 Single source current drive patterns for electrical impedance tomography IEEE Instrumentation & Measurement Technology Conf. Proc. *(Austin, TX, 3–6 May)* pp 1477–80

[58] Correia T, Gibson A, Schweiger M and Hebden J 2009 Selection of regularization parameter for optical topography *J. Biomed. Opt.* **14** 034044

[59] Hansen P C 1990 The discrete Picard condition for discrete ill-posed problems *BIT Numer. Math* **30** 658–72

[60] Strang G 2015 7.4 Laplace Equation, MIT OCW RES.18-009 Learn Differential Equations: Up Close with Gilbert Strang and Cleve Moler https://www.youtube.com/watch?v=-D4GDdxJrpg

[61] Adler A 2017 Sensitivity of EIT and reconstruction - sensitivity of EIT in 2D https://eidors3d.sourceforge.net/tutorial/EIDORS_basics/sensitivity_map.shtml

[62] Kauppinen P, Hyttinen J and Malmivuo J 2006 Sensitivity distribution visualizations of impedance tomography measurement strategies *Int. J. Bioelectromag.* **8** 63–71

Chapter 5

Effects of the hyperparameter

Regularization is used to allow the creation of an approximate electrical impedance tomography (EIT) image in the presence of noise, but it comes at a cost to resolution and amplitude, and, arguably more importantly, these effects have strong spatial non-uniformity. Our motivating question in this chapter is, how does the hyperparameter, which controls the extent of regularization, affect tactile images? A small value of noise is utilized to isolate the effects of regularization from the effects of noise, since the two are intimately related and therefore often confounded. The distortions to EIT images are quantitatively examined, from the point of view of tactile imaging, as the hyperparameter λ is increased. The effects of regularization are first addressed by examining several image metrics for one injection–measurement (I–M) pattern in order to show which image characteristics are affected, where, and by how much. Using a reduced set of metrics, the study is then expanded to a small set of additional I–M patterns to probe the generality of these findings. The roles of the number of electrodes and target characteristics are then taken up, to deepen understanding of the effects of regularization on tactile imaging. Finally, we address the question of how the hyperparameter can be chosen for tactile imaging applications. These studies are done through simulations employing the Gauss–Newton 1-step algorithm implemented in EIDORS; simulations allow the exploration of a large number of configurations. The performance metrics of most interest are, in order, the absence of artefacts, uniformity of performance over the sensor area; amplitude, resolution, and feature volume; and position error. Image spectra $|\mathbf{V}^{\mathrm{T}}\boldsymbol{\sigma}|$ are employed to provide insight and to understand differences in performance at small and large hyperparameters: the rate at which $|\mathbf{V}^{\mathrm{T}}\boldsymbol{\sigma}|$ coefficients are diminished as a function of hyperparameter is shown. The priors affect the EIT images in different ways, with the Laplace prior being favorable for tactile imaging based on four key metrics. Next the dependence of key metrics on λ and on the position of a tactile contact, or target, are determined, and the relationship between

doi:10.1088/978-0-7503-5402-8ch5

loss of amplitude and coarsening of resolution is shown. The impact of the I–M pattern is then discussed with respect to the properties of the sensitivity matrix. In addition, the dependence of performance metrics on the number of electrodes is quantified, showing that practitioners should consider reducing the number of electrodes from the usual 16. lastly, the effects of the hyperparameter depend strongly on target size as well as on the number and positions of the targets, which has not previously been examined.

5.1 Qualitative effects of regularization

A central topic of EIT is regularization, which enables imaging in the inevitable presence of noise. As discussed in chapter 4, regularization is essentially a smoothing or filtering operation applied during image reconstruction. The amount of regularization, controlled by the hyperparameter λ, must be raised as noise increases. Even surprisingly, small amounts of noise may require a fairly large λ for successful image reconstruction, leading to extensive distortion as shown below. (Noise is examined in chapter 6.) Regularization coarsens resolution and lowers peak amplitudes because it removes not only the high-frequency noise but also the high-frequency image features. The effects of regularization are spatially dependent, being most pronounced at the center of the sensed area, which can be an even more serious problem.

The effect of the hyperparameter were first introduced in section 4.4.3. While the extensive mathematical discussions of EIT methods have proven to be an obstacle for some experimentalist newcomers, the open-source code for performing EIT, EIDORS [1–3], is user-friendly and thus presents little barrier for beginners. The code can, as a consequence, be used as a black box. It is therefore not unusual for the tactile imaging literature to omit the reconstruction conditions, since the focus of that work is on the sensor materials or new applications (chapter 2). This chapter takes a look under the hood, so to speak, using simulations to review the role and closely examine the effects of the hyperparameter.

Since the EIT images and effects of regularization are strongly algorithm-dependent, it is necessary to be specific: this work employed difference EIT, the Gauss–Newton (GN) 1-step algorithm, and Tikhonov regularization employing the Laplace prior, which is the default in EIDORS and are thus used by many in the tactile imaging community. General conclusions made here refer only to this reconstruction method, and results will differ somewhat for other algorithms and priors (see section 4.5). It is nevertheless helpful to understand the consequences of increasing the hyperparameter for this particular case, since it is so frequently employed.

A substantial body of prior work has focused on choosing an appropriate hyperparameter, λ (see for example [4–7]); that topic is not covered here. Section 7.1 examines the relationship between the amount of tolerable noise and λ. The issues of image break-up—due to noise—and image metrics—such as resolution—are related, but not identical. *Therefore, in this chapter low noise is used to permit isolation of the effects of λ alone.*

Table 5.1. Simulation parameters for the baseline case in this chapter.

Forward Model Parameter	**Symbol**	**Value**	**Target Parameter**	**Symbol**	**Value**
# electrodes	$N_{electrodes}$	16	# targets	—	1
injection–measurement pattern	I–M	7–1	target position	x	varies
				y	0.0
injected current	I	1×1^{-3}	target size	r_T	0.2
noise	N	1×10^{-12}	target shape	—	circle
sensor conductivity	σ_0	1×10^{-2}	target conductivity	σ_T	$0.9\ \sigma_0$ (contrast = −10%)

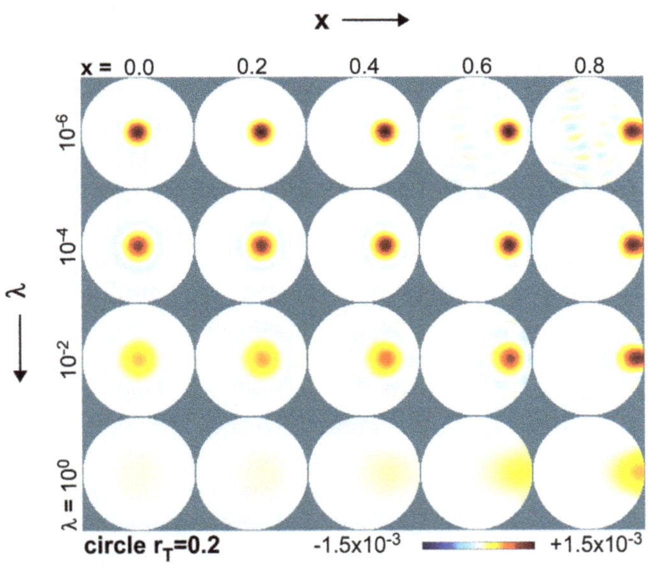

Figure 5.1. EIT images of a circular target of $r_T = 0.2$ at different x-positions for increasing values of the hyperparameter λ. Decreases in conductivity are shown as red, increases in conductivity as blue, reversed from the convention used in medical imaging. (16 electrodes, I–M = 7–1, $I = 10^{-3}$, $\sigma_0 = 10^{-2}$, $\sigma_T = 0.9\sigma_0$, $N = 10^{-12}$) ($\lambda_s = 10^{-7}$ to 10^{-1})

Simulation parameters are summarized in table 5.1 for the base case used in this chapter, around which variations were made.

5.1.1 Overview

Figure 5.1 shows the target at different x-positions for a circular target for a range of hyperparameters. Since the effects of the hyperparameter are substantially circularly symmetric [8–10], only x was varied. The smallest hyperparameter that yielded consistent successful reconstructions was $\lambda = 10^{-6}$, at which the reconstructed feature showed no qualitative dependence on position, although ringing increased as the target approached the perimeter. Increasing λ to 10^{-4} produced some blurring at the center. By $\lambda = 10^{-2}$ the reconstruction was strongly affected at the center of the sensor, with the reconstructed feature notably decreasing in amplitude and becoming broader. The feature was less affected at the perimeter because the terms used to build the center of the image are more heavily weighted by λ, as further discussed below. The physical reason for defocusing at the center is the smaller change in perimeter voltages caused by changes in conductivity at the center of the sensor, which is reflected in the sensitivity matrix, or Jacobian **J**, from the forward problem This spatial non-uniformity of resolution in reconstructions is typical of regularized linear methods; there are other methods that are more spatially uniform [11].

Cross-sections along the x-axis display the reconstructed feature's amplitudes and widths in the radial direction (again of value because the system is substantially circularly symmetric). Figure 5.2 shows, for two I–M patterns, the dependence on λ for a target at $x = 0$ (red curves), where the effect of λ is greatest, as well as the dependence on x for a fixed $\lambda = 10^{-2}$ (blue curves). The blue curves illustrate how much more, even for a medium level of regularization, features at the center are broadened ('defocused') compared to those closer to the edge: the peak amplitude at the center was half what it was at $x = 0.7$ when using I–M = 7–1 (figure 5.2a). The spatial dependence differed using another I–M pattern: for 3–3 (figure 5.2b) the height was level between $x = 0.0$ and 0.3, at two thirds of its height at $x = 0.7$. The red curves illustrate that at small hyperparameters the amplitudes were the same for the two I–M patterns, and that they were the same at the center and the edge. However, with increasing λ the feature defocused to such a degree that by $\lambda = 10^0$ the reconstructed feature filled much of the sensor area. These curves show how the hyperparameter controls the blur radius $R_{\text{blur}}(x,\lambda)$, and how that is spatially dependent. (Note that the shapes of the cross-sections resemble the intensity from a single slit diffraction, or Airy disk, and they can be well fit by that model; the upper halves of the peaks can be well approximated as Gaussians.)

As discussed in section 4.4.4 regarding the numerical values of λ, the regularization strength for a given system depends on the injected current and the sensor background conductivity: it scales linearly with current but as the inverse square of the conductivity. For a 10x decrease in injected current I, a hyperparameter 10x smaller is required to provide the same influence on the EIT image, as illustrated by the cross-sections in figure 4.14 (see also appendix E.1). For a decrease in sensor conductivity σ_0 of 10x (an increase in resistivity of 10x), a hyperparameter 100x larger has the same effect on the feature width (see appendix E.2). Thus, we can consider the values of λ to be per $(\text{S/cm})^2/\text{A}$. For example, for $\lambda = 10^{-2}$, if I and σ_0 are both raised by 10x, the equivalent λ becomes $10^{-2}*10/100 = 10^{-3}$. (A difference in the relative conductivity of the target, $\Delta\sigma_T$, reduces the peak height by 10x but leaves the peak width unchanged. Target amplitude impacts the signal to noise ratio but not the scaling.) We can employ a scaled hyperparameter as in chapter 4, equation (4.13), $\lambda_s = \lambda\sigma_0^2/I$, to allow comparisons across different settings.

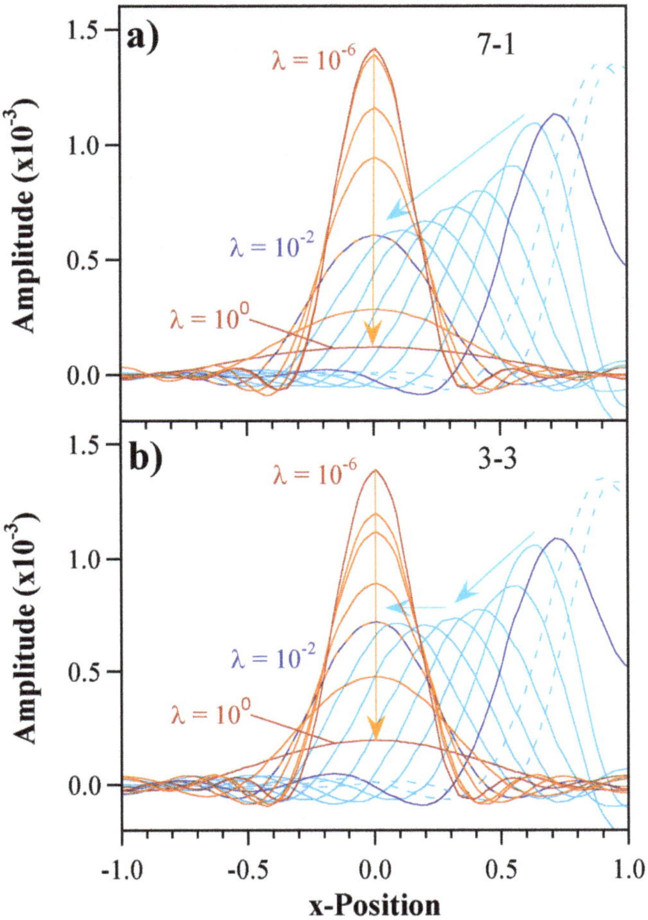

Figure 5.2. Cross-sections at $y = 0$ showing the dependence of the reconstruction on λ for a circular target at $x = 0$ (red and orange lines, λ decreasing by a factor of 10 with each line) and the dependence on target position at $\lambda = 10^{-2}$ (blue lines) ($\lambda_s = 10^{-3}$) for (a) I–M = 7–1 and (b) 3–3. Dashed lines indicate positions at which the target touched or extended beyond the perimeter, $x = 0.8$ and 0.9. (16 electrodes, $r_T = 0.2$, $I = 10^{-3}$, $\sigma_0 = 10^{-2}$, $\sigma_T = 0.9\sigma_0$, $N = 10^{-12}$)

5.1.2 $|\mathbf{V}^T\boldsymbol{\sigma}|$ spectra

To illustrate the workings of the hyperparameter, it is helpful to examine the product $\mathbf{V}^T\boldsymbol{\sigma}$, where $\boldsymbol{\sigma}$ is the image vector. Chapter 4 reviewed the singular value decomposition (SVD) of the sensitivity matrix, or Jacobian **J**, into $\mathbf{J} = \mathbf{USV}^T$, where **S** is a diagonal matrix of singular values $s_i = \mathbf{S}_{ii}$ and i is the singular value index. **J** can be expressed as the sum of r matrices $s_i\mathbf{u}_i\mathbf{v}_i^T$, where r is the rank of **J**, and $\mathbf{u}_i$ and $\mathbf{v}_i$ are orthonormal bases ($\mathbf{U}^T\mathbf{U} = \mathbf{I}$, $\mathbf{V}^T\mathbf{V} = \mathbf{I}$, where **I** is the identity matrix). The s_i couple the two bases and are sorted from largest to smallest. The $\mathbf{v}_i$ are eigen-images that are summed to form the EIT image; the coefficients C_i associated with the $\mathbf{v}_i$ used in that sum are given by $\mathbf{V}^T\boldsymbol{\sigma}$ [12], in which the $\mathbf{v}_i$ are each multiplied by the image.

Another way to conceptualize this explanation is that the feature is constructed from a series of basis functions, which for a circular sensor have the appearance of drumhead modes (see figure 4.8). (Note that it is necessary to use the same mesh for the forward and inverse problems to obtain this product.)

The absolute values of $\mathbf{V}^T\boldsymbol{\sigma}$ for a circular target at $x = 0.5$ for I–M = 7–1 are shown in figure 5.3(a) at four values of λ, ordered by the index i. Also shown are several of the $\mathbf{v}_i$ that contribute to the final image. These spectra serve as a fingerprint of the reconstructed image and are the translation of the underlying physics into the mathematical representation used in the reconstruction, including

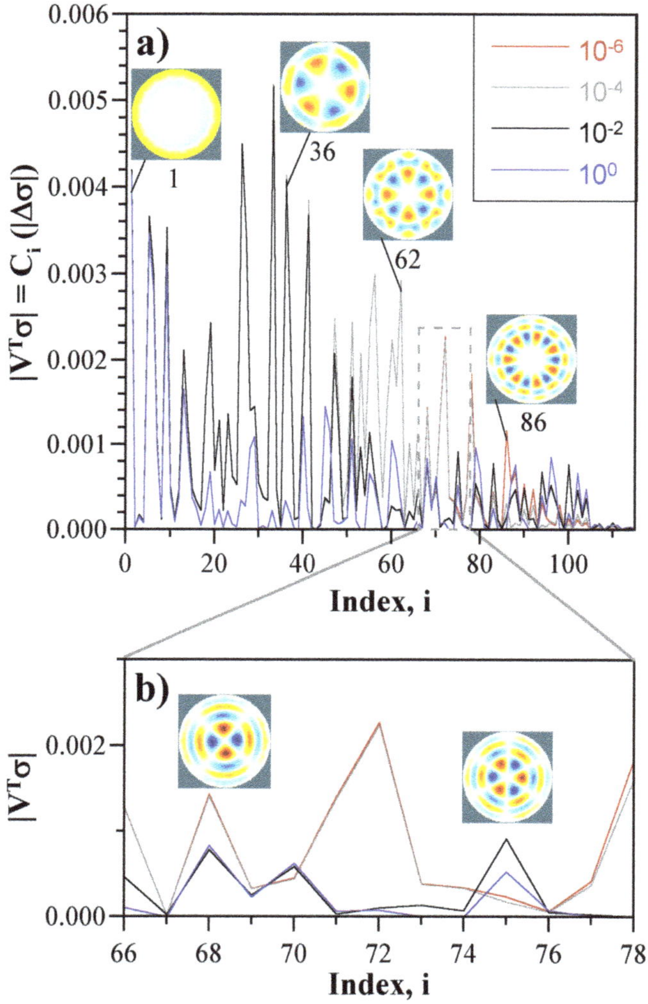

Figure 5.3. (a) The absolute values of $\mathbf{V}^T\boldsymbol{\sigma}$ at increasing values of λ for a circular target at $x = 0.5$. Where two spectra coincide only the uppermost, belonging to the largest λ, is visible (e.g. since the spectrum at 10^{-6} (red) is bottom-most, it is not visible below $i = 70$, where the overlying spectrum at 10^{-4} (gray) is coincident). Several $\mathbf{v}_i$ are shown for illustration (colorbar ±0.01). (b) A close-up of the fingerprint spectrum in (a). (16 electrodes, I–M = 7–1, $r_T = 0.2$, $I = 10^{-3}$, $\sigma_0 = 10^{-2}$, $\sigma_T = 0.9\sigma_0$, $N = 10^{-12}$)

the regularization. The spectra reflect the sensitivity at the electrodes (without considering sign) to conductivity differences at various positions on the sensor. For a given target, the $\mathbf{v}_i$ change for different I–M patterns because of the differing dot products between injection and measurement fields, which are highest when the fields are parallel [13]. For a given I–M pattern the $|\mathbf{V}^T\boldsymbol{\sigma}|$ spectrum changes with the target. Looking at the spectra provides insight. For example, if the C_i at small i are large, then conductivity changes are easy to detect [12].

For $i > 104$ (the rank of $\mathbf{J}$ for this system), the $|\mathbf{V}^T\boldsymbol{\sigma}|$ coefficients C_i are negligible; they are only nonzero due to rounding errors in solving the inverse problem. For $i \leqslant 104$, the spectra for $\lambda = 10^{-6}$ (red) and 10^{-4} (gray) coincided until approximately $i = 77$; for larger i, the C_i for $\lambda = 10^{-4}$ were reduced. (Since the gray line overlies the red one, the latter becomes visible above $i = 77$.) Thus, eigen-image $\mathbf{v}_{86}$, which played a significant role in the image at $\lambda = 10^{-6}$ (red peak) did so no longer. The spectrum for $\lambda = 10^{-2}$ (black) diverged sooner, starting near $i = 50$. Thus, $\mathbf{v}_{62}$, which still contributed at $\lambda = 10^{-4}$, contributed far less at $\lambda = 10^{-2}$. The spectrum for $\lambda = 10^0$ (blue) was diminished starting at even smaller i, so the EIT image did not have a contribution from $\mathbf{v}_{36}$. All spectra had strong contributions from $\mathbf{v}_1$. Note that the spatial frequency of the eigen-images generally increases with i [14], consistent with the loss of detail, or coarser resolution, with increasing λ in figure 5.1. (A demonstration of the loss of image resolution with solution components was given in [15] using a hollow-circle target.)

Thus, the hyperparameter behaves analogously to a low-pass filter with the index i playing the role of frequency. However, the overall trend of spatial frequency increasing with i did not hold strictly true. Furthermore, while there was an overall downward trend of the C_i with increasing i, there were variations in the diminution, as shown in the close-up in figure 5.3b. For example, while the amplitude of $\mathbf{v}_{68}$ dropped monotonically with λ, the amplitude of $\mathbf{v}_{75}$ instead increased. Other examples can be seen in figure 5.3(a), such as the amplitude increase of $\mathbf{v}_{60}$ for $\lambda = 10^{-2}$ compared to $\lambda = 10^0$. These variations occur because this reconstruction employed the Laplace prior, which reduces the amplitudes of the $\mathbf{v}_i$ using a weighting scheme, as discussed in section 5.1.4.

5.1.3 Diminution of $|\mathbf{V}^T\boldsymbol{\sigma}|$ peaks and singular values

Tikhonov regularization is described as filtering out components for which $s_i^2 < \lambda^2$ [15] or, alternatively, as damping the eigen-images $\mathbf{v}_i$ by $s_i^2/(s_i^2+\lambda^2)$ [14]. The singular values s_i are shown as a function of index i in figure 5.4 (× symbols) for I–M = 7–1 and 3–3. (This plot is another way of displaying information in the sensitivity maps that were shown in figure 4.6. For 7–1, the s_i were previously plotted in figure 4.9.) As has been explained previously, the s_i decrease with i. Over most of the range, log (s_i) dropped linearly with i, but for small i, $i < 24$, they fell less rapidly with index. Also, at small index, $i < 15$, the s_i were higher for 3–3 than for 7–1. The result is consistent with the smaller amount of regularization at large λ shown in the cross-sections of figure 5.2(b) compared to figure 5.2(a).

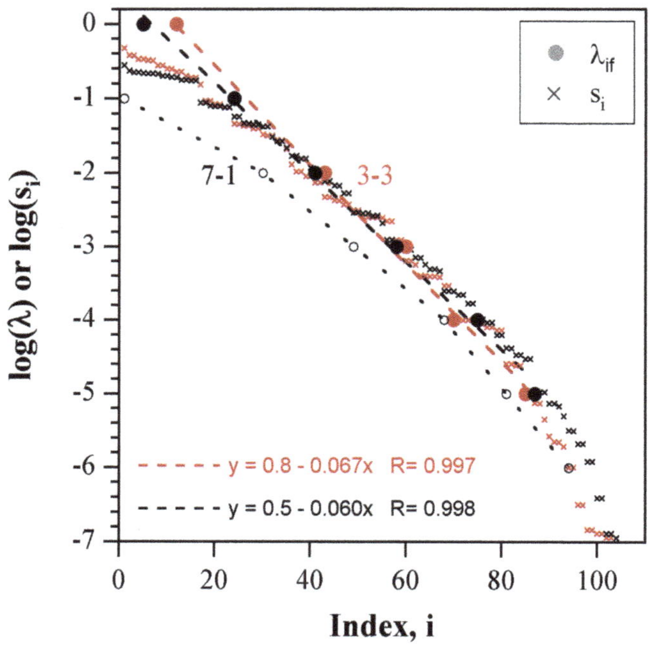

Figure 5.4. $\log(s_i)$ as a function of index i (× symbols) for I–M = 7–1 (black) and 3–3 (red), and $\log(\lambda)$ as a function of i_f (large filled circles) for a circular target at $x = 0.5$. Also shown is $\log(\lambda)$ as a function of i_f obtained from $s_i^2/(s_i^2+\lambda^2)$ at various λ for I–M = 7–1(open circles). (16 electrodes, $r_T = 0.2$, $I = 10^{-3}$, $\sigma_0 = 10^{-2}$, $\sigma_T = 0.6\sigma_0$, $N = 10^{-12}$)

Also shown in figure 5.4 (large filled circles) are the indices i_f at various λ of a circular target at $x = 0.5$. At i_f the most significant $\mathbf{v}_i$ were first lowered by more than 5% relative to their values at $\lambda = 10^{-6}$, where the most significant contributors to the final image were defined as those having $C_i > 2 \times 10^{-4}$. The i_f are a measure of the 'reach' of λ toward lower-index eigen-images: the smaller the i_f at a given value of λ, the greater the effect of λ on the image. For hyperparameters between 10^{-5} and 10^0 the relationship between $\log(\lambda)$ and i_f was linear. This relationship allows one to estimate the number of coefficients C_i affected at a given λ. *This relationship did not depend on target position or shape, but it did depend on I–M.* For this target, the slope was steeper and the intercept larger for I–M = 3–3 than for 7–1, again showing that at large λ, 3–3 experienced less defocusing.

Comparing $\log(\lambda)$ at i_f with $\log(s_i)$, the two sets of curves overlay each other between $\lambda = 10^{-1}$ and $\lambda = 10^{-5}$. For larger λ, however, the 'reach' of the regularization was reduced below that expected from the filtering relationship $s_i^2 < \lambda^2$. The damping was less than expected. For example, for 7–1 at $\log(\lambda) = 0$, $\mathbf{v}_1$ was unaffected (remaining at 99% of its amplitude at $\lambda = 10^{-6}$), despite the singular values being considerably smaller than λ there.

Finally, figure 5.4 (small open circles) shows the indices at which $s_i^2/(s_i^2+\lambda^2)$ was reduced by more than 5% for different values of λ for 7–1; this expression is the filter factor for Tikhonov regularization [16]. This curve showed an even stronger damping (leftward shift) than the actual C_i from the simulations did. In these simulations, there was instead a linear relationship between the index i_f at which damping started to occur and $\log(\lambda)$. Thus, the filter factors do not tell the entire story.

5.1.4 Discussion

For experiments with high noise, it is not uncommon to require a large λ [17], which can result in substantial distortion of the touch signal. It is thus essential to reduce noise as much as possible when using EIT so that λ can be kept to values small enough to allow reasonably accurate visualization of tactile input, the required accuracy depending on the application.

5.2 Quantitative effects of the hyperparameter

Some relationships between various performance metrics and λ have been described previously, but a comprehensive discussion for tactile imaging has been missing, and often the effects of regularization have been comingled with the effects of noise. By separating the effects of the problem—noise—from the cure—regularization—this chapter explicitly and quantitatively shows the damage wrought by increasing the amplitude of the cure, completely aside from problems in the image caused by noise, focusing on scenarios that may be encountered in tactile imaging. We illustrate that the energy of reconstructed features is conserved while the amplitude of the features drops as $\log(\lambda)$ and the resolution coarsens as $1/|\log(\lambda)|^{1/2}$.

As pointed out in [18], even if an EIT image is not faithful, it can still be useful. A better understanding of how reconstructions differ from faithfulness can help experimentalists to determine the usefulness of the information the images provide and to make tradeoffs in their system to balance that with the costs of noise rejection [19]. We examine how λ affects the reconstructed images depending on various target properties and measurement conditions, where *target* refers to the input contrasts, or spatial pattern of conductivity change. Section 5.3 examines how the generality of these effects with regard to various current injection and voltage measurement patterns. Sections 5.4 and 5.5 explore the question, how does the effect of regularization change with the number of electrodes and with the size and position of conductivity changes?

As discussed previously, tactile imaging applications seek the number, locations, and strengths of touches, but the hyperparameter λ results in undesirable spatial dependences in the reconstructions. To quantify the effects on EIT images, metrics were obtained as functions of both λ and radial position for a circular target; positions were varied along x, since prior simulations have shown symmetry up to distances of $x = 0.7$ for a target of radius of 0.2 [10]. Since most metrics have been developed for a circular target, results for a 1-circle target of $r_T = 0.2$ are presented first. While this has been the most usual target employed in simulations, it is also particularly relevant for finger-touches on tactile sensors of 10–20 cm diameter (chapter 2, section 2.6.1.4). The primary I–M pattern used in this section is I–M = 7–1; for comparison I–M = 3–3 is also examined in some cases. (All the bipolar I–M patterns are compared in section 7.2.)

5.2.1 Size metrics

Figure 5.5 shows four metrics relating to the size of the reconstructed feature, allowing one to see relationships between height, peak width, and total volume. Beyond $x = 0.8$, indicated by the gray shading, the target extended beyond the perimeter.

Amplitude is linked to detectability in the presence of noise. For small λ, the peak amplitude of the reconstructed feature was greater than that of the target (figure 5.5(a)), as expected from figure 3.2(b,c). The amplitude error (figure 5.5(b)), obtained from the average amplitude of the half-amplitude set, was actually somewhat negative even for small λ, also as would be expected from figure 3.2(b,c): the amplitude error depends on the threshold f, and for half-maximum the sum of amplitudes is slightly smaller than that of the cylindrical target. The peak and average amplitude tracked each other closely until $x \geqslant 0.8$. It is clear from figure 5.5(a,b) that to achieve the most uniform response to a tactile signal, the hyperparameter must be kept as small as possible. For $\lambda = 10^{-1}$, the

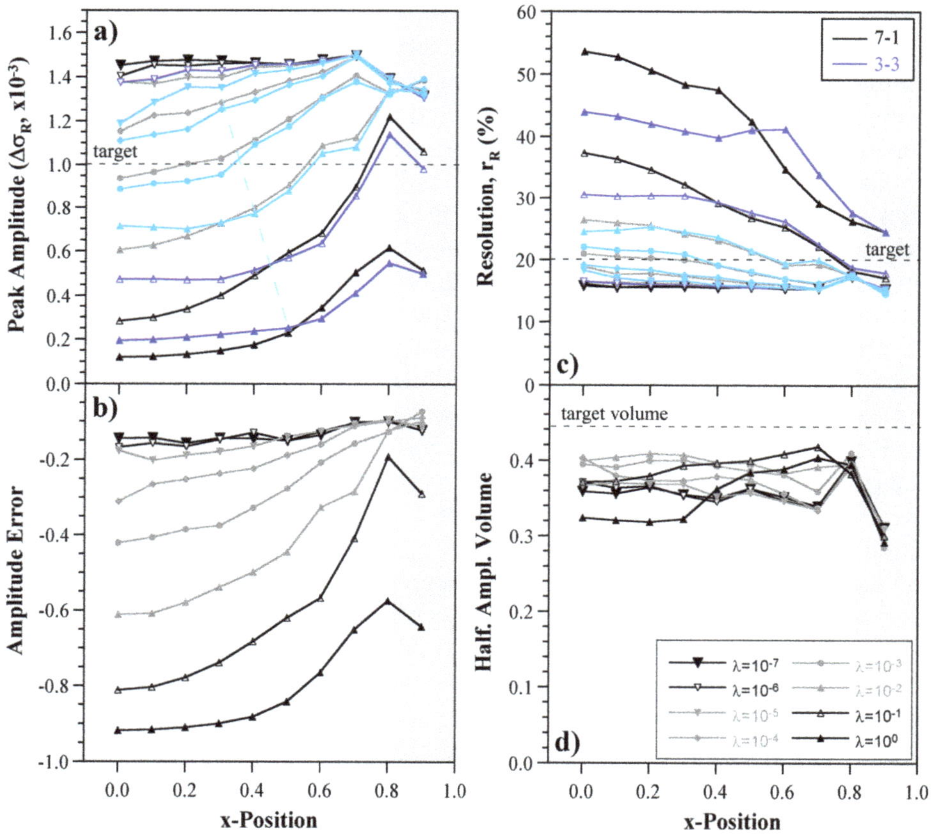

Figure 5.5. Size-related metrics for a circular target as a function of position for different hyperparameters λ: (a) maximum peak amplitude, $\Delta\sigma_R$, (b) amplitude error (chapter 3, equation (3.3)), (c) resolution (chapter 3, equation (3.6)), and (d) feature volume (chapter 3, equation (3.11)). Black lines are for I–M = 7–1 and blue lines for 3–3. Gray shading indicates positions where the target extends partly outside the sensor area. (16 electrodes, $r_T = 0.2$, $I = 10^{-3}$, $\sigma_0 = 10^{-2}$, $\sigma_T = 0.9\sigma_0$ (−10% target contrast), $N = 10^{-12}$, $\lambda_s = 10^{-8}$ to 10^{-1})

average amplitude was 80% of the target's at $x = 0.8$, but at the center it was down to less than 20%, giving an amplitude uniformity of only 0.25.

The resolution or radius of the reconstructed feature, r_R, given as a percentage of the sensor radius, determines target resolvability, meaning the ability to distinguish one target from a neighboring one. As shown in figure 5.5(c), r_R underwent a corresponding increase with λ as the amplitude fell. Due to the choice of the threshold $1/f = 0.5$, the resolution was finer than that of the original target at small λ.

The volume of the target (figure 5.5(d)) was, however, comparatively constant with position at all λ: the 'energy' in the feature was largely preserved across the sensor until the feature exited the sensor at the perimeter. This uniformity is a known advantage of regularized linear algorithms [11]. There were relatively small variations with λ, but not in a consistent direction. For $\lambda = 1$, a value so high that the regularization behavior changes (figure 5.4), features at the center lost energy. This conservation-of-feature-energy was also seen consistently in other cases examined below. In principle, this information could be used, together with knowledge of dependences such as shown in figure 5.5, to partially correct images by post-processing for touches at different locations [10,20]. (Additional size metrics are shown in appendix E.4.)

5.2.1.1 Amplitude Fits

It is of interest to know how amplitude and resolution depend on x and λ. For 7–1 the dependence of the amplitude error on position x and hyperparameter λ could be approximated for $\lambda \geqslant 10^{-4}$ and $x \leqslant 0.6$ by:

$$\text{Amplitude Error} = [a \log \lambda + b]x^2 + [c \log \lambda + d] = [ax^2 + c]\log \lambda + [bx^2 + d] \quad (5.1)$$

This relationship did not hold for smaller hyperparameters, at which there was little effect of regularization. The hyperparameter exerted an effect on the amplitude error that went as the square of the radial position and the log of λ. (Further information on the curve fits is given in appendix E.3.). As shown in figure 5.5, the peak amplitude curves had the almost the same shape as the amplitude error curves, and they could be fit by an equation of the same form.

For 3–3, this relationship held regarding $\log(\lambda)$ but not regarding the x-position. To the right of the slanted blue dashed line in figure 5.5(a), the curves for 3–3 and 7–1 were similar, but to the left they diverged. Rather than being substantially parabolic, the blue curves flattened in the center. The extent of the flattening moved rightward, toward the perimeter, with increasing λ. For example, at $x = 0.7$, the amplitudes for $\lambda = 10^{-6}$, 10^{-5}, and 10^{-4} were all 1.5, whereas at $x = 0.1$ the amplitudes dropped linearly with $\log(\lambda)$.

The differences in behavior between 7–1 and 3–3 are the result of the differences in singular values (figure 5.4), which reflect differences in the sensitivity matrix **J** (see e.g. figure 4.6 and appendix C) for different I–M, which are in turn are due to differences in the current flow at the center of the sensor. Such observations motivate our subsequent comparisons of I–M patterns (section 7.2). However, there is no evidence that superior performance in the center of the sensor meant reduced performance at the edge; rather, the two patterns had similar performance at the edge until λ reached very high values.

5.2.1.2 Resolution fits

The resolution determines how close two touches can be. For other image reconstruction algorithms, resolution across the image was theoretically predicted to vary as $1/(1-x^2)$ [21] or $R_c(1-\alpha x^2)$ [22], where R_c is the resolution at the center of the image and α is related to the I–M pattern. However, the curves in figure 5.5(c) did not have this relationship for I–M = 7–1. In fact, the finding of a nearly constant feature volume requires that the product of the peak height and the square of the resolution (area A_R) be constant. Therefore, since the amplitude for 7–1 increased as x^2, resolution was expected to decrease as x. Such fits accounted well for the data in figure 5.5(c) between $\lambda = 10^{-1}$ and 10^{-4} and between $x = 0$ and 0.7. The slopes and intercepts went as $1/\ |\log(\lambda)|^{0.5}$.

$$\left[a'\sqrt{\left|\frac{1}{\log\lambda}\right|}+b'\right]x+\left[c'\sqrt{\left|\frac{1}{\log\lambda}\right|}+d'\right] \tag{5.2}$$

At first glance, this may seem to be a strange dependence, but the area of the curve then has a dependence on $1/\log\lambda$, which counters the $\log\lambda$ dependence of the amplitude to maintain constant volume. For 3–3 the resolution could also be reasonably well fit by $1/|\log(\lambda)|^{0.5}$ for any given value of x, but there was no simple relationship with target position.

Thus, there was no general relationship between x and the peak amplitude or resolution that held true for all the I–M patterns. The effect of regularization at different positions on the sensor varied among the patterns, although it was always greater in the center than at the perimeter. However, one can estimate for a given x-position that the hyperparameter, once it is large enough, will decrease the amplitude approximately as $\log(\lambda)$ and increase the resolution approximately as $\sqrt{|1/\log\lambda|}$.

5.2.1.3 Uniformity

Figure 5.6 presents the amplitude and resolution uniformity as defined in chapter 3 equations (3.4) and (3.8). Very roughly, the uniformity decreased as $\log\lambda$ between $\lambda = 10^{-5}$ and 10^{-1}, with amplitude having a stronger dependence than resolution, as expected from the foregoing. This relationship held for both 7–1 and 3–3, but the slopes were higher for the former.

5.2.2 Other metrics

Figure 5.7(a) shows the position error (chapter 3, equation (3.12)). It was independent of hyperparameter until $\lambda = 10^{-1}$, when the size of the target became so large that the amplitude from one side of the feature to another was strongly

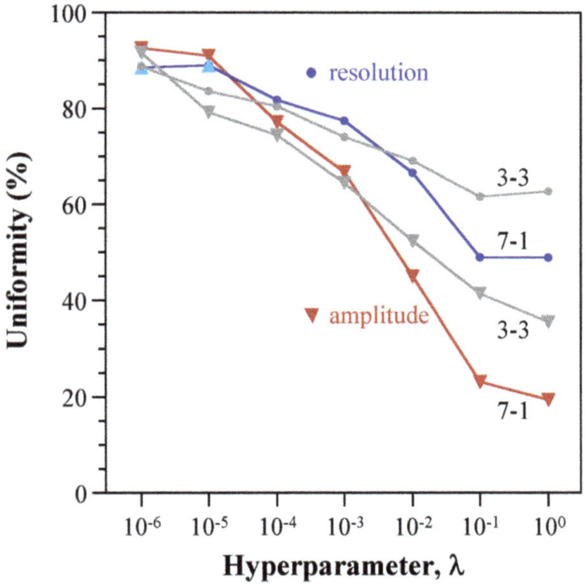

Figure 5.6. Uniformity of the peak amplitude (triangles) and resolution (circles) for a circular target, excluding the points at $x = 0.9$, for I–M = 7–1 (color points) and 3–3 (gray points). For resolution, upward-pointing light blue triangular points indicate that the maximum value occurred at $x = 0.8$ (see figure 5.5(c)), while circular points indicate that the maximum was at $x = 0$ (e.g. coarsest resolution at the center). (16 electrodes, $r_T = 0.2$, $I = 10^{-3}$, $\sigma_0 = 10^{-2}$, $\sigma_T = 0.9\sigma_0$, $N = 10^{-12}$)

asymmetric and a significant fraction of the feature was outside the sensor (figure 5.1). Even then, the error was less than 5% for $\lambda = 10^{-1}$ and less than 10% for $\lambda = 1$. For smaller hyperparameters, the position error was relatively independent of position before $x = 0.8$. For all λ the position error was high at the edge, where the feature first stretched outward, as can be seen in figure 5.1 and as has been noted by others [23], and then as it left the sensor.

Figure 5.7(b) shows the ringing (chapter 3, equation (3.17)), which could be seen getting stronger in figure 5.1 as the target approached the edge. This error was most pronounced for small λ: it is associated with the inclusion of high-frequency $\mathbf{v}_i$ to reconstruct the target. Already by $\lambda = 10^{-5}$, the ringing was largely removed. Ringing can be eliminated from tactile sensor images by applying a threshold to the display, as in figure 3.2, so it is not typically a concern. While ringing might pose a problem for the detection of small peaks if an experimental system could operate at such a small λ, this possibility is usually unrealistic in the presence of real-world noise.

Two shape metrics are presented in figure 5.8. As would be expected, for all λ the shape error (chapter 3, equation (3.13)) was highest at the perimeter, on the order of 10%, due to the aforementioned stretching as the feature first touched, and then extended beyond, the edge. Shape errors remained below a few percent for $x < 0.8$ until λ reached 10^{-1} (figure 5.8(a)), at which point the target became so

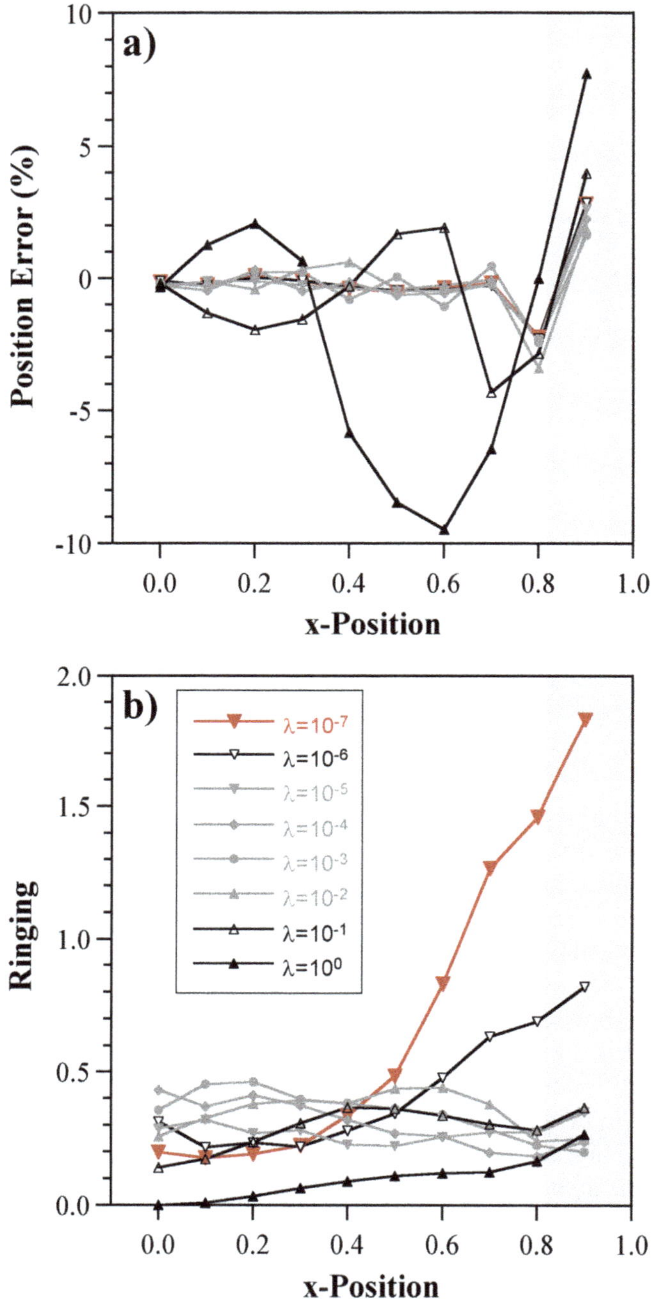

Figure 5.7. (a) Position error (chapter 3, equation (3.12)) and (b) ringing (chapter 3, equation (3.17)) for a circular target using I–M = 7–1 as a function of position and hyperparameter. (16 electrodes, $r_T = 0.2$, $I = 10^{-3}$, $\sigma_0 = 10^{-2}$, $\sigma_T = 0.9\sigma_0$, $N = 10^{-12}$)

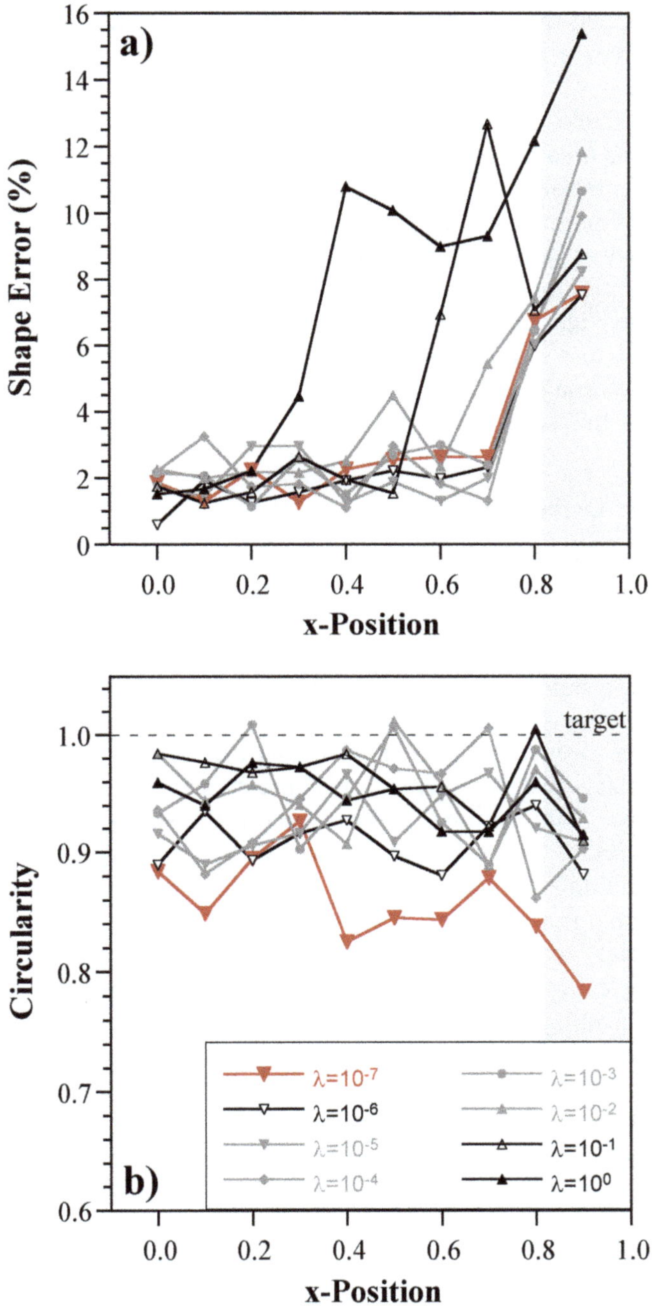

Figure 5.8. (a) Shape error (chapter 3, equation (3.13)) and (b) circularity (chapter 3, equation (3.14)) for a circular target using I–M = 7–1 as a function of position and hyperparameter. (16 electrodes, $r_T = 0.2$, $I = 10^{-3}$, $\sigma_0 = 10^{-2}$, $\sigma_T = 0.9\sigma_0$, $N = 10^{-12}$)

large that it touched the edge even at smaller x. The features became stretched in the y-direction (parallel to the perimeter) and were cut off in the x-direction (radially).

For a perfect circle, circularity = 1. The circularity of the reconstructed features (figure 5.8(b)) was on average smaller, near 0.95, even for the smallest λ because the pixelated representations were slightly rough: this lowered the circularity by raising the length of the perimeter. For the two smallest λ, the circularity dropped even further, since they experienced the least smoothing.

Since the four metrics of this section showed no strong, systematic dependence on λ, aside from the edge-induced distortions for high λ, since for the most part these errors were small, and since position inaccuracy has been found to be mainly caused by the presence of image artifacts [23], we shall not examine these metrics further in the remainder of this book.

5.2.3 Metrics for tactile contacts

Table 5.2 repeats table 3.1 from chapter 3. It summarizes the most critical characteristics of tactile contacts and the associated metrics required for capturing each of them. All depend on the absence of artefacts, which translates to a required minimum hyperparameter for a given system at a given noise level. This relationship is clarified in chapters 6 and 7, but it must be kept in mind here because the required λ determines the extent of image distortion. The performance measures also depend on the uniformity of the distortions caused by regularization: non-uniformity masks the presence of contacts near the center, misrepresents the relative sizes of contacts, distorts the shape of the features, misleads about the strength and intensity of the touch, and contributes to position error. Since non-uniformity can result in masking when there are multiple simultaneous touches, particularly of touches having different strength, uniformity is a significant metric for tactile imaging. Correct determination of the number, size, and shape of contacts further depend on having sufficiently fine resolution. To detect low-strength contacts, where strength means either pressure or displacement depending on the sensor, loss of amplitude of the reconstruction must be minimized. To correctly represent high-strength contacts requires good performance of the algorithm when changes in conductivity are high, when the linearity assumption begins to fail. Because EIT performance is severely degraded by regularization, the elimination of noise to allow the use of a small hyperparameter must be a primary emphasis of an experimental set-up.

Table 5.2. Characteristics of tactile contacts and the key associated metrics.

<table>
<tr><th>number</th><th>area</th><th>shape</th><th>strength</th><th>intensity</th><th>location</th></tr>
<tr><td colspan="6">absence of artefacts</td></tr>
<tr><td colspan="6">uniformity of amplitude and volume over the sensor</td></tr>
<tr><td colspan="3">resolution</td><td>amplitude</td><td>volume</td><td>position error</td></tr>
<tr><td>ringing</td><td>size error</td><td>shape error</td><td>ringing</td><td></td><td></td></tr>
</table>

5.3 Effects of the hyperparameter for different injection–measurement patterns

We now turn to the question of how I–M patterns other than 7–1 and 3–3 are affected by λ: how are the dependences found in the previous section altered? Among other things, we show how symmetry dominates the performance of I–M patterns at low hyperparameter, but sensitivity dominates at large hyperparameter. This topic is taken up again in section 7.2., where the effects on all I–M patterns are fully examined.

Three additional patterns are compared here, 1–1, 4–4, and 8–8, for the following reasons. Regarding 1–1, it is known from prior work that the small dot product between the injection and measurement fields of 1–1 (adjacent) results in a greater influence of λ. Regarding 4–4 and 8–8, the rank of **J** is lower for some I–M patterns based on symmetry, and general observations about the inferior performance of low-rank patterns have been made. While patterns 1–1, 3–3, and 7–1 have rank $r = 104$ for a 16-electrode system, 4–4 has only $r = 62$ and 8–8 only $r = 28$.

5.3.1 Overview

Reconstructions for a circular target at two positions are shown in figure 5.9 for the lowest $\lambda = 10^{-6}$ and for $\lambda = 10^{-2}$ and $\lambda = 10^{-1}$. At $\lambda = 10^{-6}$, the three full-rank patterns resulted in the same images. However, the high-symmetry 4–4 and 8–8 differed, with 4–4 having a small inverse mirror 'ghost' feature for $x > 0$ and 8–8 having an equal-size positive ghost. In addition, the amplitudes for both were smaller at $x = 0$. These features are a consequence of their low rank.

At the more experimentally meaningful $\lambda = 10^{-2}$, the three full-rank patterns still looked similar. The reconstructions for 4–4 began to resemble them, with a comparable amplitude and resolution and its ghost disappearing. However, 8–8 retained the mirror and the stronger defocusing.

With even stronger regularization at $\lambda = 10^{-1}$, the pattern 1–1 became more defocused than 3–3, 4–4, and 7–1. The pattern 3–3 retained more focus at $x = 0$ than 7–1, but was comparable at $x = 0.5$. The 8–8 pattern kept its poor performance.

Thus, for full-rank I–M patterns, at small hyperparameters all had substantially the same performance. The relatively poor performance of 1–1 did not appear until the hyperparameter became large. The rank-deficient patterns were problematic at small hyperparameters, but for one of them the performance equalized as λ was increased.

5.3.2 Size metrics

The peak amplitudes and the resolutions of the five I–M patterns are plotted as a function of λ for two x-positions in figure 5.10. At $x = 0$, as anticipated from figure 5.9(a), both high-symmetry patterns, 4–4 and 8–8, showed markedly lower amplitudes than the others at small λ (figure 5.10(a)). In fact, their amplitudes had no dependence on λ at all until $\lambda = 10^{-4}$ and $\lambda = 10^{-2}$, respectively, whereas the others

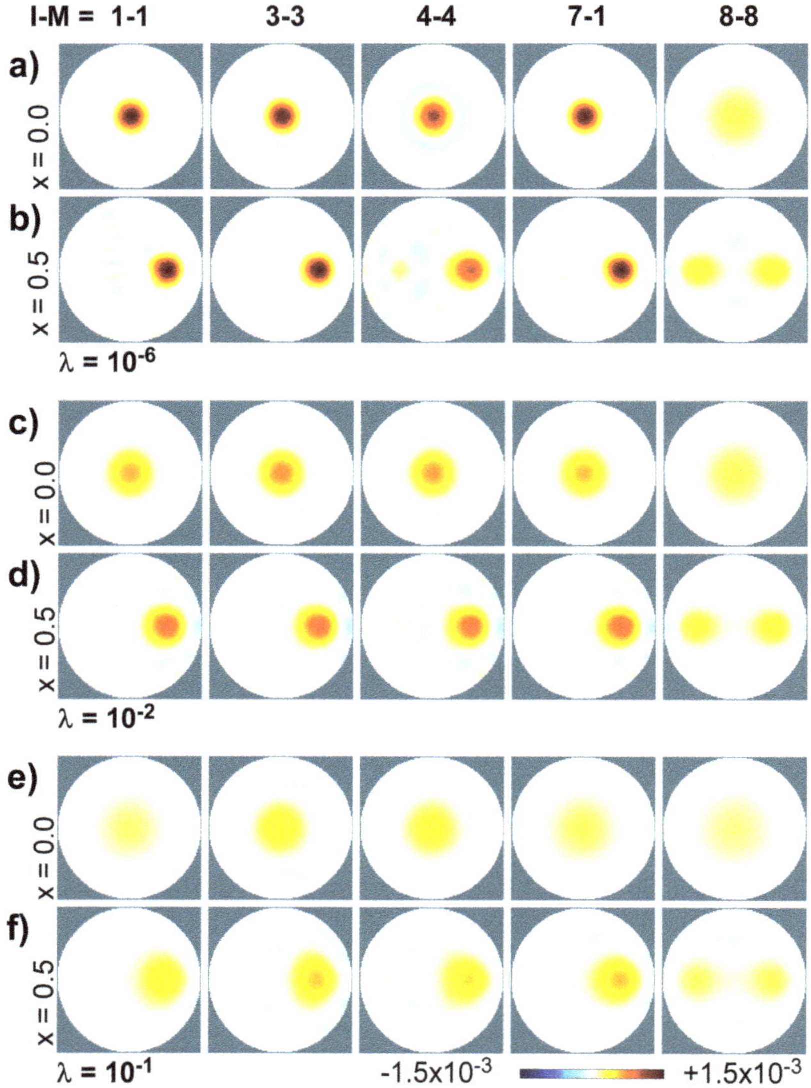

Figure 5.9. EIT images from five I–M patterns with a circular target at $\lambda = 10^{-6}$ for (a) $x = 0.0$ and (b) $x = 0.5$, at $\lambda = 10^{-2}$ for (c) $x = 0.0$ and (d) $x = 0.5$, and at $\lambda = 10^{-1}$ for (e) $x = 0.0$ and (f) $x = 0.5$. (16 electrodes, $r_{\mathrm{T}} = 0.2$, $I = 10^{-3}$, $\sigma_0 = 10^{-2}$, $\sigma_{\mathrm{T}} = 0.9\sigma_0$, $N = 10^{-12}$)

began to show a significant dependence on λ at $\lambda = 10^{-5}$. At $\lambda = 10^{-2}$, there was a cross-over of the 4–4 curve, which thereafter had a somewhat higher amplitude than the others. The 3–3 curve started with 1–1 and 7–1 at 10^{-6}, then dropped more quickly, then subsequently joined 4–4 to cross over them, and then remained higher. The behavior of 8–8 was similar to 4–4 but delayed, with the cross-over not occurring until λ increased beyond 10^{-1}. The 1–1 pattern was virtually the same as 7–1 until it separated above $\lambda = 0.1$, dropping dramatically downward to have a near-zero peak amplitude at $\lambda = 1$. Note that at $\lambda = 10^{-2}$ the amplitudes of all the

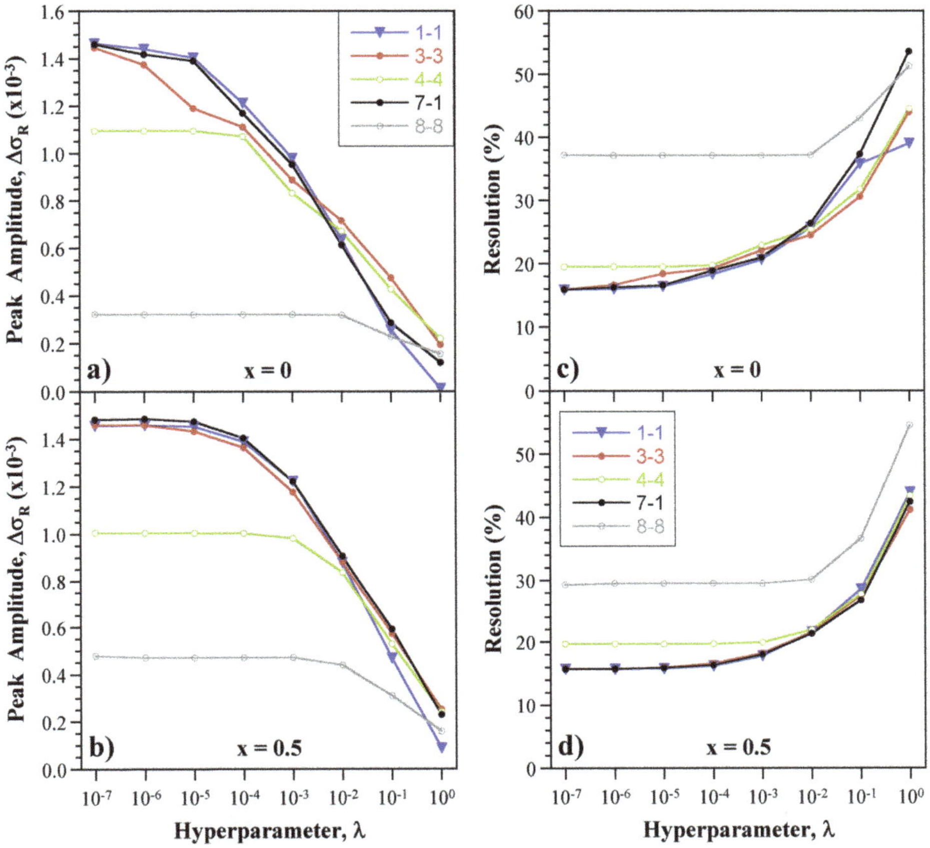

Figure 5.10. Peak amplitude as a function of hyperparameter for the indicated injection-measurement (I–M) patterns for circular targets at positions (a) $x = 0$ and (b) $x = 0.5$. High symmetry I–M are indicated by open symbols. (16 electrodes, $r_T = 0.2$, $I = 10^{-3}$, $\sigma_0 = 10^{-2}$, $\sigma_T = 0.9\sigma_0$, $N = 10^{-12}$)

patterns except 8–1 were similar. Turning to the resolution (figure 5.10(c)), the results were consistent with the expectation of constant volume: the same trends appeared, but with resolution going up (coarsening) instead of down. One exception was a finer resolution for 1–1 at $\lambda = 1$ despite its lower amplitude, discussed below.

At $x = 0.5$, the behaviors of the five patterns were broadly similar to those at $x = 0$. The curves for 1–1, 3–3, and 7–1 were again similar, until after $\lambda = 10^{-2}$, when 1–1 dropped faster. Again, the amplitudes for 4–4 and 8–8 were flat and lower at small λ. However, the onset of the effects of regularization was delayed to higher λ for $x = 0.5$ with respect to $x = 0$. Again, regularization had the greatest effect in the center of the sensor.

It is clear that for a circular target, $x = 0$ is a special case, so it is of interest to examine the spatial dependence of the metrics as a function of λ more carefully. The peak amplitudes and resolutions are shown as a function of position for three values of λ in figure 5.11.

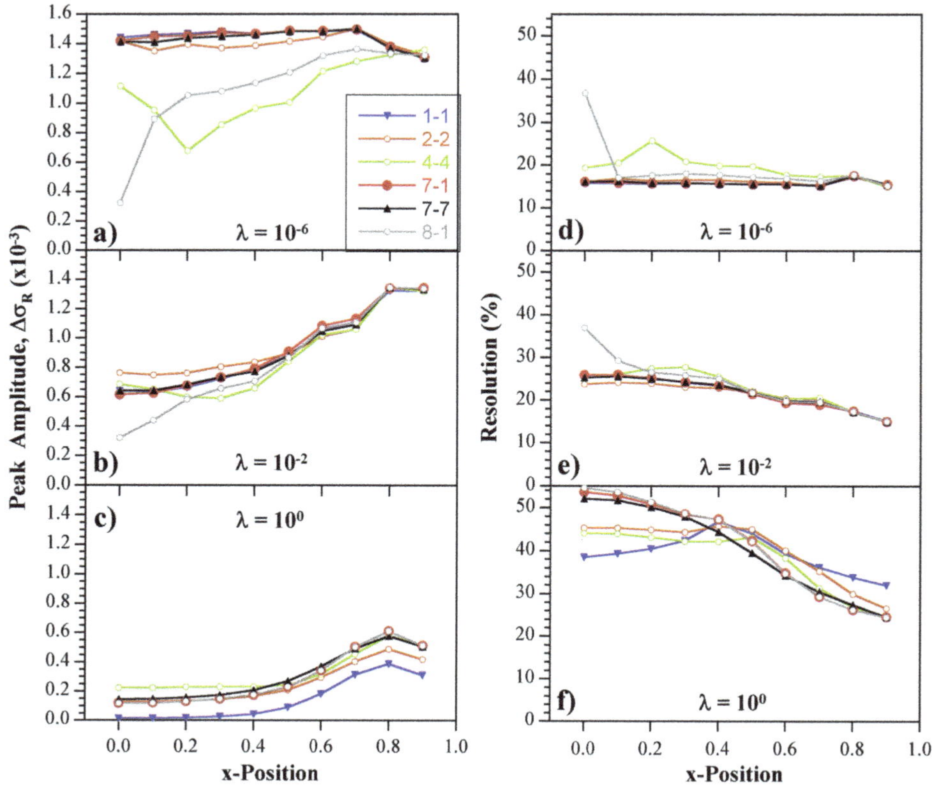

Figure 5.11. (a–c) Peak amplitude and (d–f) resolution as a function of target position for different injection-measurement patterns at three hyperparameters, (a,d) $\lambda = 10^{-6}$, (b,e) $\lambda = 10^{-2}$ and (c,f) $\lambda = 1$. (16 electrodes, $r_T = 0.2$, $I = 10^{-3}$, $\sigma_0 = 10^{-2}$, $\sigma_T = 0.9\sigma_0$, $N = 10^{-12}$)

At the small $\lambda = 10^{-6}$ the amplitudes of 1–1, 7–1, and 7–7 were constant with position, but the amplitudes for 4–4 and 8–1 varied with x due to the mirror 'ghosts' (figure 5.9(b)). The crossover of 4–4 and 8–1, mentioned above, was shown clearly: the amplitude of 4–4 was a minimum at $x = 0.2$. For 2–2, there was a small decrease in amplitude when $0 < x < 0.7$. At the perimeter all the patterns had nearly the same amplitude. Turning to the resolutions, they were again consistent with the maintenance of a constant volume of the feature.

For $\lambda = 10^{-2}$, the spatial dependence of all six patterns was similar, and all showed the parabolic dependence on x found for 7–1 above, except for 8–1, which climbed almost linearly from the small amplitude at $x = 0$. The 4–4 pattern again showed a minimum, which occurred at $x = 0.3$. Resolutions were once more as would be predicted from the peak amplitude behaviors.

At the largest $\lambda = 1$, other than 4–4 and 1–1, and curves for I–M were similar. As seen for 7–1, at this large hyperparameters the parabolic dependence on x was flattened at the center, which was most pronounced for 4–4. 1–1 had the smallest amplitudes everywhere, followed by 2–2. The resolutions followed more complex trajectories. 1–1, 2–2, and 4–4 had better resolutions at the center than the other three, which were comparable. The anomalously small resolution of 1–1 was previously attributed to the relatively small contributions of low-resolution eigen-images. Above $x = 0.5$, the resolution of all six configurations became finer.

Looking over the data in this section, the hyperparameter did affect most I–M patterns the same way, with the amplitude decreasing as $\log(\lambda)$ and having an x^2 dependence on target position. However, some I–M patterns were affected differently. The number of eigen-images contributing to the reconstruction depend on the I–M's symmetry and rank, as well as the steepness of the index versus λ curve. The pattern 1–1, which has the smallest field line dot product at the center of the sensor, had the greatest number of additional $\mathbf{v}_i$ affect by each tenfold increase in λ. It thus suffered at the larger λ, which are of the most interest in real-world measurement systems. The high-symmetry, low-rank I–M performed more poorly at small λ, but that is not of importance for most tactile imaging applications: for $\lambda \geqslant 10^{-2}$, their performance equaled the others. The effect of I–M pattern on reconstructions will be further examined in chapter 7, but these data already suggest that high symmetry patterns and 1–1 should probably be avoided for tactile imaging: they offer no obvious advantages, and there are many other patterns that do not suffer from the drawbacks that these do.

5.3.3 $|\mathbf{V}^{\mathrm{T}}\boldsymbol{\sigma}|$ spectra

Insight into the differences seen in figure 5.10 among the I–M patterns can be obtained by examining the $|\mathbf{V}^{\mathrm{T}}\boldsymbol{\sigma}|$ spectra in figure 5.12 (expanded here from chapter 4, figure 4.22). The most significant coefficients C_i are shown as peaks in the plot. For a circular target at $x = 0.0$, EIT images made at $\lambda = 10^{-6}$ (blue curves) using the full-rank patterns comprised six circularly symmetric $\mathbf{v}_i$. The indices i for these $\mathbf{v}_i$ varied with the I–M pattern. At $\lambda = 1$ (red curves overlying the blue ones for small i) these C_i were diminished at higher i. Unlike for the other patterns, for 1–1 the first coefficient was located not at $i = 1$ but at $i = 8$ (corresponding eigen-images shown in figure 4.7), and its amplitude was small. Furthermore, the amplitude damping experienced by 1–1 was more severe; comparing the red curves for 1–1 and 3–3, for 1–1 the height of $\mathbf{v}_8$ was reduced to 64%, while for 3–3 there was no reduction of $\mathbf{v}_1$ and $\mathbf{v}_{17}$ was reduced to only 77%. Both factors account for the smaller amplitude seen in figure 5.10(a) for $\lambda = 1$. Physically, this behavior is determined by the current paths and electrical fields for the I–M patterns, and since less information is available at the electrodes from the center of the sensor for 1–1 than for 3–3, the algorithm makes greater utilization of prior information there. The prior information is generally a uniform conductivity σ_0, so substituting that into the image results in peak broadening.

For 4–4 and 8–8, the low rank is clear from the spectra in figure 4.22, which terminated at smaller i. For 4–4 there were five circularly symmetric $\mathbf{v}_i$ instead of six, so for the target at $x = 0$ it took a larger λ for the image to be affected, accounting for the flatness of the curve at small λ in figure 5.10(a). I–M = 8–8 had only three circularly symmetric $\mathbf{v}_i$, so λ needed to be even larger to have an effect. Previewing section 5.4, the amplitude and resolution curves for 4–4 resembled those for an eight-

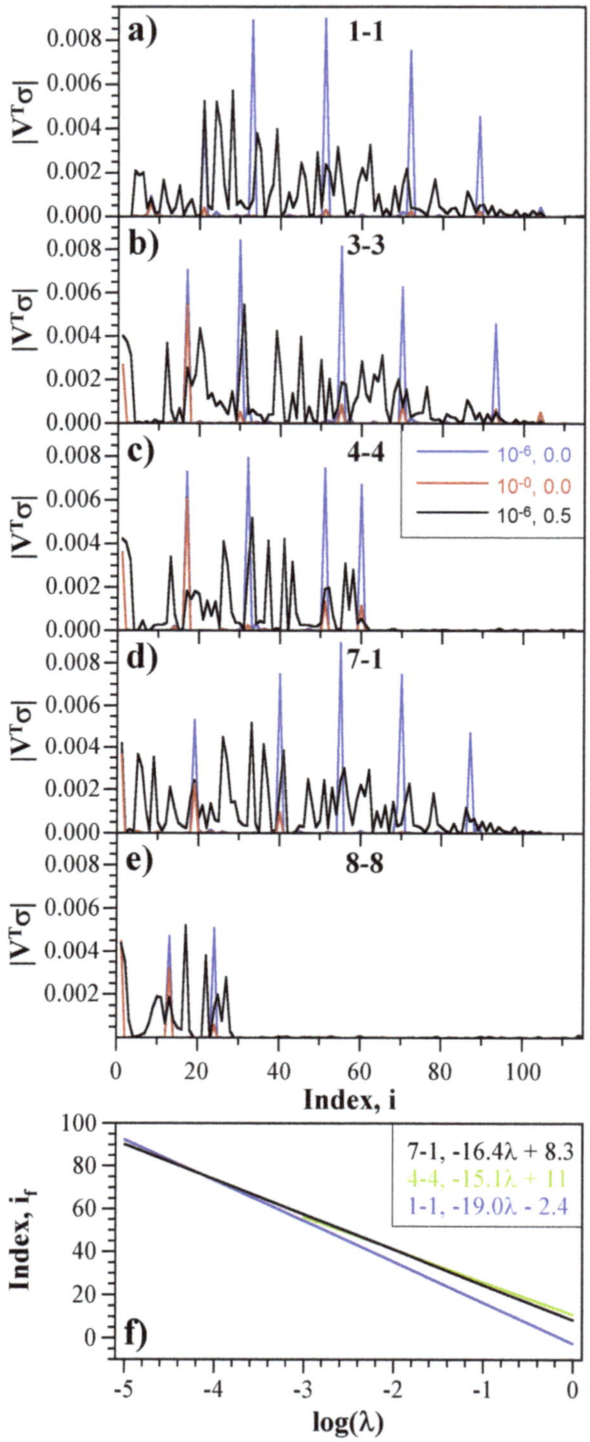

Figure 5.12. The absolute values of $V^T\boldsymbol{\sigma}$ for a circular target at $x = 0.0$ for $\lambda = 10^{-6}$ (blue) and $\lambda = 10^0$ (red) and at $x = 0.5$ for $\lambda = 10^{-6}$ (black) for (a) 1–1, (b) 3–3, (c) 4–4, and (d) 7–1, and (e) 8–8. (f) Index i_f as a function of λ for three I–M patterns. (16 electrodes, $r_T = 0.2$, $I = 10^{-3}$, $\sigma_0 = 10^{-2}$, $\sigma_T = 0.9\sigma_0$, $N = 10^{-12}$)

electrode system, which also has reduced rank. This similarity arises because in both cases a small number of eigen-images (fewer basis functions) contribute to the final EIT image at small λ.

For a circular target at $x = 0.5$ (black curves) the singular value indices i_f were found at which spectrum values greater than 2×10^{-4} were first lowered by more than 5% from their values at $\lambda = 10^{-6}$, for hyperparameters between 10^{-5} and 10^{0}. The points were fit to the form $i = -a\log(\lambda) + b$, which accounted well for the data, once λ was large enough to affect the coefficients (this onset was delayed for 4–4 and 8–8). The fits are shown in figure 5.12(f) for three of the I–M patterns. One curve stood out from the others: 1–1. Not only did it have a steeper slope, showing a more rapid advance over i with λ, but it also had a negative intercept, showing that even the first coefficient was affected at $\lambda = 1$. This dependence was reflected in the peak amplitude (figure 5.10(b)). The slope for 4–4 was slightly lower than that for 7–1, once λ was large enough to have a regularizing effect.

At small λ, the resolution of 1–1 (figure 5.10(c,d) was comparable to that of 3–3 and 7–1, since a similar number of $\mathbf{v}_i$ were used. Consistent with the ranks and symmetries discussed previously, 8–8 had the worst resolution at small λ since the image was built from only a few small-index $\mathbf{v}_i$, corresponding to low spatial frequencies (figure 5.3(a)). What accounts for the anomalously fine resolution of 1–1 at $x = 0$, $\lambda = 1$? Examining the blue curves in figure 4.22, the largest contributions to the images for 4–4 and 8–8 were from the lowest spatial resolution $\mathbf{v}_1$, with the next highest from $\mathbf{v}_{17}$ and $\mathbf{v}_{19}$, respectively. On the other hand, 1–1 had approximately equal size, albeit small, contributions from all six of the circularly symmetric $\mathbf{v}_i$. Thus, the sum was narrower.

This section does not address the question, is the same hyperparameter needed for different I–M patterns? That is determined by the noise susceptibility, which is addressed in chapter 6. As shown there, 7–1 is more noise immune than 1–1, so it would require a smaller λ and its resolution in use would actually be better than suggested here using the same hyperparameter. The 'apples to oranges' nature of the comparison of I–M patterns at the same λ, as was done here, is the reason that the necessary λ is normally found for a given set of experimental parameters to balance the noise artefacts in the image (perturbation error) and resolution (regularization error).

From the data presented in this section, one can conclude that the amplitude and resolution dependences on the hyperparameter are, indeed, generalizable to other bipolar I–M patterns, provided that the rank of the sensitivity matrix $\mathbf{J}$ is large enough that there are image components that can be affected by λ. As shown in figure 5.3a, the effects of λ move from right to left, from large i to smaller i, as λ increases. Until λ is large enough to affect a contributing eigen-image, there is no dependence on λ. The rate of movement from right to left depends on the I–M pattern.

It has been said that differences in the performance of different injection-measurement patterns are accounted for by rank, but this is only the case for small λ. The amplitude and resolution were similar for the various I–M patterns (excepting 8–8) near $\lambda = 10^{-2}$. For higher λ, a low-rank I–M may actually outperform a full rank I–M, as was the case for 4–4. For experimentally encountered large hyperparameters, it is the slope and intercept of the i_f-λ relationship as well as the indices and amplitudes of the $\mathbf{v}_i$ contributing to the particular feature that determine performance. For example, in the case of 1–1 for a target near the center the high index of the first significant eigen-image and the large damping by λ at that index combine to give its singularly poor performance starting near $\lambda = 10^{-2}$, below which 1–1 performed similarly to 7–1.

5.4 Effects of the hyperparameter for different numbers of electrodes

This section clarifies how different size targets are affected differently by the hyperparameter. It is well known that the number of electrodes limits the best achievable spatial resolution. It has also been pointed out that for measurements containing significant noise, for which a large hyperparameter is required, all that more electrodes accomplish is to better resolve the noise [30]: the quality of the image will not increase with additional electrodes. While the most frequently used number of electrodes in tactile imaging is 16, it is of interest to examine how the effects of the hyperparameter differ for systems with more or fewer electrodes. This investigation is important because the greater the number of electrodes, the greater the hardware cost and complexity, the longer the measurements take (the number of measurements increases by approximately a factor of 4 for every doubling of the number of electrodes), and the greater the computational overhead; noise may also increase with the number of electrodes [31]. This section examines the relationship between feature size metrics and the number of electrodes at different λ. We demonstrate that for tactile imaging the use of a smaller hyperparameter in a system with fewer electrodes may offer comparable resolution while mitigating masking.

5.4.1 Overview

Reconstructions of a circular target of $r_T = 0.2$ at $x = 0.5$ are compared in figure 5.13 using three hyperparameters and 8, 12, 16 and 32 electrodes. Simulations were identical but for the number of electrodes, and all used the pseudo-polar, or 'nearly opposite', I–M pattern. The configurations were 3–1 for eight electrodes, 5–1 for 12, 7–1 for 16, and 15–1 for 32. The ranks of $\mathbf{J}$ were 20, 54, 104, and 430, respectively.

Looking from top to bottom, as expected from the smaller rank at all λ the peaks for eight electrodes were noticeably reduced and broadened compared with 16 electrodes, whereas for 32 electrodes the peaks were taller and narrower. Looking from left to right, increasing λ produced qualitatively similar effects for 8, 12, 16, and 32 electrodes.

5.4.2 Size metrics

It has been reported that spatial resolution, as a percentage of sensor size, is given by $\sqrt{1/N}$, where N is the number of independent measurements; $N = 104$ for 16 electrodes, which would give a resolution of 10%, and N = 430 for 32 electrodes,

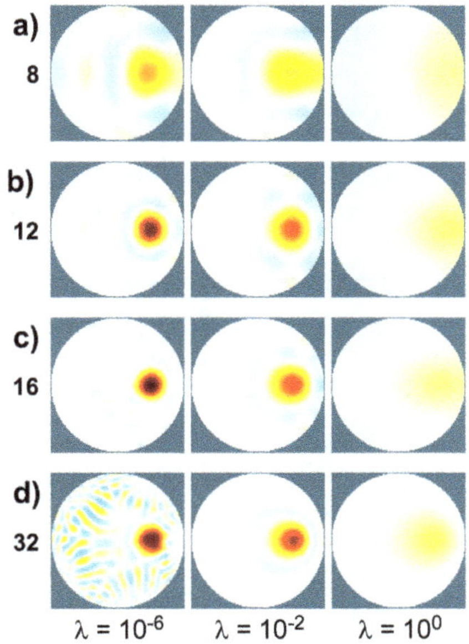

Figure 5.13. Reconstructions using nearly opposite (pseudo-polar) configurations of a circular target at $x = 0.5$ for (a) 8, (b) 12, (c) 16, and (d) 32 electrodes using three hyperparameters, $\lambda = 10^{-6}$, 10^{-2}, and 10^{0}. (Fixed color scales ±0.0015) ($r_T = 0.2$, $I = 10^{-3}$, $\sigma_0 = 10^{-2}$, $\sigma_T = 0.9\sigma_0$, $N = 10^{-12}$)

giving an expected resolution of 5%. These values would be the ultimate resolution in response to a point contrast using a small hyperparameter. At larger λ, the position-dependent blur radius would need to be considered. The reason for this $\sqrt{1/N}$ dependence is that the number of independent pixels cannot be greater than the number of independent measurements; a square image would then have a resolution equivalent to, at best, that of a 10×10 array [18]. To quantify the improvements with increasing numbers of electrodes for 7–1, the peak amplitude and resolution are shown as a function of λ in figure 5.14.

For $r_T = 0.2$ (filled symbols), both amplitude and resolution for 12, 16, and 32 electrodes were close to each other, with amplitudes decreasing and resolutions increasing starting at $\lambda = 10^{-5}$. At $x = 0$, the three amplitude and resolution curves became identical above $\lambda = 10^{-3}$, but for $x = 0.5$, 32 electrodes maintained a somewhat better performance than 16, and 16 better than 12. Specifically, at $x = 0.5$, between $\lambda = 10^{-4}$ and $\lambda = 10^{-1}$ the peak heights for 16 electrodes were 87%–96% of those for 32, and those for 12 electrodes were 76%–83% of those for 32. In contrast, for eight electrodes at small λ the peak amplitude was markedly lower, at half the height of that for 16 electrodes, and the resolution was coarser. Further, the action of λ was delayed, kicking in above $\lambda = 10^{-3}$. The curves for eight electrodes were similar to those for the low rank I–M = 4–4 and 8–8 (compare figure 5.10).

For $r_T = 0.2$ at $x = 0.5$, resolutions were 3%–9% larger for 16 electrodes than 32 and 14%–17% larger for 12. (The anomalously lower amplitude and coarser

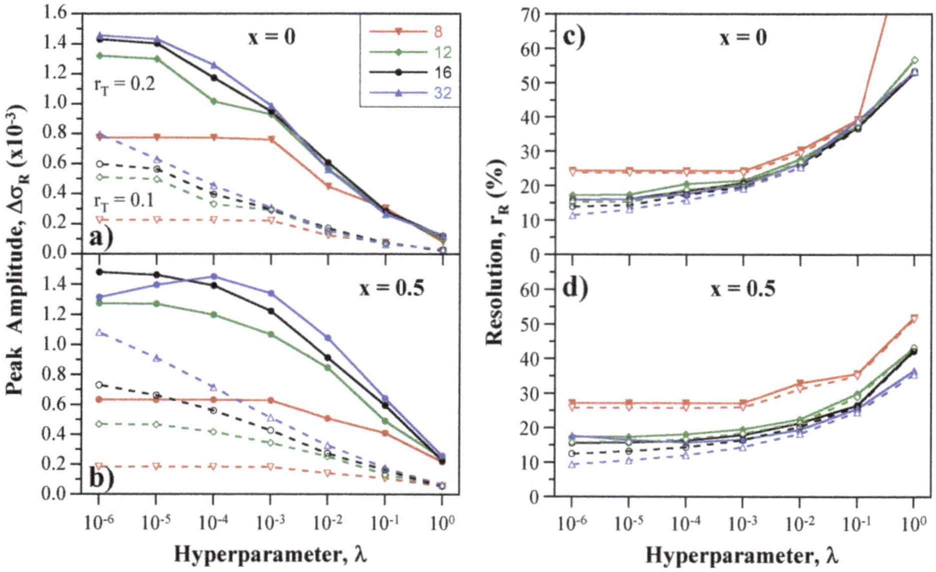

Figure 5.14. (a,b) Peak amplitude and (b,d) resolution for reconstructions of circular targets of $r_T = 0.2$ (solid symbols) and $r_T = 0.1$ (open symbols) at two positions, $x = 0.0$ (a,c) and $x = 0.5$ (b,d) using the pseudo-polar-adjacent pattern with eight (I–M = 3–1), 12 (5–1), 16 (7–1), and 32 (15–1) electrodes. ($I = 10^{-3}$, $\sigma_0 = 10^{-2}$, $\sigma_T = 0.9\sigma_0$, $N = 10^{-12}$)

resolution with 32 electrodes for small λ at $x = 0.5$ was due to image instability (figure 5.13(d)). These resolution improvements were considerably smaller than expected. Also, for a non-point target, it is critical to note that increasing the number of electrodes does little to counteract the coarsening of resolution with λ.

For $r_T = 0.1$ (open symbols in figure 5.14), the resolution was a little finer for all four systems than at $r_T = 0.2$. Reductions in radius beyond this value, for example to $r_T = 0.02$, did not result in further improvements in resolution; the values in figure 5.14(c,d) represent lower limits, consistent with figure 5.19. Once again, the differences in resolution for different numbers of electrodes were not as sizeable as might have been expected. Nevertheless, the relative differences were more pronounced at small λ, with differences diminishing at higher λ. The amplitudes, however, continued to decrease with radius, as in figure 5.19. Differences in amplitude among 8, 12, 16, and 32 electrodes were appreciable at small λ, going from a factor of almost 4 at $x = 0$ to over 5 at $x = 0.5$ for $\lambda = 10^{-6}$. These differences also vanished as λ increased to 1.

These results demonstrate the prior conclusion from the literature that using more electrodes is worthwhile only for small hyperparameter (low noise) conditions; the advantages disappear with increasing λ. The results further suggest that the tradeoff between resolution and speed, linked to the number of electrodes, not only strongly favors 16 electrodes instead of 32, but likely favors a further reduction to 12 (or 13, as shown in chapter 7). The shorter time required to collect a frame of data and perform the reconstruction using a smaller number of electrodes could be traded for a larger number of data points taken at each frame position, reducing noise and thus reducing the size of the required hyperparameter. The gain in resolution and amplitude from a smaller λ may be more significant than can be achieved with more electrodes and a larger λ. Perhaps more importantly, a smaller hyperparameter reduces non-uniformity (figure 5.6), improving the ability to detect multiple contacts.

5.4.3 $|\mathbf{V}^T\boldsymbol{\sigma}|$ spectra

To provide insight into the performance of the four systems, the $|\mathbf{V}^T\boldsymbol{\sigma}|$ at $x = 0.5$ are shown in figure 5.15(a–c) for three hyperparameters. Figure 5.15(d) shows the number of $\mathbf{v}_i$ affected as a function of λ, the latter obtained as in figure 5.4. For eight electrodes, there was no diminution of the coefficients until λ reached 10^{-2}, as expected from figure 5.14. Since the rank was only 20, below that there were no $\mathbf{v}_i$ to be affected. Even at the largest $\lambda = 10^0$, the first several coefficients remained unaffected (compare red and blue curves), leading to a positive intercept in figure 5.15(d). Since there were so few coefficients, the slope in figure 5.15(d) was shallow. With increasing numbers of electrodes, the slopes in figure 5.15(d) became steeper as the number of $\mathbf{v}_i$ affected with each decade increase in λ grew. Correspondingly, the index i at which a given λ first acted increased. For 32 electrodes, only a partial set of coefficients can be shown using the same scale for the x-axis. Figure 5.15(d) illustrates that already at $\lambda = 10^{-5}$ roughly half of the 430 $\mathbf{v}_i$ were diminished. Thus, a large fraction of the $\mathbf{v}_i$ were unused even at the lowest hyperparameters. From figure 5.13(d), it is clear why the resolution was only marginally better for 32 electrodes than 16: a much smaller hyperparameter would be needed to improve the resolution further, yet for $\lambda = 10^{-6}$ the reconstructions had already started to be corrupted by this small level of noise ($N = 10^{-12}$). Theoretical minimum resolution is unachievable at realistic minimum hyperparameters, which eliminate hundreds of eigen-images that supply the finest detail.

Comparing the red curves in figure 5.15(a–c), the larger number of terms contributing to the images at $\lambda = 10^0$ for more electrodes resulted in higher resolution. However, at first glance it is puzzling that with i going to over 100 for $\lambda = 10^{-2}$, the resolution for 32 electrodes was not far finer than for the maximum $i = 54$ for 12 electrodes. The answer lies partly in the large number of near-zero-amplitude C_i for 32 electrodes as well as the specific eigen-images used to make up the reconstruction. At $\lambda = 10^{-2}$ for 32 electrodes, there were 18 $C_i > 5 \times 10^{-4}$, while for 12 there were 17 such C_i.

The results in this section showed that the hyperparameter's effects on reconstructions were similar in nature regardless of the number of electrodes, provided that the hyperparameter was large enough to affect the $\mathbf{v}_i$; this was not the case for eight electrodes until $\lambda > 10^{-3}$. Also, there is little advantage, based on peak amplitude and resolution under conditions of moderate regularization, to using 32 electrodes, since resolution was only marginally improved over 16 electrodes. Likewise, EIT images for 12 electrodes were only marginally reduced in quality from 16, suggesting that 12 may be a good choice for tactile sensors since it would cut the data collection time nearly in half as well as reduce the image processing

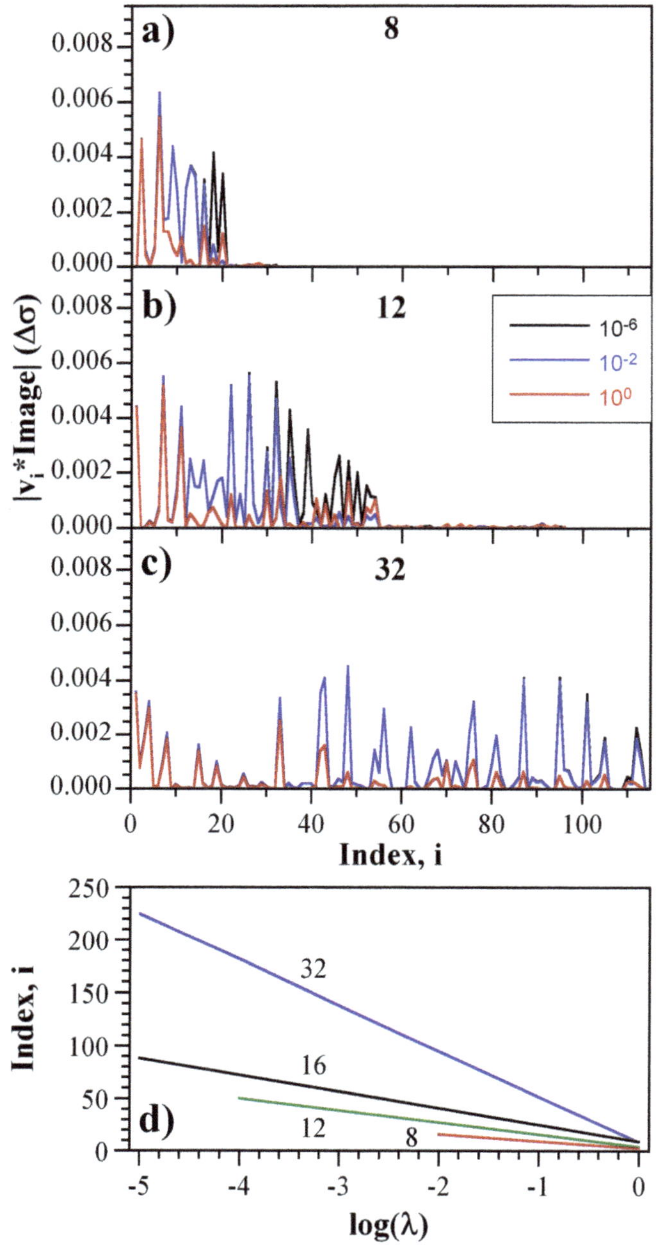

Figure 5.15. The absolute values of $\mathbf{V}^{\mathrm{T}}\boldsymbol{\sigma}$ for a circular target at $x = 0.5$ for $\lambda = 10^{-6}$ (red), 10^{-2} (blue), and 10^{0} (black) for (a) eight electrodes, (b) 12 electrodes, and (c) 32 electrodes. (d) Curve fits to the lowest index value at which λ affected the $|\mathbf{V}^{\mathrm{T}}\boldsymbol{\sigma}|$ spectra as function of $\log(\lambda)$. (Pseudo-polar, $r_{\mathrm{T}} = 0.2$, $I = 10^{-3}$, $\sigma_0 = 10^{-2}$, $\sigma_{\mathrm{T}} = 0.9\sigma_0$, $N = 10^{-12}$)

time, allowing either faster operation, or alternatively, a greater number of samples to be taken at each electrode to reduce noise. However, the performance of eight electrodes was markedly worse, even at large hyperparameters, and should be avoided.

5.5 Effects of the hyperparameter for different sizes and numbers of targets

With an understanding having been established of how the 'standard' target was affected by λ, this section turns to target variations, beginning with target size and then moving to multiple simultaneous targets. The 7–1 I–M pattern is again utilized for these illustrations.

5.5.1 Circular targets of different size

This section shows how the effects of λ change if the target is smaller than the narrowest eigen-peaks employed in the reconstruction (figure 5.16(a)), as well as if the target is so large that it requires multiple eigen-peaks to render (figure 5.16(b)). It has been noted that the linearization of the inverse problem is a reasonable approximation if the size of the object is no greater than 50% of the size of the sensed region [31].

5.5.1.1 Overview

Figure 5.16(a) shows reconstructions using I–M = 7–1 for a circular target of radius $r_T = 0.1$ with the target x-position increasing left to right and λ increasing from top to bottom. Even at the smallest hyperparameter $\lambda = 10^{-6}$, the feature did not reach the amplitude of figure 5.1. Figure 5.16(b) shows reconstructions for a target of $r_T = 0.4$. Five narrow peaks made up the reconstruction at $\lambda = 10^{-6}$, clearly visible at $x = 0.6$. They merged together as λ increased, with merging being strongest at the center of the sensor, as expected from the foregoing.

To quantify the information in figure 5.16, cross-sections are shown in figure 5.17 for $r_T = 0.1$, 0.2, and 0.4 at three hyperparameters. The cross-sections for $r_T = 0.1$ were nearly the same shape and width as those for $r_T = 0.2$ at the same λ, but they were shorter. The curves for $r_T = 0.1$, which acts as a point-target in this system, give the blur radius at that hyperparameter. The curve for $r_T = 0.4$ at $\lambda = 10^{-5}$ showed multiple peaks; the feature was too wide for its flat top to be successfully represented by the narrower eigen-peaks. At $\lambda = 10^{-3}$ the eigen-peaks merged into a single broad peak of comparable amplitude to the one for $r_T = 0.2$ at $\lambda = 10^{-5}$. For $\lambda = 10^{-1}$, peaks for all three radii had essentially the same widths, but different amplitudes. The amplitude and resolution for $r_T = 0.4$ showed a much smaller dependence on λ than those for $r_T = 0.2$.

Figure 5.18 (repeated here from chapter 4, figure 4.13) shows additional cross-sections at two hyperparameters for a range of r_T, from 0.01 to 0.9, illustrating the blur radius and how additional peaks are recruited with increasing r_T for the 1–1 adjacent pattern (7–1 gives similar results) using noise-free simulations and a small

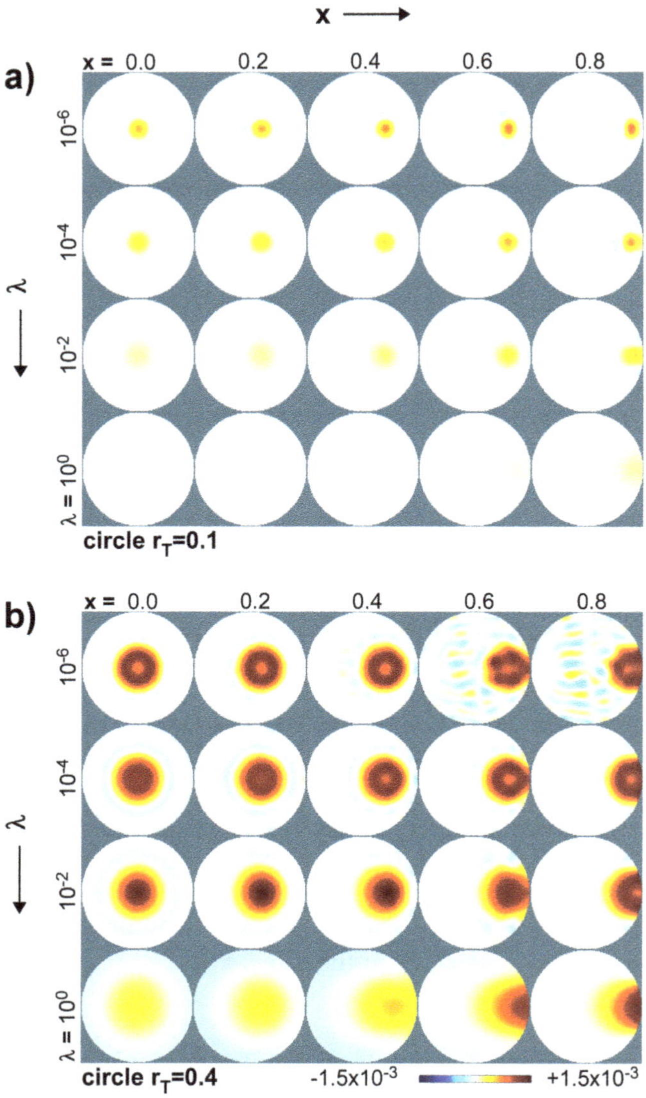

Figure 5.16. EIT images for circular targets of radius (a) 0.1 and (b) 0.4 at four λ, increasing top to bottom, and at five x-positions, increasing left to right. (16 electrodes, I–M = 7–1, $I = 10^{-3}$, $\sigma_0 = 10^{-2}$, $\sigma_T = 0.9\sigma_0$ (−10% target contrast), $N = 10^{-12}$)

$\lambda = 4 \times 10^{-8}$. In figure 5.18(a) the target is again at $x = 0$. It should be noted that these curves illustrate how targets are built up from basis functions with fixed width and position, so that narrow targets are represented as smaller, larger-area targets and the edges of reconstructed features have a given slope.

Below a target radius of $r_T = 0.1$, the reconstructed peak decreased in amplitude but did not decrease significantly in width; for $r_T = 0.1$, the full width at quarter max

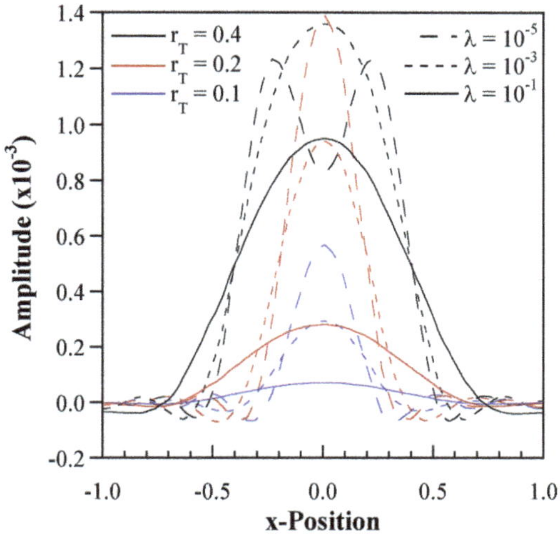

Figure 5.17. Cross-sections of reconstructions of circular targets at $x = 0$ with $r_T = 0.1$ (blue), 0.2 (red), and 0.4 (black) for $\lambda = 10^{-5}$ (large dash), 10^{-3} (small dash), and 10^{-1} (solid line). (16 electrodes, I–M = 7–1, $I = 10^{-3}$, $\sigma_0 = 10^{-2}$, $\sigma_T = 0.9\sigma_0$, $N = 10^{-12}$)

FWQM = 0.15. For larger targets, the eigen-peaks are clearly visible, which have, along the x-axis, fairly constant width and position. Since the center of the feature was sometimes a local minimum, the maximum value cannot in general be used to identify the center of the target and to find its position the centroid must be calculated. Simplifying the display to show only values above a threshold eliminates the rippled representation, but doing so may hinder distinguishability of closely positioned touches.

When the target was off center (figure 5.18(b)) the reconstructed feature became increasingly asymmetric with target size, even under optimal conditions with small λ and no noise. Beyond a certain radius (in this example, at $r_T = 0.6$) the reconstruction was unsuccessful. This issue was also seen for a two-circle target when both circles were near the perimeter (figure 5.25(d,f)). Thus, reconstructions of large targets at the edge of the sensor are problematic. Such stimuli might occur during tactile imaging [33, 34].

5.5.1.2 Size metrics

Figure 5.17 and figure 5.18 raise the question, how do the amplitude and resolution of the reconstructed feature depend on λ for different size targets? Point targets, for example of radius 0.01, are used as inputs to obtain the point spread function or blur radius and have been used to compare the performance of reconstructions (see e.g. [11]). Figure 5.19 shows, for several r_T, the dependence of amplitude error and resolution on position, together with curve fits, at a single hyperparameter, $\lambda = 10^{-2}$.

For $r_T \leqslant 0.2$ the parabolic dependence of amplitude error on position for 7–1 (equation (1)) still held but depended linearly on r_T: amplitude error

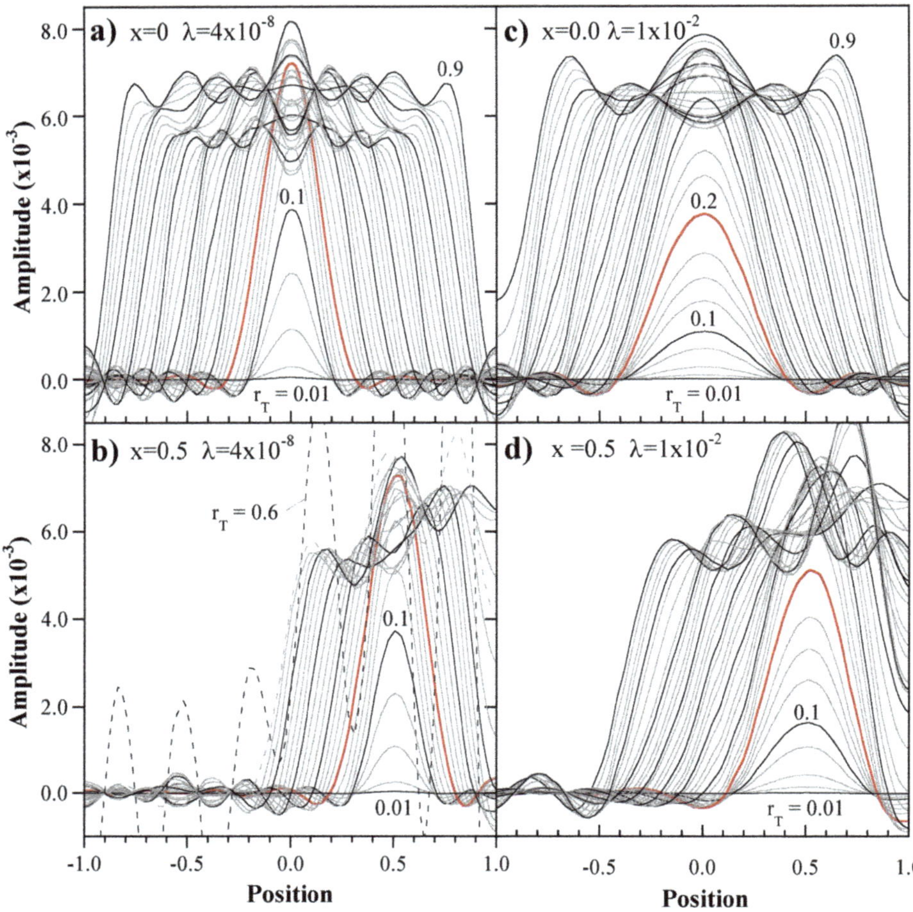

Figure 5.18. Cross-sections taken along the x-axis of reconstructed EIT images for the ADJ–ADJ pattern (I–M = 1–1). (a) At the smallest hyperparameter, a target at the center of the sensor. (b) The same as (a) but with the target at $x = 0.5$. (c) The same as (a) but with a larger hyperparameter. (d) The same as (c) but with the target at $x = 0.5$. Black lines show $r_T = 0.01$ and multiples of 0.1, the red line shows the base case of $r_T = 0.2$, and gray lines show intermediate sizes, while dashed lines show problematic reconstructions. (16 electrodes, I–M = 1–1, $I = 3 \times 10^{-3}$, noise-free $N = 0$, $\sigma_0 = 10^{-2}$, $\sigma_T = 0.6\sigma_0$, $\lambda = 4 \times 10^{-8}$)

$\sim (ar_T\text{-b}) + (cr_T - d)x^2$. The error was larger for smaller r_T. The inability to accurately represent small-area targets resulted, due to conservation of target volume, in greater loss of peak height. On the other hand, for larger radii, the position dependence of the amplitude was gradually lost, with large radius features having no loss of amplitude at the center of the sensor.

The resolution dependence showed a different pattern: for small radii the resolution was the same as that for $r_T = 0.15$, which is the blur radius. As expected from figure 5.17, even though the target had a smaller radius, the reconstructed radius could not decrease since resolution was limited by the radii of the smallest eigen-peaks. For targets of $r_T > 0.2$, the resolution increased with target size, since additional eigen-peaks could be used to form the feature. Like the amplitude, the resolution had little dependence on position for large r_T—until the target reached the perimeter, indicated by the gray shading; in this region the size of the feature appeared to decrease as it moved off the sensor.

The target of size $r_T = 0.2$ occupied a special place between these limiting behaviors. Perhaps coincidentally, this is a typically studied size. The results presented in figure 5.19 shows that one must be careful in drawing general conclusions from this size.

Figure 5.20 examines the size metrics for targets with $r_T = 0.1$ and 0.4 at multiple hyperparameters, incrementing by factors of 10. The amplitude error for $r_T = 0.1$ (blue lines) increased steadily with λ (the amplitude decreased) while the resolution correspondingly increased, as had been the case for $r_T = 0.2$. The amplitude curve was fairly flat, and the curve lowered but did not become appreciably more curved for higher λ, unlike for $r_T = 0.2$. In contrast, for $r_T = 0.4$ there was little dependence of amplitude on the hyperparameter below $\lambda = 0.1$. Above that, features at the center of the image began to be affected by regularization. By $\lambda = 1$, the feature had been diminished in size even close to the perimeter.

For the small target, the resolution increased with λ, just as for $r_T = 0.2$. The resolution behavior was more complex for the large target: it actually decreased initially with λ, corresponding to the peak merger seen in figure 5.17 (a single broad eigen-peak did a better job of representing the feature and was narrower). Then for $\lambda \geqslant 0.1$ the resolution coarsened again, corresponding to the amplitude decrease. For both radii the volume of the feature (see 0) was constant with x and λ until $\lambda = 10^{-3}$, when the volume began to drop in the center of the sensor.

The larger targets were unaffected by regularization until λ became substantial because the smoothing was small relative to their radii. Conversely, smaller targets broadened and lost amplitude even going from $\lambda = 10^{-6}$ to $\lambda = 10^{-5}$. At $\lambda = 1$, targets of $r_T = 0.1$ and 0.4 had, at the center of the sensor, the same radius. With this amount of regularization, information about the size of the touch was entirely lost since the blur radius had become so large. Repeating the lesson from above, sufficiently small hyperparameters are essential for obtaining meaningful image information, which requires making thorough efforts to eliminate noise.

For completeness, figure 5.21 shows the amplitude and resolution uniformity (chapter 3, equations (3.4) and (3.8)) as a function of λ for the set of seven target radii. The smallest radii had the lowest (worst) amplitude uniformity, at all λ. For $r_T = 0.05$ the uniformity was below 0.65 even at $\lambda = 10^{-6}$. For larger radii, the λ at which features began experiencing non-uniformity increased with r_T, moving from $\lambda = 10^{-6}$ at $r_T = 0.2$, to $\lambda = 10^{-3}$ at $r_T = 0.3$, to $\lambda = 10^{-2}$ at $r_T = 0.4$, to $\lambda = 10^{-1}$ at $r_T = 0.6$. The corresponding resolution uniformity was also worst for the smallest r_T, with the exception of $r_T = 0.6$, which suffered from high non-uniformity due to the inability of the algorithm to properly reconstruct this large feature at the perimeter. (Difficulty with large features at the perimeter is a recurring issue for EIT and is illustrated in the next section for a two-circle target.)

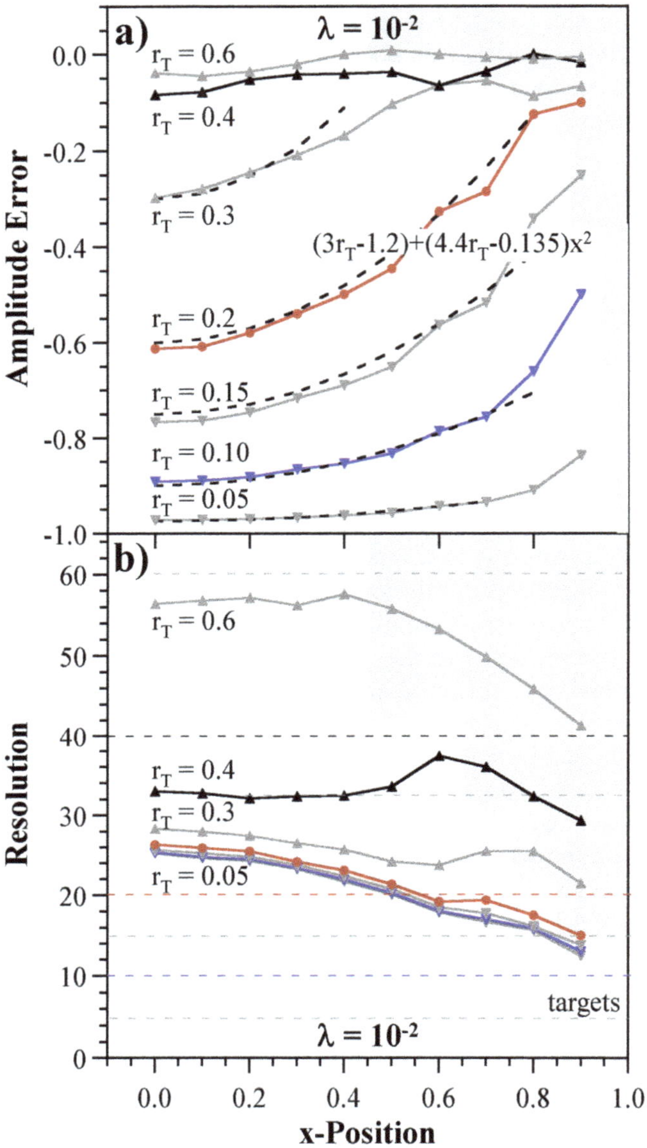

Figure 5.19. (a) Amplitude error and (b) resolution as a function of position for different target sizes between $r_T = 0.05$ and 0.6 at $\lambda = 10^{-2}$. The red line shows the base case $r_T = 02$. Dashed lines in (a) indicate curve fits; dashed lines in (b) indicate target radii. Gray shading indicates when the target began contact with the perimeter. (16 electrodes, I–M = 7–1, $I = 10^{-3}$, $\sigma_0 = 10^{-2}$, $\sigma_T = 0.9\sigma_0$, $N = 10^{-12}$)

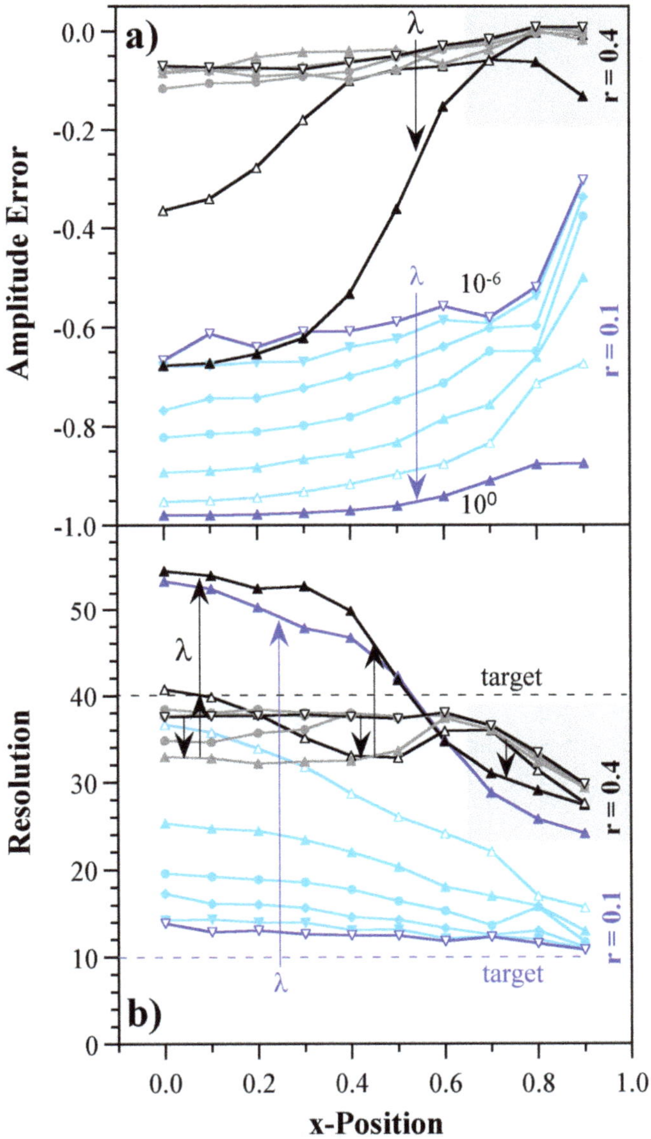

Figure 5.20. (a) Amplitude error and (b) resolution as a function of position for target sizes $r_T = 01$ (blue lines) and 0.4 (black lines) for hyperparameters between $\lambda = 10^{-6}$ and $\lambda = 10^{0}$. Arrows indicate the direction of increasing λ. Gray shading indicates when the target began contact with the perimeter. (16 electrodes, I–M = 7–1, $I = 10^{-3}$, $\sigma_0 = 10^{-2}$, $\sigma_T = 0.9\sigma_0$, $N = 10^{-12}$)

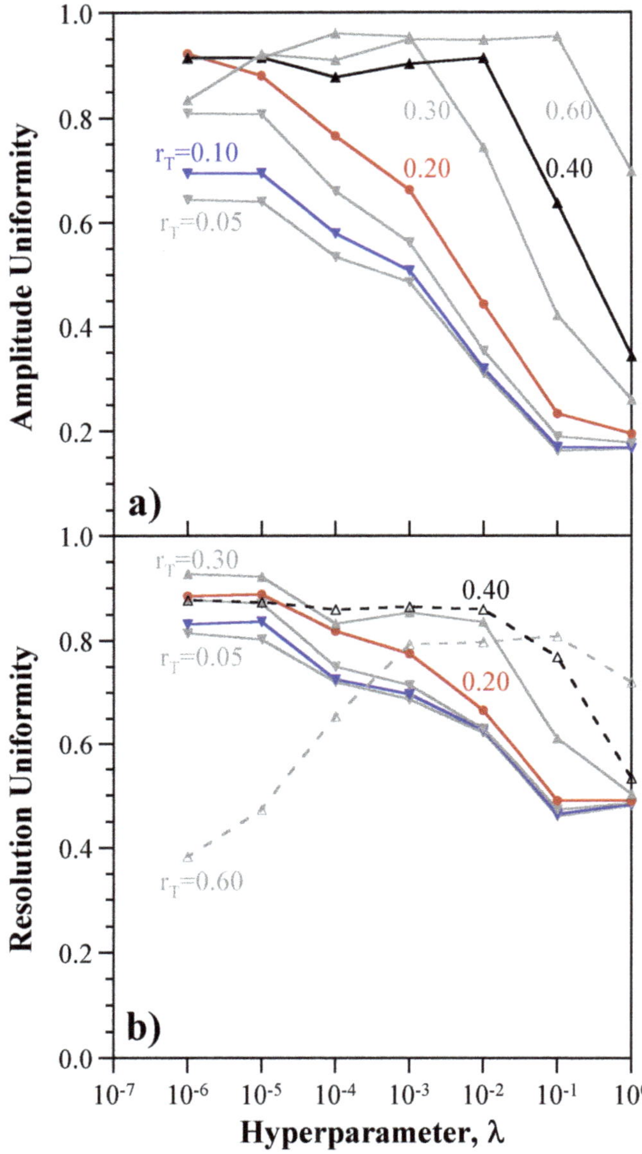

Figure 5.21. (a) Amplitude uniformity and (b) resolution uniformity as a function of λ for different target radii, calculated excluding point $x = 0.9$. (16 electrodes, $I = 10^{-3}$, I–M = 7–1, $\sigma_0 = 10^{-2}$, $\sigma_T = 0.9\sigma_0$, $N = 10^{-12}$)

5.5.1.3 Feature volume

Returning to the question, 'Does constant feature volume hold at all r_T?', figure 5.22 shows the volume as a function of x for various r_T at one hyperparameter, $\lambda = 10^{-2}$. The volumes showed little dependence on position before the target touched the perimeter, until $r_T = 0.05$, for which the volume increased for $x > 0.7$. Figure 5.23(a) shows the volume as a function of r_T at one position, $x = 0$. Volume scaled with the area, r_T^2, as expected. Figure 5.23(b) shows the volume as a function of λ. The volume increased between 10^{-6} and 10^{-4}, after which the curves plateaued; this plateau was also evident in figure 5.23(a). Thus, the energies of the targets at all radii were fairly well preserved over the sensor area, although that was accomplished for small radii by representing the features as wider and shorter than their true sizes. The energy did, however, depend on the hyperparameter for small values of λ.

Figure 5.24(a) shows the volume of large and small circular targets ($r_T = 0.1$ and 0.4) as a function of position for a series of hyperparameters; figure 5.24(b) shows a close-up of the smaller target. Volume was not conserved, as expected, once the large feature contacted the perimeter. Volume also began to be lost at the center of the sensor at $\lambda = 10^{-3}$.

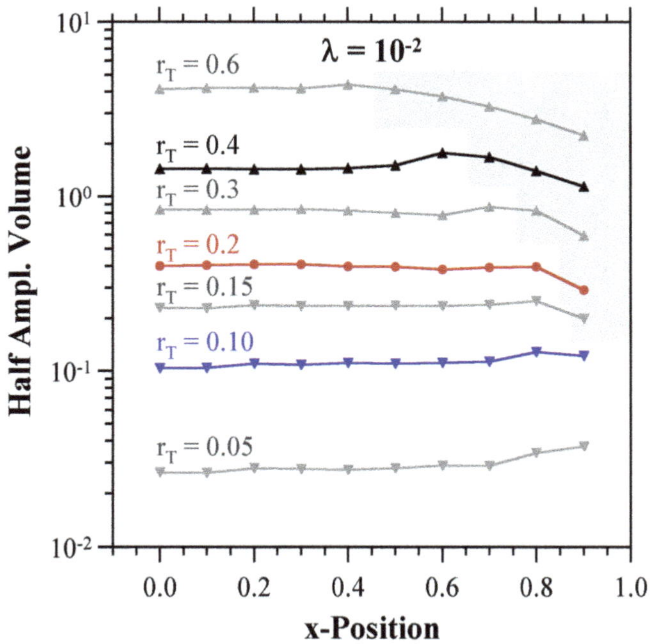

Figure 5.22. Volume of the feature as a function of position for a fixed hyperparameter, $\lambda = 10^{-2}$. (16 electrodes, I–M = 7–1, $I = 10^{-3}$, $\sigma_0 = 10^{-2}$, $\sigma_T = 0.9\sigma_0$, $N = 10^{-12}$)

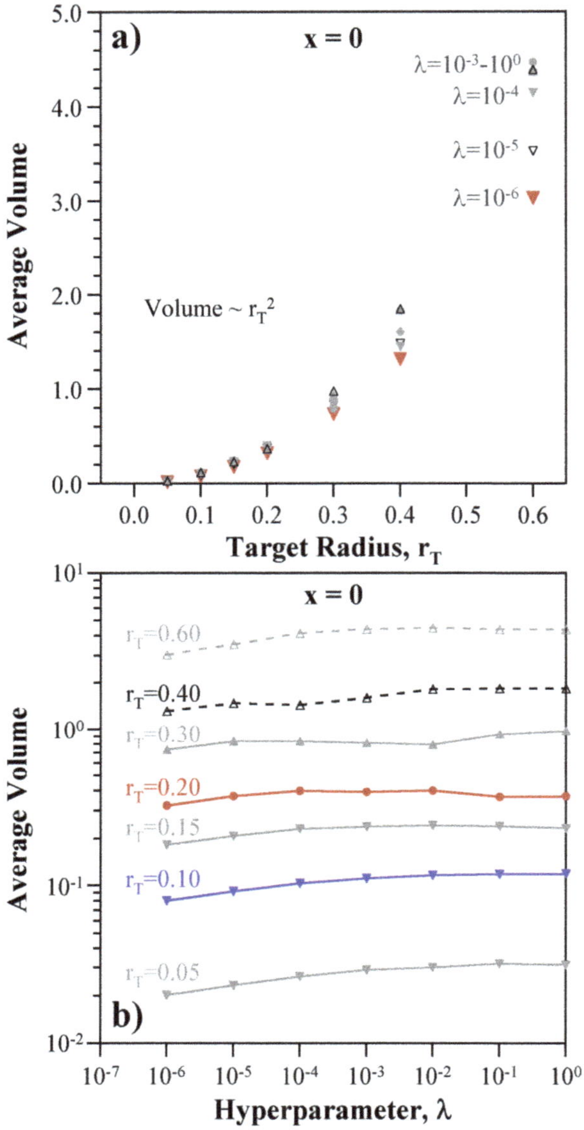

Figure 5.23. Average feature volume at $x = 0$ as a function of (a) r_T and (b) λ. (16 electrodes, I–M = 7–1, $I = 10^{-3}$, $\sigma_0 = 10^{-2}$, $\sigma_T = 0.9\sigma_0$, $N = 10^{-12}$)

5.5.2 Two-circle target

Contacts at multiple locations on the sensor surface occur frequently in tactile imaging. Here, two targets of the same radius $r_T = 0.2$ were studied at different absolute and relative positions.

In a linear imaging system, the image of two simultaneous targets is equivalent to the sum of the targets imaged separately. Figure 5.25(a,b) show two targets of equal

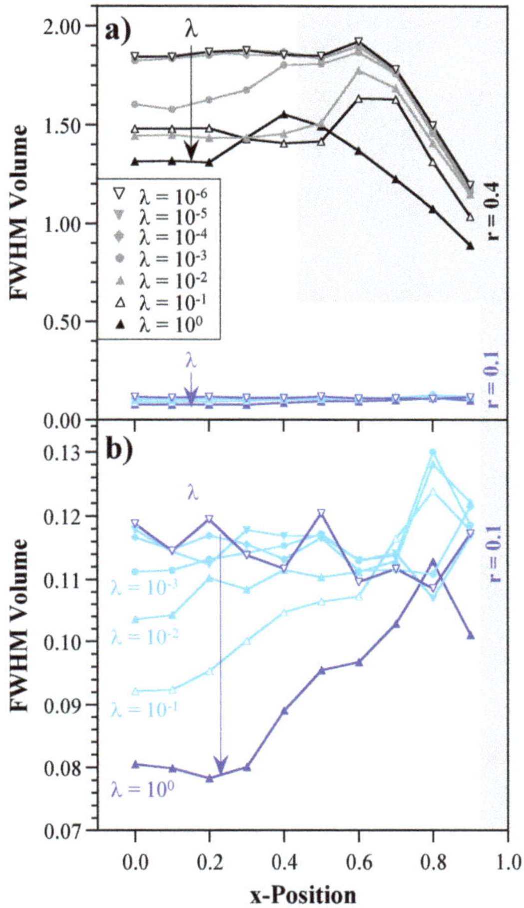

Figure 5.24. (a) Volume of the feature as a function of position for various hyperparameters for circular targets of radius 0.1 and 0.4. (b) Close-up of lower part of (a); the y-axis does not go to zero. (16 electrodes, I–M = 7–1, $I = 10^{-3}$, $\sigma_0 = 10^{-2}$, $\sigma_T = 0.9\sigma_0$, $N = 10^{-12}$)

amplitude separated by $\Delta x = 0.6$ as they move rightward together, for two values of λ. For small λ, the two targets were both represented with the same height and radius. For larger λ, centrally-located targets were strongly affected while those at the perimeter were not. The behavior is just as would have been the case if there were only a single target (compare the third row of figure 5.1). Figure 5.26 shows cross-sections when one target was at $x = 0$ for three cases: both targets introduced together, each target introduced separately, and the sum of the two separate targets. The two targets together and the sum of each separately gave exactly the same result. Thus, the superposition principle holds (provided that the eigen-peaks are not too narrow, as in figure 5.16(b).

The relative amplitude of the targets was changed next, as shown in figure 5.25(c) for $\lambda = 10^{-3}$. The target on the left had half the amplitude of the one on the right, and their separation was $\Delta x = 0.5$. These results were also as

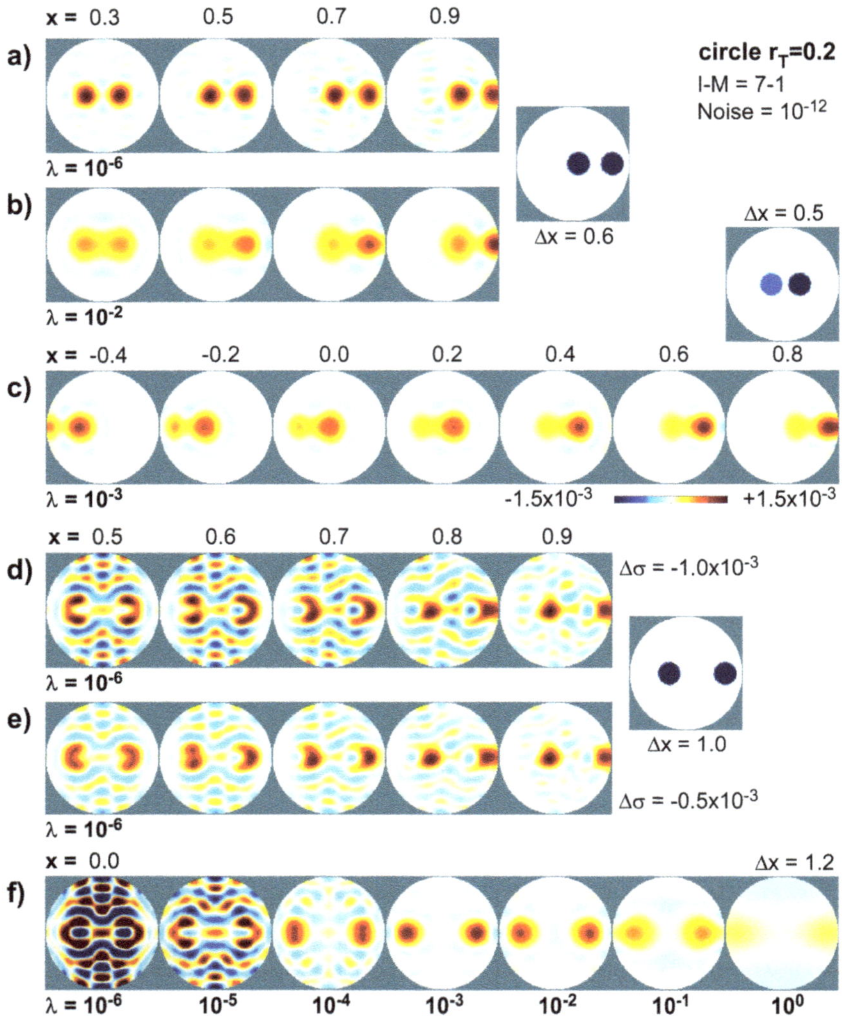

Figure 5.25. Two-circle targets at various positions and strengths. (a) Targets of equal conductivity change $\Delta\sigma$ (contrast -10%) at different x-positions, specified for the target on the right, at a) $\lambda = 10^{-6}$ and (b) $\lambda = 10^{-2}$. (c) The target on the left has half conductivity change (contrast -5%) of the one on the right; $\lambda = 10^{-3}$. (d) Targets of equal $\Delta\sigma$ (contrast –10%) with a large separation. (e) The same as (d) but with a smaller contrast (contrast –5%). (f) The same as (d) but with a larger separation, as λ increases. (16 electrodes, I–M = 7–1, $r_T = 0.2$, $I = 10^{-3}$, $\sigma_0 = 10^{-2}$, $\sigma_T = 0.9\sigma_0$ unless noted, $N = 10^{-12}$)

expected from examining the two targets separately. It has been noted previously that stronger signals mask weaker ones [35]. In this case the target with the larger $\Delta\sigma$ did not mask the smaller one, which remained detectable even at the center of the sensor, but a greater difference in strength or λ would have led to masking. The image was nevertheless dominated by the target at the perimeter. It may be advantageous to employ a color mapping that better displays the full range of

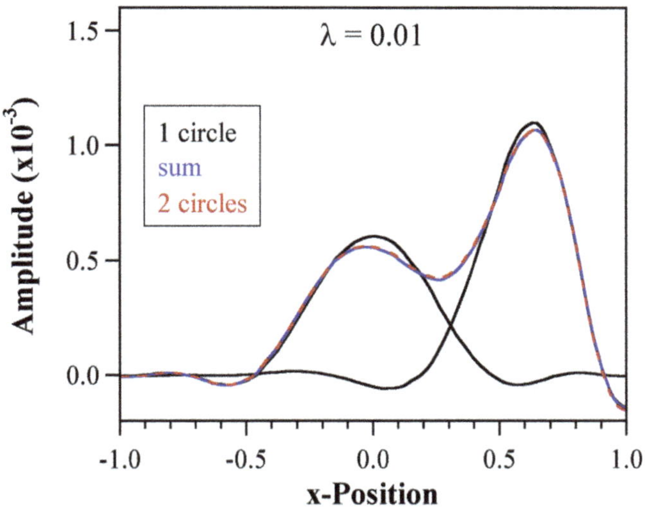

Figure 5.26. Cross-sectional views of reconstructions at $\lambda = 10^{-1}$ for a two-circle target at $x = 0.0$ and 0.6, as in figure 5.25(a,b) (red dashed line) superimposed on peaks of each circle alone (black) and their sum(blue). (16 electrodes, I–M = 7–1, $r_T = 0.2$, $I = 10^{-3}$, $\sigma_0 = 10^{-2}$, $\sigma_T = 0.9\sigma_0$, $N = 10^{-12}$, $\lambda_s = 10^{-2}$)

expected contrast ratios. Appropriate display of the information becomes increasingly challenging as larger hyperparameters are employed, increasing the spatial non-uniformity. Of course, smaller peaks will also be more easily lost in noise and ringing due to too small a hyperparameter. Amplitude and resolution correction by post-processing the image, as shown in [20], taking into account the known blur radii, could be considered. Such processing may improve the utility of EIT images in the presence of contacts having large dynamic range. However, a different, hardware-based approach to large dynamic range may be required, for example designing the sensing system so that it shows greater sensitivity at small strain or force and lower sensitivity at large strain or force [36].

Returning to targets of equal amplitude, the separation was widened to $\Delta x = 1.0$ in figure 5.25(d) with a small $\lambda = 10^{-6}$. The algorithm struggled when both targets were near the perimeter. Instability also occurred for a single large-area target at the perimeter, as shown in figure 5.18. Strong contacts at the edge of the sensor may occur during tactile imaging, which may lead to instability of the inversion. Figure 5.25(e) shows that stability was restored when the strength of the touch ($\Delta\sigma$) was reduced. Figure 5.25(f) shows that raising λ also removed the instability, as designed.

5.6 Summary and conclusions

While hyperparameter *selection* has been extensively studied in the medical EIT literature, addressing the problem of detecting small conductivity changes buried in a given level of noise, this chapter looked at the effects of regularization in the context of stimuli that may be encountered by tactile sensors.

Increases in resistivity (decreases in conductivity) with touch were simulated using difference imaging, and the Gauss–Newton one-step reconstruction algorithm was employed for reconstruction with a Laplacian prior. This combination represents a narrow slice of the available methods for performing EIT, but as it is the approach that has been most commonly used it is worthwhile examining what happens when the regularization hyperparameter is increased, and why. While previously known abstractly, the practical implications of regularization for tactile imaging have now been more fully elucidated with examples. The effect of the hyperparameter on performance metrics depends on the number of electrodes, the I–M pattern, and the location and size of the target, all of which were explored here.

5.6.1 Tactile imaging performance

Capturing the most important features of tactile contacts depends on eliminating artefacts, which determines the minimum hyperparameter needed for a given system, algorithm, and noise level. In turn, / determines the extent of image distortion: sensitivity loss at the center of the sensor, misrepresentation of relative sizes, and shape distortion. These hinder determination of the number, strength, and shape of contacts. The effects of regularization are non-uniform, which can mask simultaneous touches. Given the severity of these effects, the elimination of noise to allow the use of a small hyperparameter must be a primary emphasis of an experimental set-up.

It is also important to select appropriate parameters for image creation. Among the regularization approaches, an advantage of the Laplace prior, as shown in section 4.5, is the preservation of feature volume over much of the sensor area and over a large range of λ, which conserves the overall intensity or 'touch energy' of the contact. If the volume of the reconstructed feature is constant, then as the hyperparameter broadens, the peak height drops commensurately; the two are predictably linked. Other advantages of the Laplace prior include smooth, monotonic changes in metrics with target position and small position error.

Another source of image degradation is a violation of the assumption, in a one-step inversion, of small changes in conductivity. Such a situation occurs for high-strength contacts or for large-area contacts at the perimeter. Thus, handling dynamic range is another consideration for experimental work.

5.6.2 $|\mathbf{V}^{\mathrm{T}}\boldsymbol{\sigma}|$ spectra

A critical concept is that the EIT image can be considered to be a sum of eigen-images, with a resolution determined by the number of independent terms in that series whose amplitudes are greater than the noise. High-symmetry measurement configurations such as polar have fewer independent terms, and thus inherently lower possible resolution.

To understand the action of the hyperparameter it can thus be helpful to look at $|\mathbf{V}^{\mathrm{T}}\boldsymbol{\sigma}|$ spectra, which are alternative views of the EIT image in the form of fingerprints that show the coefficients C_i of the eigen-images that sum to produce the EIT image. The spectra reveal how the coefficients change with the particular coupling of injection and measurement pairs at different locations on the surface and with target properties. The hyperparameter controls the number of eigen-images contributing to the reconstruction; more specifically, λ controls the amplitudes of those eigen-images, which are systematically reduced in favor of prior information as λ increases. The prior information is typically a uniform background conductivity for a tactile sensor. Therefore, the features broaden and fall.

Since the $|\mathbf{V}^T\boldsymbol{\sigma}|$ spectra reflect the action of the hyperparameter, through the final image $\boldsymbol{\sigma}$, they demonstrate explicitly how smoothing occurs and show the relative rate versus index i at which increases in λ affect the coefficients. The eigen-images corresponding to the highest index singular values, which are associated with the highest spatial frequency information, are removed first. With increasing λ, the number of eigen-images contributing to the EIT image drops as $\log\lambda$. The rule of thumb that regularization removes image components for which the singular values $s_i^2 < \lambda^2$ holds for a broad range of i but breaks down at large λ. For large hyperparameters, which for the simulation conditions used in this book means $\lambda = 1$, only a handful of low-frequency eigen-images remain. Thus almost all information about the contacts is lost, including the radius. The scheme governing the details of coefficient reduction is determined by the prior that is chosen. While regularization acts broadly as a low-pass filter, where the index i plays the role of frequency, the details depend on the image filtering strategy, or prior.

Both the I–M pattern and the target characteristics determine the original coefficients in the $|\mathbf{V}^T\boldsymbol{\sigma}|$ spectra. For the simulations in this book, the coefficients were unaffected below $\lambda = 10^{-6}$. The particulars of which coefficients are large, and thus which associated $\mathbf{v}_i$ make a substantial contribution to the final image, provide insight into the reconstructions. Some I–M patterns yield no appreciable peaks at low index for a given target, while others have a peak immediately at $i = 1$. The former are thus affected at a smaller hyperparameter than the latter. These differences reflect the underlying physics: the current flowing through different locations on the sensor depends on the injection pattern. For the same reason, the I–M pattern determines the rate at which the hyperparameter advances across the spectrum of eigen-image coefficients. The steepness of that slope and the particular eigen-images contributing to forming the reconstructed feature determine the image metrics.

5.6.3 Scaling

Regarding the numerical values of λ, the regularization strength, for a given system, depends on the injected current and the sensor background conductivity: it scales linearly with current but as the inverse square of the conductivity. Given the scaling relationships for λ and the predictability of the effects of the hyperparameter, knowledge of any three of these four things, target size r_T, current I, hyperparameter λ, and sensor conductivity σ_0, permits estimation of the fourth, provided that the noise level is not too high. Since the resolution does not depend on $\Delta\sigma$, unlike the amplitude, resolution is a good metric to use for such interconversions. As an illustration, suppose an experimental measurement used a target with a radius $r_{T,exp} = 0.05$, current $i_{exp} = 3 \times 10^{-3}$, and $\lambda_{exp} = 3 \times 10^{-1}$, but the conductivity of the sensor was unknown. If the FWHM of the reconstructed peak was 25% of the diameter at $x = 0$, then that resolution corresponds to a hyperparameter in this book (figure 5.20(b)) of $\lambda_{\text{this chapter}} = 1 \times 10^{-2}$. Since $i_{\text{this chapter}} = 1 \times 10^{-3}$, the scaling to match the experimental current takes $\lambda_{\text{this chapter}}$ from 1×10^{-2} to 3×10^{-2}. This value is a factor of 10 higher than λ_{exp}. Since $\sigma_{0,\text{this chapter}} = 1 \times 10^{-2}$, the experimental sensor conductivity $\sigma_{0,exp}$ must be $\sqrt{10} = 3$ times smaller than $\sigma_{0,\text{this chapter}}$, meaning that $\sigma_{0,exp} = 3 \times 10^{-3}$. A scaled hyperparameter was therefore introduced in chapter 4, equation (4.13): $\lambda_s = \lambda\sigma_0^2/I$.

5.6.4 I–M pattern

Broadly speaking, the I–M pattern affects performance in two ways. The first is symmetry, which plays a role at small hyperparameter. Symmetry results in less information gathered despite an equal number of measurements, reflected in a reduced rank r. Rank deficiency means the following three related things, all of which have size r: a smaller number of eigen-Δ (less input information), a smaller number of singular values, and a smaller number of available eigen-images. A small r results in relatively poor resolution and small feature amplitude when regularization is minimal, except for the highest symmetry cases which are affected even for large λ. In addition, 'ghost' features can manifest themselves from the lack of information due to symmetry. Patterns such as 8–8 and 4–4 should be avoided for a 16-electrode system. In fact, as will be shown in chapter 7, any patterns with 2, 4, and 8 as I or M should be avoided for 16 electrodes, while the 3 and 5 should be avoided for 15 electrodes. Excluding the rank-deficient patterns, at small hyperparameter it makes little difference which I–M is chosen.

The second consideration applies only at large hyperparameters: low sensitivity at the center of the sensor. When regularization is high, more prior information than measured information is used to form the image, resulting in loss of resolution and amplitude. In bipolar I–M patterns, the amount of information at the periphery is always greater than in the center, so the reconstructions maintain peak amplitude and fine resolution there. The choice of pattern therefore comes down to which provides the best information coverage over the entire sensor; this question is further examined in chapter 7. Alternatively, it has been shown that adding an electrode to the center of the sensed region can substantially improve performance [24–26], although doing so defeats a key advantage of EIT: confining electrodes to the periphery. Another alternative is to use other injection electrode choices [27–29], which, however, may be more complex to implement or require advance knowledge of the target. There are also 'optimal' bipolar injection patterns that do not maintain a constant angle between the electrodes, but vary the positions to provide better coverage [26].

Comparing I–M patterns, they have (excluding the highly rank-deficient 8–8) similar amplitude and resolution at $\lambda = 10^{-2}$, which is a crossover point between patterns that perform better at low or at high λ. For example, the adjacent 1–1, which has the lowest sensitivity at the center of the sensor, performs as well as the pseudo-polar 7–1 up to that level, only falling thereafter, and 4–4, which has low amplitude, poor resolution, and an inverse mirror up to that level, surpasses 7–1 beyond it. At the point $\lambda = 10^{-2}$ regularization switches from being dominated by rank to being dominated by the sensitivity matrix.

5.6.5 Dependences on x, λ

The relationship between λ and amplitude and resolution was examined. For the simulation parameters used in this book, λ starts to have a significant effect at 10^{-4} and by 10^{0} the images are too broad to be useful. For I–M patterns without high symmetry, the amplitude is always smallest for a target at $x = 0$ and increases with radial position; the amplitude decreases with $\log\lambda$. (Recall that the number of singular values also has a $\log\lambda$ dependence.) Over some portion of the sensor the amplitude increases with the square of the distance from the center. For 7–1, the parabolic relationship held from $x = 0$ to 0.6, but for 3–3 there was little change in amplitude at the center and the parabolic relationship began at values of x that increased with λ. This plateau in height for 3–3, and resulting greater uniformity of amplitude response, is an attractive feature for an I–M pattern. Commensurately, the resolution is worst at the center and becomes finer with radial position and with $1/|\sqrt{\log \lambda}\,|$. The fixed relationship between amplitude and resolution is determined by the constant volume of the feature. Two identical touches at different places on the surface thus appear quite differently in the reconstructed image. In fact, at a particular λ it may be impossible to image a second contact, depending on its relative strength.

Other metrics, such as the position and shape errors, did not show strong, systematic dependence on λ. The greatest position error was 10% at $\lambda = 1$, at which point the resolution was too coarse for the image to be useful. The shape errors were also on the order of 10% near the perimeter for the largest λ.

5.6.6 Target characteristics

The dependences of the amplitude and resolution on position and hyperparameter were first shown for a typical target radius $r_T = 0.2$. However, the dependences vary with target size, so different target sizes are distorted differently. Given that a tactile sensor is likely to experience varying sizes of touch, this behavior should be appreciated.

For larger targets the effect of λ becomes weaker: by $r_T = 0.4$, there was no significant amplitude error or degradation of resolution at $x = 0$ until λ reached 10^{-1}. Below that amount of regularization, the smoothing, or blur radius, was small compared to the large radius of the feature. The large targets are represented as a set of overlapping narrower peaks. In optics, an image can be considered to be a sum of a large number of point spread functions, but the relatively large minimum radius of the eigen-peaks in EIT (limited by the number of measurements at the periphery) means that only a few of them can go into the sum, resulting in a ripple-topped feature. Thus, targets of radius 0.2 and greater can be properly represented, albeit with a wavy surface.

However, a target of size $r_T < 0.15$ appears to be at least 0.15 in radius, but of lower amplitude. As the target radius decreases, so does the amplitude (amplitude error decreases linearly with increasing r_T), and the loss of height becomes severe even near the perimeter. The resolution, however, reaches a lower limit a result of the eigen-images having insufficiently high spatial resolution to show a smaller feature, or put another way, the feature radius cannot shrink below the blur radius. Thus, smaller size is reflected instead as a lower amplitude. Below the blur radius, lighter contacts and smaller contacts look identical. This misrepresentation of small targets can only be partially mitigated by increasing the number of electrodes.

The volume of the features, on the other hand, remains reasonably constant with position and hyperparameter, for targets that do not make contact with the perimeter and for $\lambda > 10^{-4}$. There is a linear dependence of volume on target radius, as anticipated. Thus the intensity of the touch, the product of size and strength, is preserved.

An attractive feature of EIT is that the reconstruction of two targets introduced simultaneously is the same as their sum when introduced separately, in other words as would be expected from summing the reconstructions of the individual targets. There are no nonlinear interactions that prevent the use of standard peak-finding algorithms, which is aided by the tops of the peaks being satisfactorily fitted as Gaussians, provided that the resolution is not so high that single features are misrepresented as multiple peaks.

A challenge to be addressed in future work is the large dynamic range that may be encountered in tactile imaging. Problems may include masking of light contacts in the presence of heavier ones and instability of the inversion caused by strong contacts, particularly if they have a large area near the perimeter. Handling large dynamic range may be beyond the reach of changes to the EIT process and may require hardware solutions. For example, to enable greater dynamic range, particularly when there are two simultaneous contacts, one strong and one weak, it is possible to employ localized amplification and amplification of weak touches by tailoring the substrate underneath the sensor [17].

5.6.7 Number of electrodes

EIT has frequently been called a 'low resolution' imaging method, although the resolution is higher than would be achieved with a similar number of row and column electrodes. As mentioned previously, the resolution is limited by the size of the smallest eigen-peaks available in the reconstruction. Therefore, increasing the number of electrodes improves resolution at small λ, when higher-index $\mathbf{v}_i$ contribute to the image. *However, when the degree of regularization is high, the resolution becomes similar regardless of the number of electrodes.* Thus, it is unlikely to be time- or cost-effective, weighing the greater hardware complexity and lower speed against the marginal additional resolution and amplitude, to increase the number of electrodes on a tactile sensor from 16 to 32. In fact, depending on the particulars of the experimental system, lowering the number of electrodes from 16 to 12 or 13 may make sense.

5.6.8 Future work

If the application allows the increased computational time, resolution can be improved by using an iterative reconstruction algorithm. Experimentalists who are interested in higher resolution imaging may wish to explore reconstruction methods, such as, should it become available in an open-source code, D-bar, which maintains high resolution across the whole surface of the sensed medium even while rejecting noise [11]. Another recently proposed approach worth exploring, although it does require greater computational time, is a multi-step reconstruction that reduces the amount of regularization near probable targets. This detection of target and edge refinement (DeTER) method is available as an EIDORS plug-in and has impressive image resolution [37]. Machine learning, as discussed in section 2.6.4, may be a way to increase resolution without sacrificing reconstruction speed.

Alternatively, one potential area for additional future work is post-reconstruction image adjustment, again provided it does not lead to undue computational overhead. Such a correction is possible because the blur radius $R_{\text{blur}}(x,\lambda)$ is known and, because the reconstruction is linear, the superposition principle holds. Deconvolution is performed in optics using knowledge of the point spread function. For EIT, the point spread function is not 'shift invariant', since it depends on radial position, but this issue has been addressed (see for example [38, 39]). In fact, deblurring was demonstrated for EIT in [20], where it was noted that since the eigenpeaks could be well fitted by a Gaussian, conventional spatial frequency filtering techniques could be applied. Of course, information that has been lost, for example the shape of the target (figure 3.2(g) or the radius of a small target, could not be recovered, but masking in the presented image might be mitigated and the representation to the user made more true to life. Some tactile sensor images may be particularly amenable to rapid post-processing if they are relatively simple, for example consisting of only several finger-touches within a known, narrow range of target sizes. In such a case, full deconvolution may not be needed: a new image could instead be created with smoothed features replaced by peaks that have been appropriately narrowed. Machine learning has also been used to improve previously reconstructed images.

While it is best to keep the hyperparameter small, unfortunately that is often impossible with the level of noise typically encountered in tactile imaging. In fact, λ on the order of 10^{-2}–10^{-1} may be required which results in substantial distortion. (As discussed previously, these values are for the simulation parameters used here and must be adjusted for other conditions.) Above a certain threshold ($\lambda = 10^{0}$ here), the effects of regularization become so severe that the images are of no value for conveying actionable information about the target. Measures to increase the signal through the design of the sensor and to further limit noise must then be implemented.

References

[1] Vauhkonen M, Lionheart W R, Heikkinen L M, Vauhkonen P J and Kaipio J P 2001 A MATLAB package for the EIDORS project to reconstruct two-dimensional EIT images *Physiol. Meas.* **22** 107–11

[2] Polydorides N and Lionheart W R B 2002 A Matlab toolkit for three-dimensional electrical impedance tomography: a contribution to the Electrical Impedance and Diffuse Optical Reconstruction Software project *Meas. Sci. Technol.* **13** 1871–83

[3] Adler A and Lionheart W R B 2006 Uses and abuses of EIDORS: an extensible software base for EIT *Physiol. Meas.* **27** S25–42

[4] Hansen P C 1990 The discrete Picard condition for discrete ill-posed problems *BIT Numer. Math.* **30** 658–72

[5] Graham B M and Adler A 2006 Objective selection of hyperparameter for EIT *Physiol. Meas.* **27** S65–79

[6] Correia T, Gibson A, Schweiger M and Hebden J 2009 Selection of regularization parameter for optical topography *J. Biomed. Opt.* **14** 3

[7] Hansen P C 2010 *Discrete Inverse Problems: Insight and Algorithms, Fundamentals of Algorithms* (Philadelphia, PA: Society for Industrial and Applied Mathematics (SIAM))

[8] Tawil D S, Rye D and Velonaki M 2009 Improved EIT drive patterns for a robotics sensitive skin *Australasian Conf. Robotics and Automation (ACRA) (Sydney, Dec. 2–4)* pap112s111

[9] Tawil D S 2012 Artificial skin and the interpretation of touch in human–robot interaction *PhD Thesis* Australia School of Aerospace, Mechanical and Mechatronic Engineering, University of Sydney

[10] Chen Y 2018 Tactile sensing with compliant structures for human–robot interaction *PhD Thesis* Department of Mechanical Engineering, University of Maryland

[11] Hamilton S J, Lionheart R B and Adler A 2019 Comparing D-bar and common regularization-based methods for electrical impedance tomography *Physiol. Meas.* **40** ARTN 044004

[12] Lionheart W, Polydorides N and Borsic A 2005 Chapter 1. The reconstruction problem *Electrical Impedance Tomography: Methods, History and Applications, Series in Medical Physics and Biomedical Engineering* ed C G Orton, J H Nagel and J G Webster (Bristol: IOP Publishing)

[13] Wang M, Wang Q and Karki B 2016 Arts of electrical impedance tomographic sensing *Philosoph. Trans.* A **374** 20150329

[14] Hansen P C 2010 *DIAS 006—Discrete Inverse Problems—Day 1, slides based on Discrete Inverse Problems: Insight and Algorithms vol 2020, Fundamentals of Algorithms* (Philadelphia: Society for Industrial and Applied Mathematics (SIAM))

[15] Polydorides N and McCann H 2002 Electrode configurations for improved spatial resolution in electrical impedance tomography *Meas. Sci. Technol.* **13** 1862–70

[16] Hansen P C 2010 Chapter 4. Computational Aspects: Regularization Methods *Discrete Inverse Problems: Insight and Algorithms* ed N J Higham (Philadelphia, PA: Society for Industrial and Applied Mathematics (SIAM))

[17] Chen Y, Yu M, Bruck H A and Smela E 2018 Compliant multi-layer tactile sensing for enhanced identification of human touch *Smart Mater. Struct.* **27** 125009

[18] Seagar A D, Barber D C and Brown B H 1987 Electrical impedance imaging *IEE Proc.* **134** 201–10

[19] Braun F, Proença M, Solà J, Thiran J-P and Adler A 2017 A versatile noise performance metric for electrical impedance tomography algorithms *IEEE Trans. Biomed. Eng.* **64** 2321–30

[20] Kotre C J 1994 Eit image-reconstruction using sensitivity weighted filtered backprojection *Physiol. Meas.* **15** A125–36

[21] Seagar A D, Barber D C and Brown B H 1987 Theoretical limits to sensitivity and resolution in impedance imaging *Clin. Phys. Physiol. Meas.* **8** 13

[22] Wheeler J L, Wang W and Tang M X 2002 A comparison of methods for measurement of spatial resolution in two-dimensional circular EIT images *Physiol. Meas.* **23** 169–76

[23] Elsanadedy A 2012 Application of electrical impedance tomography to robotic tactile sensing *MS Thesis* Mechanical Engineering, Carleton University

[24] Caldwell C A, Cheney M and Isaacson D 1993 Impedance imaging using interior and exterior measurements *Physiological Imaging, Spectroscopy, and Early-Detection Diagnostic Methods, OE/LASE'93* 1887 *(Los Angeles, CA, 1993/08/27)* (SPIE) pp 271–4

[25] Tawil D S, Rye D and Velonaki M 2011 Improved image reconstruction for an EIT-based sensitive skin with multiple internal electrodes *IEEE Trans. Robot.* **27** 425–35

[26] Lee H, Park K, Kim J and Kuchenbecker K J 2021 Piezoresistive textile layer and distributed electrode structure for soft whole-body tactile skin *Smart Mater. Struct.* **30** 8

[27] Demidenko E, Hartov A, Soni N and Paulsen K D 2005 On optimal current patterns for electrical impedance tomography *IEEE Trans. Bio-Med. Eng.* **52** 238–48

[28] Kaipio J P, Seppänen A, Voutilainen A and Haario H 2007 Optimal current patterns in dynamical electrical impedance tomography imaging *Inverse Prob.* **23** 1201–14

[29] Brinckerhoff M 2018 Comparison of electrical impedance tomography reconstruction algorithms with EIDORS reconstruction software *MS Thesis* Mathematics, Clemson University

[30] Newell J 2005 Chapter 13: The Rensselaer experience *Electrical Impedance Tomography: Methods, History and Applications, Series in Medical Physics and Biomedical Engineering* ed C G Orton, J H Nagel and J G Webster (Bristol: IOP Publishing)

[31] Gaggero P O 2011 Miniaturization and distinguishability limits of electrical impedance tomography for biomedical application *PhD Thesis* Landquart, SwitzerlandNanomedecine Division, Centre Suisse d'Electronique et de Microtechnique (CSEM), University of Neuchâtel

[32] Silvera-Tawil D, Rye D, Soleimani M and Velonaki M 2015 Electrical impedance tomography for artificial sensitive robotic skin *A review IEEE Sensors J.* **15** 2001–16

[33] Vauhkonen M, Kaipio J P, Somersalo E and Karjalainen P A 1997 Electrical impedance tomography with basis constraints *Inverse Probl.* **13** 523–30

[34] Vauhkonen M, Vadasz D, Karjalainen P A, Somersalo E and Kaipio J P 1998 Tikhonov regularization and prior information in electrical impedance tomography *IEEE Trans. Med. Imag.* **17** 285–93

[35] Tawil D S, Rye D and Velonaki M 2012 Interpretation of the modality of touch on an artificial arm covered with an EIT-based sensitive skin *Int. J. Robot. Res.* **31** 1627–41

[36] Chen Y, Yu M, Bruck H A and Smela E 2018 Characterization of a compliant multi-layer system for tactile sensing with enhanced sensitivity and range *Smart Mater. Struct.* **27** 065005

[37] Ranade N V and Gharpure D C 2019 Enhancing sharp features by locally relaxing regularization for reconstructed images in electrical impedance tomography *J. Electr. Bioimp.* **10** 2–13

[38] Aguet F, Van De Ville D and Unser M 2008 An accurate PSF model with few parameters for axially shift-variant deconvolution 2008 *IEEE Int. Symp. Biomedical Imaging: From Nano to Macro* **1-4** 157–60

[39] Sastry S B 2011 Computationally efficient methods for shift-variant image restoration in two and three dimensions *PhD Thesis* Computer Engineering, Stony Brook University

Chapter 6

Noise

This chapter examines how noise on the electrical impedance tomography (EIT) voltage signals manifests itself in images, and it explains how best to consider the signal-to-noise ratio (SNR). Noise necessitates the use of regularization to stabilize the images so that they represent the tactile contacts. However, as discussed in chapter 5, the required extent of regularization, given by the hyperparameter λ, may introduce distortions so severe that they also make the images unacceptable. A large l may be needed even when the noise is orders of magnitude smaller than the measured voltage differences. Using simulations, this chapter examines noise susceptibility and how minute amounts of noise affect image stability. The reason for the extreme noise sensitivity of EIT can only be well understood by examining $|\mathbf{U}^T\mathbf{\Delta}|$spectra, or the Picard coefficients, with other signal-to-noise measures being incomplete. A noise threshold metric $N_{th}(\lambda)$, above which artefacts appear in the image, is introduced that directly addresses the need for tactile imagers to accurately determine the number of contacts. First the dependence of N_{th} on the hyperparameter is shown. Next, relationships are presented between N_{th} and system and target characteristics: sensor conductivity, target position and size, current injection and voltage measurement pattern, and number of electrodes . The challenge of detecting multiple simultaneous touches is also described. This chapter shows that the issue of noise performance is more nuanced than heretofore appreciated, and that the use of the system- and target-dependent Picard coefficients gives a more complete picture.

6.1 SNR in EIT

This chapter examines how noise on the voltage signal manifests itself in images [1] and how one needs to think about the signal-to-noise ratio (SNR) in EIT. Noise and the hyperparameter are intimately linked, and they are normally considered together. In this book, however, we separately consider the two, focusing here on noise while chapter 5 considered regularization.

doi:10.1088/978-0-7503-5402-8ch6

Table 6.1. Simulation parameters for the baseline case.

Forward Model Parameter	Symbol	Value	Target Parameter	Symbol	Value
# electrodes	$N_{\text{electrodes}}$	16	# targets	—	1
injection–measurement pattern	I–M	7–1	target position	x	0.5
				y	0.0
injected current	I	1×10^{-3}	target size	r_T	0.2
hyperparameter	λ	1×10^{-5}	target shape	—	triangular
sensor conductivity	σ_0	1×10^{-2}	target conductivity	σ_T	$0.6\ \sigma_0$ (contrast = 40%)

Full details of the simulations were given in chapter 3. Briefly, the studies were performed using the Gauss–Newton 1-step algorithm with the Laplace prior, bipolar electrode configurations, and a uniform decrease in conductivity at a target location on a 2D sensor, employing the open-source software EIDORS [2–4]. Simulation allowed us to pose a large number of scenarios, including some artificial cases and comparisons across systems, to provide insight. The simulation conditions that were used, unless specified otherwise, are given in table 6.1, and the simulations employed uncorrelated white Gaussian noise.

In this chapter, several approaches to the SNR are compared, and the advantages of an approach using the basis vectors for the measured voltages are shown. The effects of target position and size and the number of electrodes are also considered.

6.1.1 Noise and SNR in EIT

The customary definition of SNR is the mean of the signal divided by the standard deviation of the signal. In difference EIT the voltage signal is $\mathbf{\Delta} = \mathbf{V}_{\text{touch}} - \mathbf{V}_{\text{ref}}$, where the reference state $\mathbf{V}_{\text{ref}}$ is an vector of m voltages, or a 'frame', measured *a priori* without a target touch and where $\mathbf{V}_{\text{touch}}$ is a frame taken during operation, which may reflect a touch on the sensor. Δ holds all the information about target position, size, and shape (figure 6.1; for further discussion of this type of plot see section 4.2). For a piesoresistive sensor, $\mathbf{\Delta}$ is due to a strain- or pressure-induced change in conductivity at the target location. (The relationship between the strain and the conductivity change is determined by the sensor design, as reviewed in chapter 2.) The values in $\mathbf{\Delta}$ increase linearly with the conductivity change. The values in $\mathbf{\Delta}$ are small, with many of them near zero because $\mathbf{\Delta}$ is a difference between two sets of measurements, with many of them little changed by the contact.

In EIT there are several alternative meanings of the term 'signal,' and some publications lack a clear definition, complicating comparisons of prior work. $\mathbf{\Delta}$ is a series of correlated voltages of differing amplitude. In other words, the variations in $\mathbf{\Delta}$ across measurement numbers are not noise, so the customary definition of SNR cannot be used directly. Signal strength has been defined as the maximum voltage in $\mathbf{\Delta}$. It has

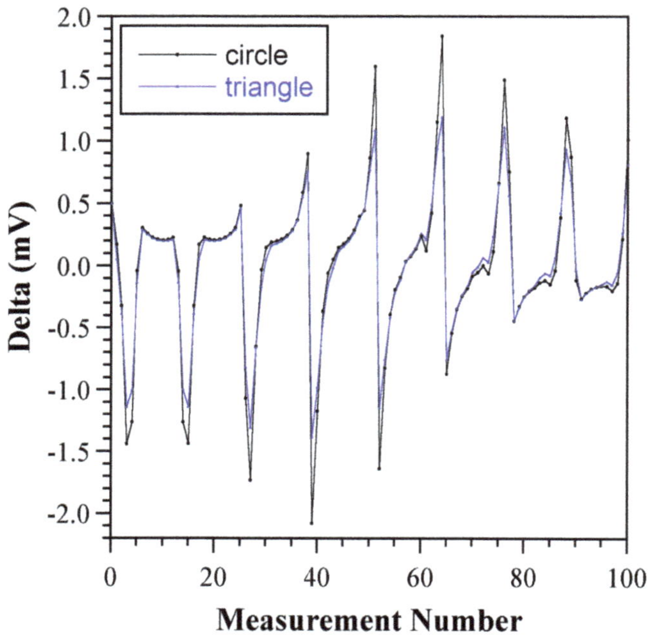

Figure 6.1. The first 100 points in a noise-free voltage signal **Δ**, of 192 total in the measurement frame for this set of parameters, for targets with the shape of circle and a triangle at position $x = 0.5$. (16 electrodes, pseudo-polar–adjacent I–M = 7–1, $\sigma_0 = 10^{-2}$, $\sigma_T = 0.6\sigma_0$ (−40% contrast), $I = 10^{-3}$, noise = 10^{-12}, $r_T = 0.2$)

also been defined as either the L1 norm of **Δ** (e.g. the average) [5, 6] or the L2 norm of **Δ** (root mean square or RMS average) [7], the latter giving more weight to large values. These norms have been referred to as 'total boundary voltage changes' [6, 8].

Because the variations in Δ are not noise, SNR must be obtained by looking at every channel, meaning at every injection and measurement electrode combination in the frame. On each channel j, n measurements of the voltage difference are taken to obtain its average $\overline{\Delta}_j$ and standard deviation, the latter being defined as the noise amplitude n_j [7]:

$$\overline{\Delta}_j = \frac{1}{n}\sum_{k=1}^{n}\Delta_{k,j}, \quad n_j = \sqrt{\mathrm{var}(\Delta_j)} = \sqrt{\frac{1}{n}\sum_{k=1}^{n}\left(\Delta_{k,j} - \overline{\Delta}_j\right)^2} \tag{6.1}$$

Then one definition of SNR for EIT, for real-valued signals, is [9]:

$$\mathrm{SNR} = \frac{\mathrm{E}(|\Delta|)}{\sqrt{\mathrm{var}(\Delta)}} = \frac{\frac{1}{m}\sum_{j=1}^{m}|\overline{\Delta}_j|}{\sqrt{\frac{1}{m}\sum_{j=1}^{n}(n_j)^2}} \tag{6.2}$$

where m is the number of measurements in the frame and E indicates the expected value or average. The absolute values $|\overline{\Delta}_j|$ are used because both positive and negative values contribute information and should not cancel each other. The noise may have contributions from both $\mathbf{V}_{touch}$ and $\mathbf{V}_{ref}$, although typically $\mathbf{V}_{ref}$ is obtained from a large number of measurements and can be treated as noise-free [7]. A channel SNR can also be found for a particular electrode combination, $SNR_{channel} = \overline{\Delta}_j / n_j$ [8, 10]. There is no direct relationship between $SNR_{channel}$ and EIT performance, since the image is reconstructed from multiple sets of data from all the electrodes, but this information can be used in a noise model as input to the reconstruction process.

While using an average signal as defined above makes intuitive sense, one drawback as shown below is that *it is not predictive of noisiness in the reconstructed images when comparing different measurement scenarios*, such as different current injection and voltage measurement (I–M) patterns or varying target positions or sizes, because $\mathbf{\Delta}$ lacks information about how the algorithms interpret the voltage data.

The above definitions of SNR, based on the voltage input signal, must be distinguished from the SNR obtained from the *image* domain, on the EIT output side. An image SNR, also known as the *distinguishability* [7, 11], has frequently been used in the literature, for example for hyperparameter selection [11, 12]. To find SNR_{image} the mean amplitude of the conductivity change within a region of interest (ROI) is calculated from reconstructions made from multiple measurement frames, and the noise amplitude is the standard deviation of those amplitudes. Typically at least ten images are used. An SNR_{image} has alternatively been obtained by comparing the signal strength of each likely target with noise in the vicinity of that target, based on a model of likely noise [12]. The ROI has often been defined as the set of points having an amplitude greater than some threshold, expressed as a fraction $1/f$ of the maximum amplitude A in the image, for example $1/f = ¼$ or ½. Detectability only within this ROI is determined in order to avoid contamination by artefacts outside the ROI [10]. Based on SNR_{image}, a noise figure NF has been defined as the ratio of the output SNR_{image} to the input SNR_{signal} [13] (for details see appendix F.2).

There is another way to consider SNR, which makes use of the singular value decomposition (SVD) of the sensitivity matrix, or Jacobian $\mathbf{J}$, where $\mathbf{J}$ relates the changes in voltages at the sensor perimeter, $\mathbf{\Delta}$, to changes in the conductivity $\boldsymbol{\sigma}$ over the sensor area: $\mathbf{J}\boldsymbol{\sigma} = \mathbf{\Delta}$ (see section 4.3). (In the inverse problem, the vector $\boldsymbol{\sigma}$ is the estimate of the conductivity changes that is displayed as the EIT image.) This approach compares the noise level to the spectrum of coefficients $|\mathbf{U}^T\mathbf{\Delta}|$ [14], where the matrix $\mathbf{U}$ is found from the SVD, $\mathbf{J} = \mathbf{USV}^T$, as discussed in chapter 4. $\mathbf{J}$ can be expressed as the sum of r matrices $s_i\mathbf{u}_i\mathbf{v}_i^T$, where r is the rank of $\mathbf{J}$, where the $\mathbf{u}_i$ and $\mathbf{v}_i$ are orthonormal bases, $\mathbf{U}^T\mathbf{U} = \mathbf{I}$, $\mathbf{V}^T\mathbf{V} = \mathbf{I}$, and where $\mathbf{I}$ is the identity matrix. The rank reflects the number of independent measurements, which is reduced from the total number of measurements by various symmetries [7, 15]. The singular values s_i link patterns of conductivity change on the sensor, expressed by the $\mathbf{v}_i$, to patterns of voltage change at the perimeter, expressed by the $\mathbf{u}_i$. The $\mathbf{v}_i$ are eigen-images that sum to form the EIT image $\boldsymbol{\sigma}$. The $\mathbf{u}_i$ are eigen-signals that sum to form the frame of measured voltages $\mathbf{\Delta}$. *Only* $\mathbf{u}_i$ *larger than the noise contribute real information to the image.* We will show that this approach is the only one of value when comparing different systems and targets.

In experimental practice, the SNR is influenced by the electronics, the amplitude of the injected current, the sensor size and its conductivity, shielding, the injection pattern, the number of electrodes, and so forth, as investigated in detail in [7]. The standard deviation of the noise may be 1–300 μV [16]. At a minimum the noise between an electrode and ground is at the level of the least significant bit of the analog-to-digital converter (ADC). The noise is typically reduced by averaging multiple readings on each measurement electrode before switching to the next position (equation (6.1)), at the cost of greater data collection time. Filtering can also be applied [17].

This chapter employs uncorrelated white Gaussian noise in the simulations. It does not examine real-world experimental noise issues such as common mode noise or capacitive coupling, noise dependence on electrode positions or separations, or noise that is correlated or not normally distributed.

6.1.2 Effect of noise on EIT images

We begin by reviewing the effects of noise on an image. Figure 6.2 shows how, for a given set of simulation parameters, an image first loses fidelity and eventually breaks up completely as the noise amplitude increases (these are so-called 'perturbation errors').

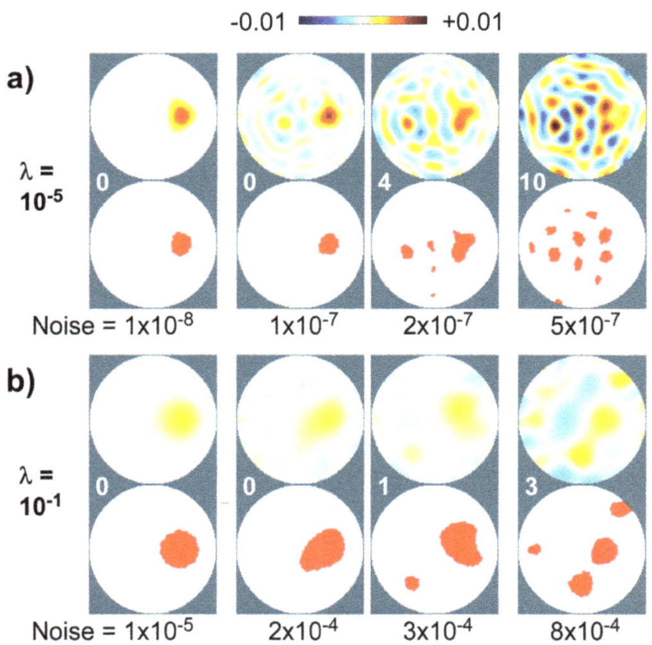

Figure 6.2. EIT images (top rows) and the corresponding HM threshold images (bottom rows) for two hyperparameters: (a) $\lambda = 10^{-5}$ and (b) $\lambda = 10^{-1}$. The noise amplitude increases from left to right; the center two images have noise levels just below and above the onset of artefacts, the number of which is indicated by the white text. The noise threshold N_{th} is the highest level of noise before image artefacts appear. Thus, for (a) $N_{\text{th}} = 1 \times 10^{-7}$ V and for (b) $N_{\text{th}} = 2 \times 10^{-4}$ V. (Decreases in conductivity are shown as red, increases in conductivity as blue, reversed from the convention used in medical imaging.) (16 electrodes, I–M = 7–1, $\sigma_0 = 10^{-2}$, $\sigma_T = 0.6\sigma_0$, $I = 10^{-3}$, triangular target, $r_T = 0.2$, $x = 0.5$)

The noise level at which perturbations appear depends on the hyperparameter λ. (Additional examples are shown in appendix F.10.) Considered in reverse, increasing the hyperparameter results in an onset of stability [18]. Figure 6.2(a) employed a small hyperparameter, $\lambda = 10^{-5}$; the top row shows the EIT images and the second row shows the corresponding $1/f = 1/2$ threshold, or half max (HM), images (HM images were defined in figure 3.2). The onset of artefacts occurred over a narrow noise range; for this case between $N = 1 \times 10^{-7}$ and 2×10^{-7} V. A noise threshold N_{th} is here introduced, defined as the highest level of noise before image artefacts appear. N_{th} was thus 1×10^{-7} at this λ. Above N_{th} the images varied substantially from one simulation run to the next (as shown in appendix F.10 with additional images for circular and triangular targets at 10 x-positions and various levels of noise and hyperparameter).

Near but below N_{th} the shape of the target was distorted, but its size and location were approximately correct. Near but above N_{th}, shortly after the onset of artefacts, the target remained technically 'detectable' in the sense that there was still a peak at the target location. Nonetheless, since in tactile imaging there is no *a priori* knowledge of target numbers and locations, the images became essentially unusable (without further information or processing) above N_{th}. For example, in figure 6.2(a) just above N_{th} there appear to be two targets. Increasing the noise even further, the images broke up into many small peaks, all of which were artefacts.

Figure 6.2(b) employed, using the same target, the much larger hyperparameter $\lambda = 10^{-1}$, and N_{th} was thus orders of magnitude higher. As discussed in chapter 4 and chapter 5, larger λ results in a loss of concentration of the image energy, meaning the

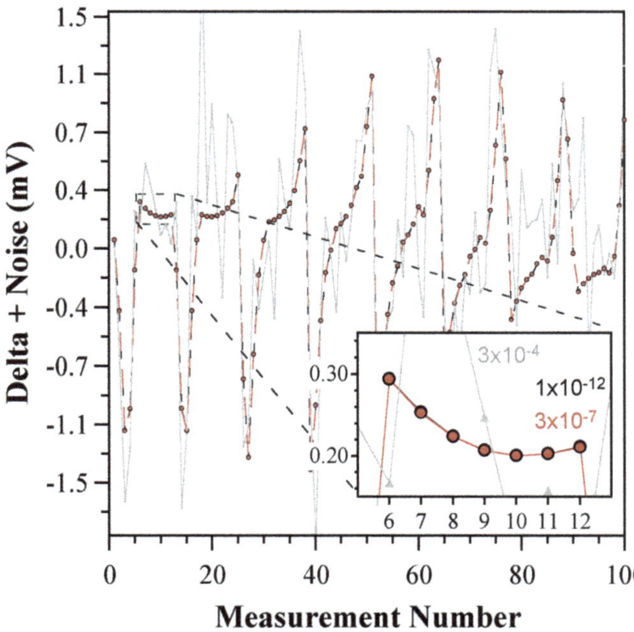

Figure 6.3. The first 100 terms (of 192) of the vector of voltage differences $\mathbf{\Delta} = \mathbf{V}_{touch} - \mathbf{V}_{ref}$ for the target of figure 6.2 with varying amounts of noise, indicated in the inset, which shows a close-up of the region enclosed by the dashed rectangle. (16 electrodes, I–M = 7–1, $\sigma_0 = 10^{-2}$, $\sigma_T = 0.6\sigma_0$, $I = 10^{-3}$, triangular target, $r_T = 0.2$, $x = 0.5$)

feature broadens and reduces in amplitude (these are so-called 'regularization errors'), which is evident in figure 6.3(b). Again there was a narrow range, relative to the greater noise amplitude, over which artefacts began to appear. Again the target was identifiable, although distorted, below N_{th}, but above N_{th} it was unclear how many targets there were. The artefacts were larger at the higher λ since the eigen-images available for reconstruction were of lower spatial frequency as discussed in chapter 5.

To provide some context for the size of the noise values in figure 6.2, figure 6.3 shows white noise added to the voltage signal $\mathbf{\Delta} = \mathbf{V}_{touch} - \mathbf{V}_{ref}$ (black points are the same as the blue curve in figure 6.1). On this plot noise of $N = 3 \times 10^{-7}$ V, which leads to break-up of the image at $\lambda = 10^{-5}$, cannot be distinguished from the case with virtually no noise, 1×10^{-12} V, even in close-up; the noise-free (black) and noisy (red) points coincide on this scale. This level of noise is 1000 times smaller than the values of $\mathbf{\Delta}$ shown in the inset (0.3 μV on top of measurements of 0.2–0.3 mV). This example illustrates the problem that small perturbations in the data can lead to large perturbations in the solution, so large, in fact, that the solution does not resemble the target at all: the EIT image is not even approximately correct (figure 6.2(a)). For experimentalists familiar with noise on other types of data (e.g. from voltage divider circuits), this extreme noise sensitivity may come as a surprise. Thus, for tactile imaging it is unrealistic to expect that hyperparameters as small as 10^{-5} can be used. A noise amplitude of 3×10^{-4}, which is high but in some cases realistic, would result in artefacts even using $\lambda = 10^{-1}$ of figure 6.2(b). This amount of noise is comparable to the values in $\mathbf{\Delta}$ and is readily obvious in looking at the voltage data. The large value of λ required to suppress artefacts in this case results in regularization errors that are so large as to confound the detection of multiple touches, as shown in chapter 5.

6.1.3 Signal-to-noise ratio

The results presented above were for a particular combination of forward problem parameters. A question to be asked by new tactile imaging experimentalists is then, 'in general what is the required SNR?' Answering this question first requires an understanding of what the SNR is for EIT, which means understanding what the 'signal' is. The definition of noise is well accepted and the amount of noise is known, in principle, since it can be obtained by taking repeated measurements at the electrodes. This sub-section then addresses the issue of *how* miniscule amounts of noise, relative to the measured voltages, can create such havoc in the images, continuing the discussion from section 4.6.

6.1.3.1 Smallest Values of Δ

It has been said that the smallest values in $\mathbf{\Delta}$ determine the quality of the image since they are the most changed by noise [6], and it has been pointed out that the value of a large voltage can be measured more precisely than that of a small one [19]. This assertion would appear to be logical: the smaller the voltage difference, the relatively more a perturbation will change it.

To test the assertion, noise was added selectively to the lowest (red points in figure 6.4(a)) and highest (blue) 20% of voltage values in $\mathbf{\Delta}$. The approach is illustrated

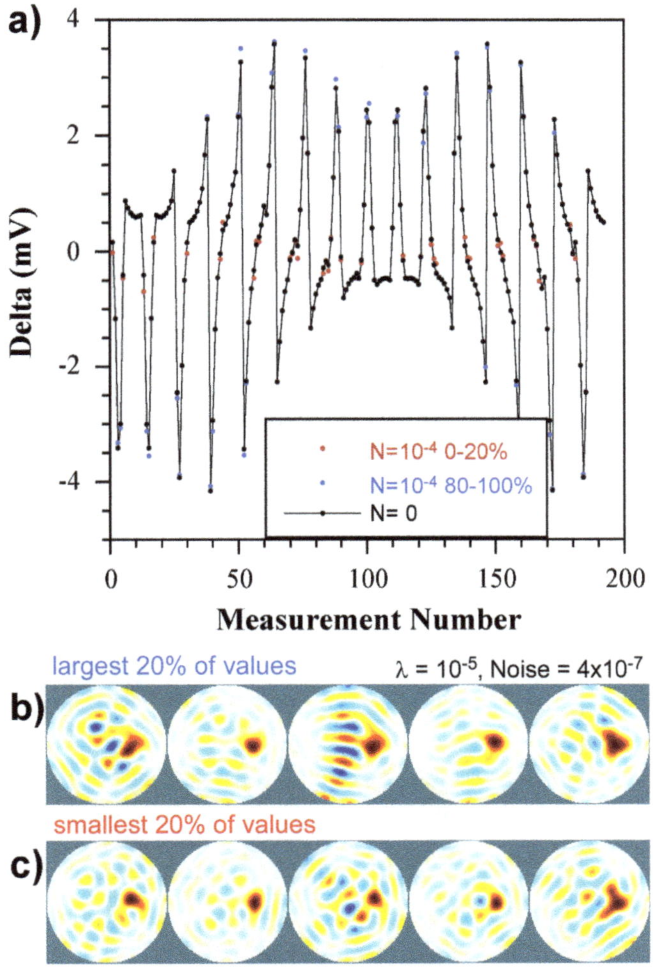

Figure 6.4. (a) Illustration of the method of selectively adding noise. The vector of voltage differences **Δ** with noise added selectively to the smallest (red) and largest (blue) 20% of measurements, compared with measurements without added noise (black). A large value of noise, $N = 10^{-4}$,was used to allow visualization of the method. (b) Using $\lambda = 10^{-5}$, the effect on a set of five EIT images of a smaller amount of noise, $N = 4 \times 10^{-7}$, added to the largest 20% of values in **Δ**. (c) The effect of the same amount of noise added to the smallest 20% of values in **Δ**. (16 electrodes, I–M = 7–1, $\sigma_0 = 10^{-2}$, $\sigma_T = 0.6\sigma_0$, $I = 3 \times 10^{-3}$, triangular target $r_T = 0.2$, $x = 0.5$) (Color bars approximately ±0.009, varying between images.)

in figure 6.4(a) for noise of 10^{-4} V, employing a large value to allow the deviations to be clearly visible in the plot. The effect on EIT images is shown in figure 6.4(b,c) for a smaller value of noise ($N = 4 \times 10^{-7}$); five runs are shown to indicate the reproducibility.

While adding noise to only 20% of the points in **Δ** improved the image stability compared to adding it to 100% of the points, it made no substantial difference whether it was added to largest or smallest voltages in the frame (compare figure 6.4(b) and (c)). Thus, the smallest voltage differences in **Δ** do *not* determine noisiness in the image.

6.1.3.2 Average value of Δ

It has been suggested in the literature that experimental configurations with overall larger **Δ** should be more immune to noise [6–8]. Also, the noise figure NF, defined as the ratio of the voltage SNR to the image SNR [20, 21], utilizes the L1 norm $E(|\boldsymbol{\Delta}|) = ||\boldsymbol{\Delta}||_1 = \sum|\Delta_i|$, the average of the absolute values of **Δ**. The distinguishability metric utilizes the L2 norm $||\boldsymbol{\Delta}||_2 = \sqrt{\sum(\Delta_i)^2}$, and it was proposed that this be used as the definition of signal strength [7].

For a given sensor configuration (here 16 electrodes and I–M = 7–1) *and target* (here triangular at $x = 0.5$), the overall size of **Δ** was a good estimate of the signal, as demonstrated by N_{th} increasing proportionally with $E(|\boldsymbol{\Delta}|)$. Figure 6.5 shows N_{th} and $E(|\boldsymbol{\Delta}|)$ as a function of target contrast and sensor background conductivity; both increased linearly with the contrast. Note that for different sensor conductivities, the hyperparameter was scaled as specified in table 4.2 to provide the same extent of regularization (effective hyperparameter). Again, N_{th} was well predicted by $E(|\boldsymbol{\Delta}|)$. Note that lowering the sensor conductivity improved the noise immunity, even

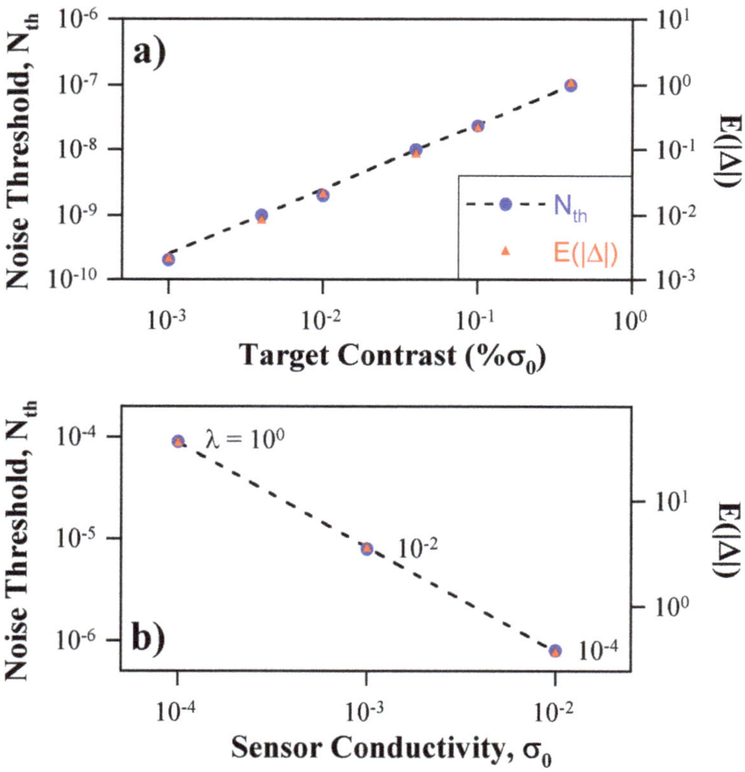

Figure 6.5. (a) The maximum noise before artifacts appear, N_{th}, and the average value of the measured voltages, $E(|\Delta|)$, as a function of target contrast ($\lambda = 10^{-5}$, $\sigma_0 = 10^{-2}$, $\sigma_T = 0.6\sigma_0$ to $0.999\sigma_0$ for contrast −40% to −0.1%). (b) N_{th} and $E(|\Delta|)$ as a function of sensor conductivity σ_0 ($\sigma_T=0.6\sigma_0$, contrast −40%). The hyperparameter was scaled as in table 4.2. (16 electrodes, I–M = 7–1, $I = 10^{-3}$, triangular target, $r_T = 0.2$, $x = 0.5$)

though the absolute contrast decreased (the relative contrast was constant) since higher resistivity increases the signal through Ohm's law.

Measured voltage differences increase with the target distance from the center, or x-position, as shown in figure 6.6(a), since more current passes through areas of the sensor near the edge than near the center. Noise thresholds at two levels of regularization are shown in figure 6.6(b,c). At small λ, N_{th} showed no clear dependence on x-position, with N_{th} near 1×10^{-7} V everywhere. At larger λ a dependence emerged: for $\lambda = 10^{-2}$, N_{th} increased from 3×10^{-5} V near the center to 7×10^{-5} V at the perimeter. *The information one can obtain from* E(|**Δ**|) *is thus incomplete, insufficient for predicting noise susceptibility if the target changes.*

Another question to be addressed is, does the metric E(|**Δ**|) allow comparison across systems? Prior work has found that noise depends on the I–M pattern, an issue taken up in detail in chapter 7. For a fixed current, placing current injection or voltage measurement electrodes on opposite sides of the sensor (position 8 for a 16-electrode system; see figure 4.2) or nearly opposite sides (position 7) yields the largest voltage differences, due to higher resistive drops (see section 4.2.2) compared to placing electrodes in adjacent positions (position 1), which yields the smallest voltage differences. Thus, the pseudo-polar–adjacent combination 7–1 was deemed to have the best

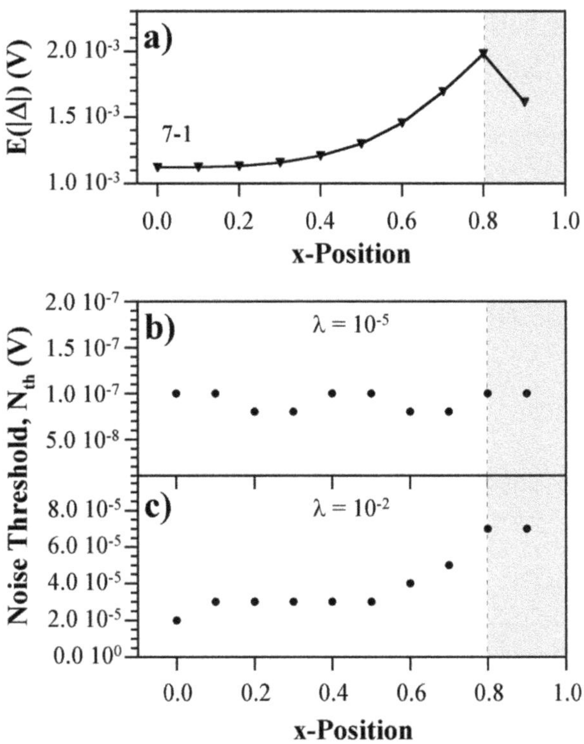

Figure 6.6. (a) Average of the absolute value of **Δ** as a function of target x-position. Noise threshold as a function of x-position at hyperparameters of (b) $\lambda = 10^{-5}$ and (c) $\lambda = 10^{-2}$. The gray areas indicate where the target extends beyond the sensor perimeter. (16 electrodes, I–M = 7–1, $\sigma_0 = 10^{-2}$, $\sigma_T = 0.6\sigma_0$, $I = 10^{-3}$, triangular target, $r_T = 0.2$)

noise performance based on an experimental resistor model [6]. In a study of the noise immunity of four I–M patterns using an undefined disturbance identification metric, the pseudo-polar pattern withstood six times more noise than the adjacent pattern [6]. Based on distinguishability, 7–1 outperformed other #–1 patterns [11], where # indicates an unspecified injection position. Using resolution as a metric, it was found that 7–1 outperformed 1–1 using a fixed hyperparameter and fixed level of noise [17]. It must be pointed out that the latter result also reflected the effect of λ on resolution, not just its effect on noise.

Figure 6.7 shows E(|**Δ**|) for a target at positions between $x = 0$ and 0.9 for three injection–measurement patterns: 1–1, 7–1, and 7–7. (The **Δ** are shown in appendix F.1.) The averages were significantly different, as has been shown in prior work [7, 8]. On the basis of figure 6.7 one would expect 7–7 to have by far the best noise performance because its E|**Δ**| is so much larger, as just discussed. At $x = 0.5$, E(|**Δ**|) is five times larger for 7–1 than 1–1, and for 7–7 it is 17 times larger. (All bipolar I–M patterns are compared in depth in chapter 7.) At $x = 0.0$ the relative differences are even larger, by factors of 7 and 25, respectively. Also shown in the figure are the L2 norms and the maximum values in **Δ**. The former had the same behavior as E(|**Δ**|), but with the larger values amplified. For 1–1 the differences between the maximum values at the center and the edge were proportionally the largest. Physically, this difference occurs because little of the current flows through the center of the sensing area, flowing instead predominantly between peripheral electrodes (see figure 4.2). For 7–1, the maximum

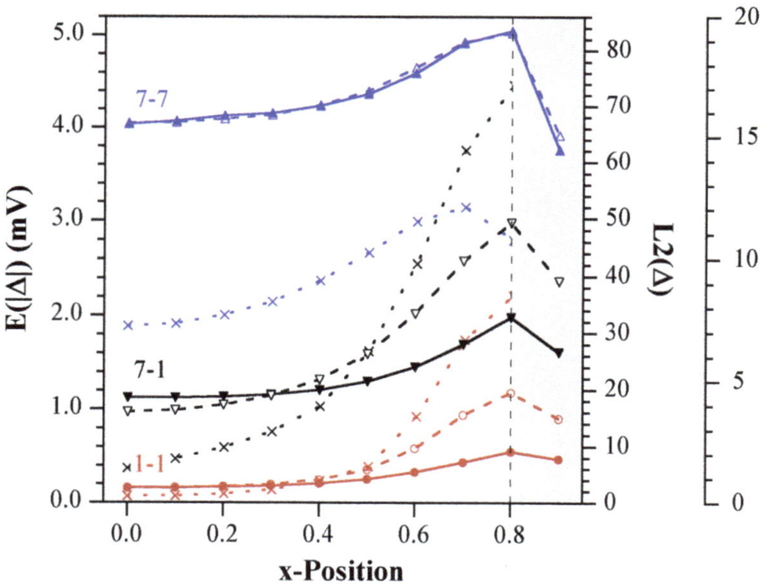

Figure 6.7. The average of the absolute values of **Δ** (solid symbols), E(|**Δ**|), as a function of position along the x-axis for a circular target for the 1–1 (red, adjacent), 7–1 (black, pseudo-polar), and 7–7 (blue, pseudo-polar–pseudo-polar) I–M patterns. Also shown are the L2 norm (root mean square) of **Δ** (open symbols) and maximum values of **Δ** (× symbols). The shaded area on the right indicates where the target extended beyond the sensing area. (16 electrodes, $\sigma_0 = 10^{-2}$, $\sigma_T = 0.6\sigma_0$, $I = 3 \times 10^{-3}$, circular target, $r_T = 0.2$)

values were actually higher than those for 7–7. The most uniformity in values was found in 7–7. A small dynamic range of the voltage values has been said to be the most favorable for SNR [6], and it has been pointed out that a large dynamic range requires a better data acquisition system [19]. Thus, 7–7 would also be expected to be highly favored regarding noise immunity.

Figure 6.8 compares five replicate reconstructions for a target at $x = 0.5$ from the three I–M patterns at two noise levels using $\lambda = 10^{-5}$ (corresponding to N_{th} and $2N_{\text{th}}$ for I–M = 7–1). *The images do not show the large differences in SNR performance that were expected* on the basis of thinking about signal strength in terms of average **Δ**. Instead, all three patterns gave similar reconstructions for the same noise. As shown below, there were measurable differences among the patterns, but they were substantially smaller than the differences in **Δ**. Small differences between the patterns may be detected by running a large number of trials, and such a statistical approach has been used in the medical EIT literature to justify the use of one pattern

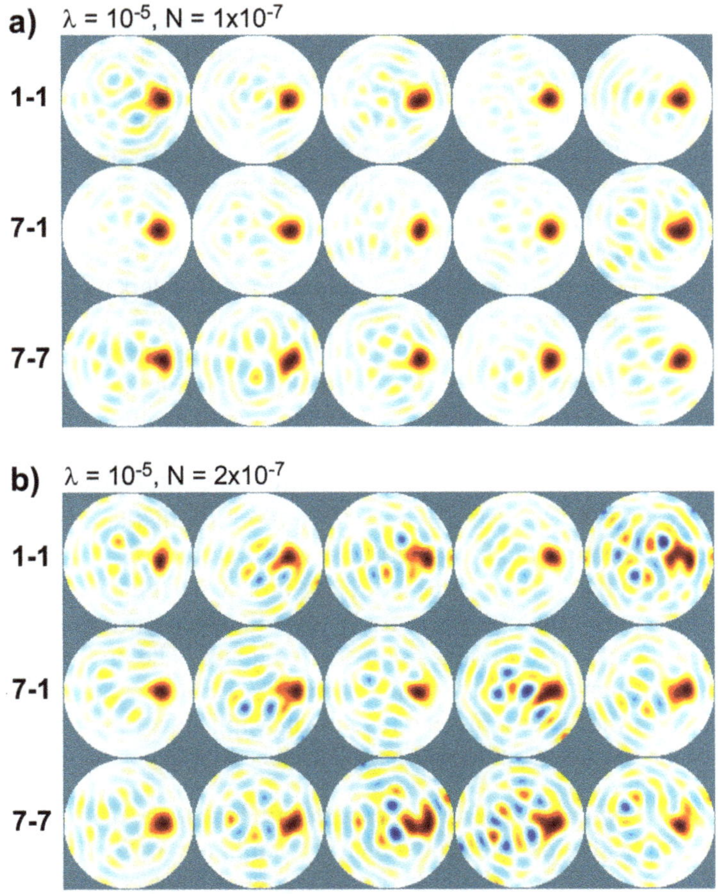

Figure 6.8. Reconstructions using $\lambda = 10^{-5}$ for a circular target at $x = 0.5$ for three I–M patterns, indicated on the left, with two levels of noise: (a,c) N = 1×10^{-7} and (b,d) at $N = 2 \times 10^{-7}$. (16 electrodes, $\sigma_0 = 10^{-2}$, $\sigma_T = 0.6\sigma_0$, $I = 3 \times 10^{-3}$, $r_T = 0.2$, $\lambda_s = 3 \times 10^{-7}$) (color scales ±0.007)

over another [11]. However, to those interested in the question of how many tactile targets there are and where, EIT images from all three I–M patterns began to lose practical value at broadly similar levels of noise. Thus, once again, the use of E(|**Δ**|) as a measure of the signal strength is seen to be incomplete: it is missing critical system information. (Peak amplitude was also examined to determine whether there was a significant difference in performance among the three patterns with noise at N_{th}, as shown in appendix F.6; there was not.)

6.1.3.3 $U^T\Delta$ and $V^T\sigma$

As mentioned in section 6.1.1, there is another conceptualization of 'signal' that can be compared with noise for EIT [14, 22, 23]. The voltage vector **Δ** can be expressed in terms of a set of basis vectors $\mathbf{u}_i$, where i is the singular value index. The $\mathbf{u}_i$ with small i correspond to the largest singular values s_i, and they carry most of the information about the touch. (Examples of the component vectors $\mathbf{u}_i$ are shown in appendix F.3.) In this approach the 'signal' is a weighted sum of the $\mathbf{u}_i$ or 'eigen-Δ'. The weights are given by the product $|\mathbf{U}^{\mathrm{T}}\boldsymbol{\Delta}|$, which yields a spectrum of coefficients $P_i = |\mathbf{u}_i^{\mathrm{T}}\boldsymbol{\Delta}|$ known as Picard coefficients [24] (also termed Fourier coefficients [25]). (The P_i can be found by adapting the Matlab EIDORS code; our codes are available upon request.) The P_i indicate the importance of the contribution of a particular $\mathbf{u}_i$ to the signal. The P_i have units of volts and can be compared to the noise. The $\mathbf{u}_i$ depend only on the system forward problem parameters, such as the I–M pattern and number of electrodes.

Thinking of the signal in terms of $|\mathbf{U}^{\mathrm{T}}\boldsymbol{\Delta}|$ adds system information, via the $\mathbf{u}_i$. Since intrinsic resolution can be formulated as the number of independent measurements that contribute meaningful information at a given noise level [3, 7], also phrased as the number singular values that are useful in the reconstruction, this conceptualization of the signal directly connects to the issue of the required regularization.

Noise has alternatively been compared to the singular values s_i when discussing noise immunity. The two spectra have similar appearance (see appendix D.6). However, the s_i pertain to **J** and therefore only reflect the measurement system, whereas the product $|\mathbf{U}^{\mathrm{T}}\boldsymbol{\Delta}|$ also carries information about the current, the target, and other factors through the measured voltage differences **Δ**.

The s_i, $\mathbf{u}_i$, and $\mathbf{v}_i$ at the singular value index i are linked. Chapter 5 made extensive use, on the image side, of the analogous spectra $|\mathbf{V}^{\mathrm{T}}\boldsymbol{\sigma}|$ [14], which show the contributions of particular eigen-images $\mathbf{v}_i$ to the final reconstructed image. The product $\mathbf{SV}^{\mathrm{T}}\boldsymbol{\sigma}$ can also be found. It is equivalent to $\mathrm{U}^{\mathrm{T}}\boldsymbol{\Delta}$ at small λ, since $\mathbf{J}\boldsymbol{\sigma} = \mathbf{USV}^{\mathrm{T}}\boldsymbol{\sigma} = \boldsymbol{\Delta}$. Unlike $\mathrm{U}^{\mathrm{T}}\boldsymbol{\Delta}$, $\mathbf{SV}^{\mathrm{T}}\boldsymbol{\sigma}$ (via $\boldsymbol{\sigma}$) is affected by the hyperparameter (as shown in appendix F.8). In fact, $C_i = P_i/s_i$ at small λ [23]; at larger λ the C_i at higher i are dampened.

6.1.3.3.1 Picard coefficients, noise, and component Eigen-signals $\mathbf{u}_i$

Figure 6.9(a) (duplicated here for convenience from figure 4.19(a)) shows the first 50 coefficients P_i without noise for circular and triangular targets, plotted in order of their singular value index i. Referring back to the corresponding plot of **Δ** in figure 6.1, differences in **Δ** for the two targets are translated into differences in P_i. *The largest P_i dominate E(|**Δ**|).*

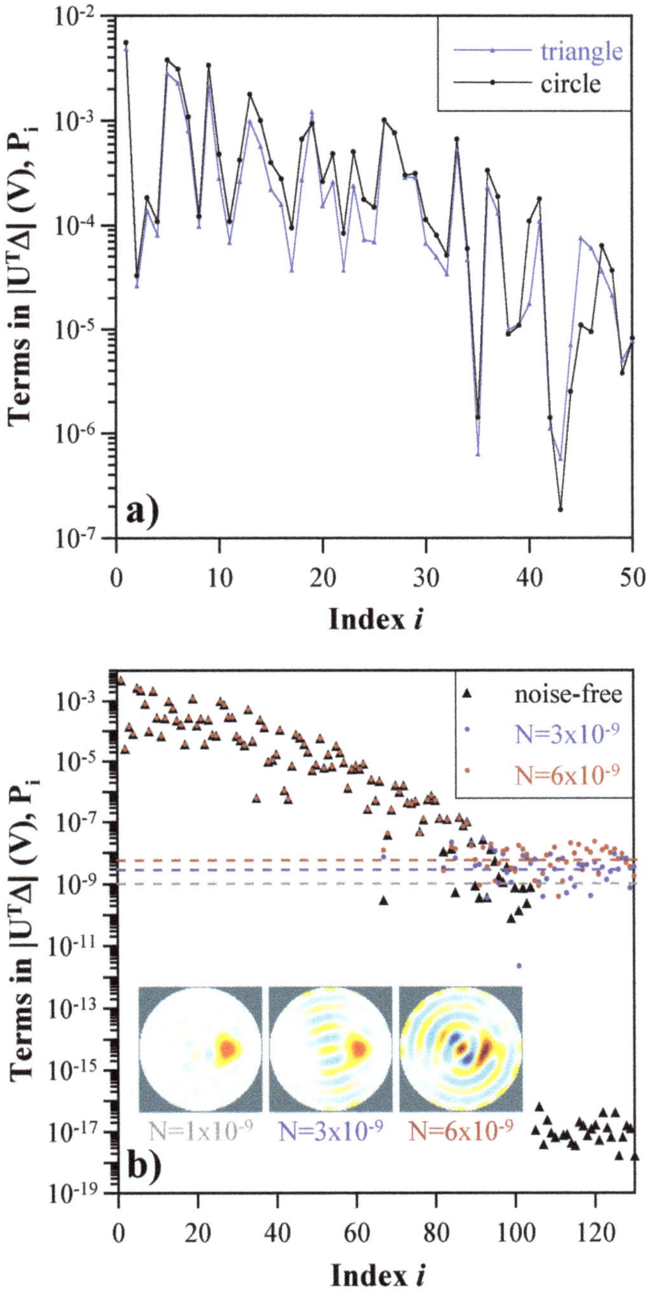

Figure 6.9. (a) The first 50 $|\mathbf{U}^T\mathbf{\Delta}|$ terms, or Picard coefficients P_i, as a function of singular value index i for triangular and circular targets at $x = 0.5$, without added noise. (b) The first 130 $|\mathbf{U}^T\mathbf{\Delta}|$ terms for a triangular target without noise and with noise at two levels. The corresponding EIT images at $\lambda = 10^{-7}$ are included. (16 electrodes, I–M = 7–1, $\sigma_0 = 10^{-2}$, $\sigma_T = 0.6\sigma_0$, $I = 1 \times 10^{-3}$, $r_T = 0.2$)

Figure 6.9(b) shows the first 130 P_i for the triangular target when two levels of noise were added, indicated by the dashed horizontal lines. Below the noise, the coefficients were perturbed. (Coefficients somewhat larger than the average noise values were also affected, due to the standard deviation of the noise.) Using the smallest hyperparameter at which reconstructions could be reliably created using these simulation parameters, $\lambda = 10^{-7}$, the noise threshold was found to be $N_{\text{th}} = 3 \times 10^{-9}$ V (see EIT image insets). At $N = 6 \times 10^{-9}$ V, the images showed artefacts. Terms beyond position 104 (the rank of **J**), which are nominally zero but are actually small values near 10^{-17} V due to numerical noise, did not play a role in the reconstruction: raising their values by 8 orders of magnitude by adding $N = 1 \times 10^{-9}$ V, which is larger than the smallest of the 104 contributing terms, did not interfere with the creation of a good image.

Noise creates incorrect images because of these incorrect amplitudes of the $\mathbf{u}_i$. Corrupted terms are used when they should be disregarded, known as 'over-fitting'. The P_i associated with the signal decay with i and then level off at the noise level. The index i at which leveling occurs is the Picard threshold. When using truncated SVD for regularization, the truncation is chosen to start at the index i at which the P_i begin to flatten due to noise [26].

As noise increases, the number of eigen-images $\mathbf{v}_i$ that can be usefully employed in the reconstruction decreases. The $\mathbf{v}_i$ corresponding to P_i in the noise plateau should be ignored as shown in the next section, 6.1.3.3.2, which is done by increasing λ. Regularization results in smoothing because image information, expressed by the $\mathbf{v}_i$, above a certain i is replaced by 'prior information', which is by default taken to be a uniform conductivity everywhere. (The correct background conductivity profile σ_0 must be employed. A mistaken assumption of a homogeneous background conductivity may result in substantial errors, as has been shown for medical imaging [27, 28]. That is also the case for tactile sensors that have a spatially-varying sensor baseline conductivity σ_0 [16].) Raising λ increases the number of $\mathbf{v}_\text{i}$ that are diminished.

The P_i can be compared with the singular values. If the P_i decay to zero faster than the s_i, then the regularized solution to the inverse problem is guaranteed to be approximately correct [25]. Known as the discrete Picard condition, it holds for those i below which P_i/s_i takes a positive slope [22, 23], which is essentially where the noise plateau begins. In other words, if $\mathbf{v}_\text{i}$ corresponding to P_i that are corrupted by noise are used in the reconstruction, instead of being eliminated by regularization, the image breaks up and is no longer an approximation of the target.

Scaling was discussed above with respect to the required hyperparameter (section 4.4.4). Changing injection current, sensor conductivity, and contrast produces proportional up or down shifting of the $|\mathbf{U}^\text{T}\boldsymbol{\Delta}|$ spectra (shown in appendix F.4) because $\boldsymbol{\Delta}$ is linearly proportional to contrast and current and inversely proportional to conductivity (figure 6.5). (The basis functions $\mathbf{u}_i$ are unaffected by these parameters.) Downward shifts, such as due to higher conductivity, make the system more susceptible to noise.

6.1.3.3.2 *Eigen-images, the spectrum $V^T\sigma$, and noise*

It is instructive, to gain an intuitive understanding of how noise affects EIT images, to examine the spectrum $\mathbf{V}^{\mathrm{T}}\boldsymbol{\sigma}$, sorted by the index *i*. This spectrum of coefficients C_i gives the amplitudes of the eigen-images $\mathbf{v}_i$ that form the image, with the smallest *i* correspond to the lowest frequency components $\mathbf{v}_i$ of the image, and the highest *i* to the highest frequency $\mathbf{v}_i$. Figure 6.10 (duplicated here for convenience from figure 4.20) shows spectra at $\lambda = 10^{-6}$ at increasing noise levels, as well as a spectrum at $\lambda = 10^{-5}$ at the top noise level. The corresponding EIT images above the plot show the outcomes of negligible noise, noise just at N_{th}, noise just above N_{th}, and noise above N_{th} with a lager hyperparameter. The amplitudes of the eigen-image $\mathbf{v}_{101}$ are shown in the inset.

Below index $i = 80$, all four spectra were identical. With negligible noise (black line), at high *i* (up to 104) the coefficients were of comparable amplitude as those at lower *i*, and the EIT image was a good approximation to the target. With increasing noise *N*, the

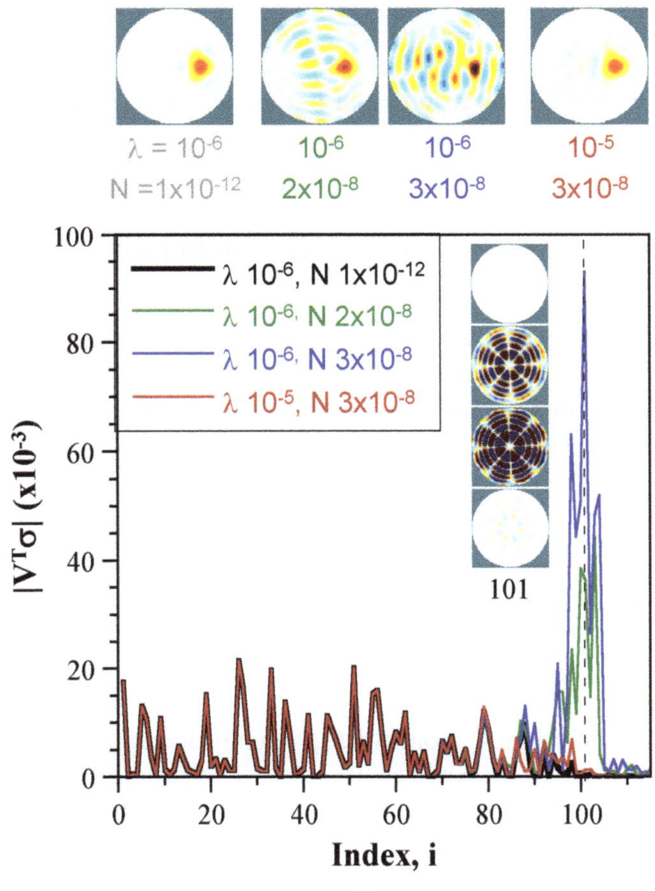

Figure 6.10. The effects of increasing noise and λ on the $\mathbf{V}^{\mathrm{T}}\boldsymbol{\sigma}$ spectrum (coefficients C_i) of a triangular target at $x = 0.5$. The corresponding EIT images are included at the top. Also shown are the $\mathbf{v}_{101}$ for each case, ordered top to bottom in the same way as the legend. (16 electrodes, I–M = 7–1, $\sigma_0 = 10^{-2}$, $\sigma_{\mathrm{T}} = 0.6\sigma_0$, $I = 1 \times 10^{-3}$, $r_{\mathrm{T}} = 0.2$)

spectra began to show increasing, unpredictable contributions from the high-index eigen-images $\mathbf{v}_i$, due to the disturbance of the corresponding $\mathbf{u}_i$ by noise, as illustrated in figure 6.9(b). For example, the amplitude of $\mathbf{v}_{101}$ was virtually zero at $N = 10^{-12}$ V and increased in intensity with increasing N. At $N = 2 \times 10^{-8}$ V (green line) the EIT image developed strong ringing, although it still had no artifacts. At $N = 3 \times 10^{-8}$ V, with the incorrect Picard coefficients being even larger, the EIT image developed artifacts. Above a certain noise level, contributions of the high-frequency eigen-images dominate the final image, resulting in a solution that is no longer approximately correct. (It has alternatively been stated that the singular values s_i must be above the Picard threshold.) Raising λ to 10^{-5}, the amplitudes of terms above $i = 87$ were dampened, effectively eliminating those eigen-images from the sum and thereby removing artefacts from the image. Thus, the noise threshold, and any other measure of noise susceptibility, is directly related to how many $\mathbf{v}_i$ affected by noise are removed, which depends on the slope of the λ versus i curve (see section 5.1), which in turn depends on the I–M pattern. Of course, with increasing λ the resolution of the image is reduced, since the high-frequency components of the solution are removed. (For illustrations see [29] and section 5.1.) (The $\mathbf{U}^{\mathrm{T}}\mathbf{\Delta}$, $\mathbf{V}^{\mathrm{T}}\boldsymbol{\sigma}$, and s_i are compared in appendix F.5.)

This example illustrated how the EIT images are corrupted by small levels of noise and how regularization works. It also illustrated how not all eigen-images are equally sensitive to noise: that is determined by the corresponding P_i, as shown in figure 6.9(b).

6.2 Dependence of noise susceptibility on measurement conditions and target characteristics

Given the understanding from section 6.1 that SNR can be understood by examining the Picard coefficients, this chapter presents the effects of various measurement conditions and target characteristics on noise susceptibility.

6.2.1 I–M pattern

To shed light on the noise sensitivity of the three I–M patterns considered in figure 6.7 and figure 6.8, their $|\mathbf{U}^{\mathrm{T}}\mathbf{\Delta}|$ spectra are shown in figure 6.11(a). The three I–M patterns have the same number of non-negligible terms (same rank), $r = 104$.

For 7–7, the largest coefficients P_i at small i were above the largest for 7–1, and both were far above those for 1–1. As mentioned previously, the largest P_i dominate $\mathrm{E}(|\mathbf{\Delta}|)$, and they account for the high measured voltages seen in figure 6.7 for 7–7 compared to 1–1. However, the differences among the P_i gradually disappeared moving rightward, until by the 50th position the coefficients for all three patterns were similar. At even higher index the amplitudes of the spectra actually reversed, with 1–1 having the largest P_i. Figure 6.11(a) also indicates noise at $N = 1 \times 10^{-7}$ V (horizontal line), which for a hyperparameter of 10^{-5} was the noise threshold for 1–1. This plot clarifies why the three patterns had the same noise performance at that N and λ (figure 6.8(a)). At $N = 3 \times 10^{-7}$ V the reconstructions failed at $\lambda = 10^{-5}$ (figure 6.8(b)): a larger λ is required to handle that amount of noise.

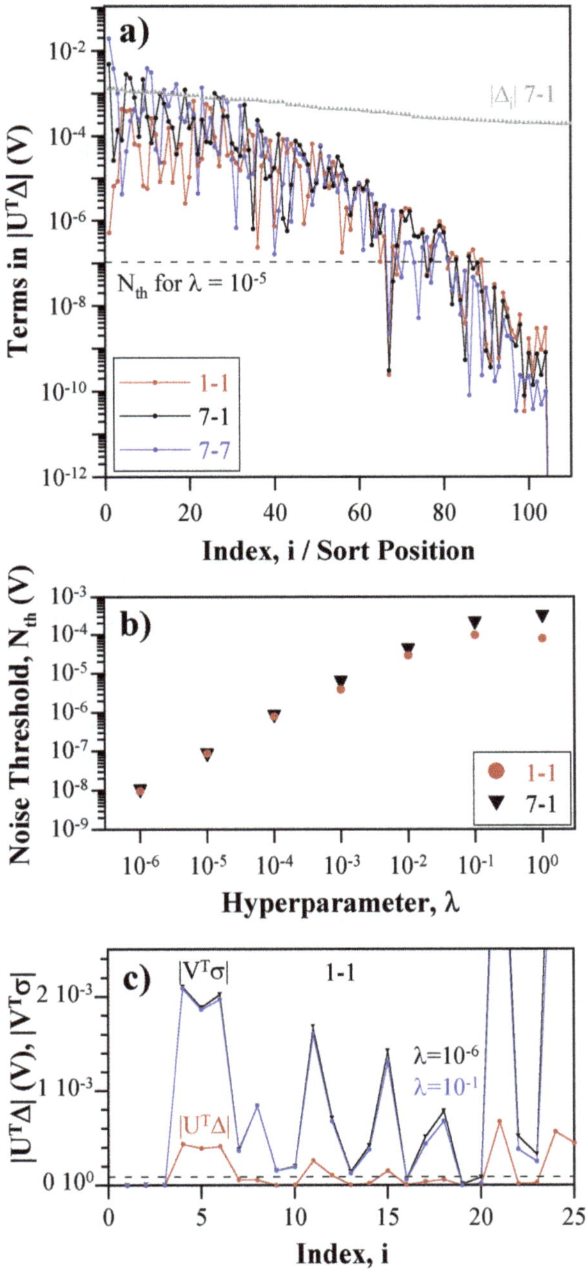

Figure 6.11. (a) The sorted absolute values of the P_i, without noise, for three injection–measurement patterns, I–M = 1–1, 7–1, and 7–7, with a triangular target at $x = 0.5$ (color symbols). The horizontal line indicates noise of 1×10^{-7} V, corresponding to figure 6.8(a). For $\lambda = 10^{-5}$, this level is the noise threshold N_{th} for 1–1. Also shown are the absolute values of the voltage differences Δ_i, sorted by amplitude, for 7–1 (gray triangle symbols). (b) Noise thresholds as a function of hyperparameter for I–M = 1–1 and 7–1. (c) Shown on a linear scale, a close-up of the $|\mathbf{U}^{\text{T}}\mathbf{\Delta}|$ and $|\mathbf{V}^{\text{T}}\boldsymbol{\sigma}|$ spectra (the P_i and C_i, respectively) for 1–1, the latter at two hyperparameters. $N = 10^{-4}$ V is indicated by the horizontal dashed line. (16 electrodes, $\sigma_0 = 10^{-2}$, $\sigma_{\text{T}} = 0.6\sigma_0$, $I = 1 \times 10^{-3}$, $r_{\text{T}} = 0.2$)

For comparison, the $|\Delta_i|$ without noise for 7–1 are also shown in figure 6.11(a) (gray triangles), sorted by their size. Most of the Picard coefficients P_i are much smaller than the Δ_i, graphically illustrating why the EIT images are so sensitive to noise and why averages of $\boldsymbol{\Delta}$ do not serve as a guide to noise performance when system parameters change. This curve is also a reminder that the number of independent terms (104) is smaller than the number of measurements (192 for 7–1 and 208 for 1–1 and 7–7).

Figure 6.11(b) compares the noise thresholds for I–M = 1–1 and 7–1. Up to a noise level of $N = 10^{-6}$ V ($\lambda = 10^{-4}$) their N_{th} were the same, consistent with their $|\mathbf{U}^{\mathrm{T}}\boldsymbol{\Delta}|$ spectra. By $N = 10^{-5}$ V ($\lambda = 10^{-3}$), the N_{th} started to separate. The N_{th} for 7–1 had grown to 2x and 4x larger at $\lambda = 10^{-1}$ and 10^{0}, respectively. Comparing with figure 6.11(a), the N_{th} and P_i followed each other closely. For example, at low i the P_i for 1–1 flattened at 10^{-4}, and N_{th} was limited to 1×10^{-4} V. The $|\mathbf{U}^{\mathrm{T}}\boldsymbol{\Delta}|$ spectra thus allow comparison of different electrode configurations.

Figure 6.11(c) shows a noise-free close-up of the first 25 P_i for 1–1, along with the C_i at two values of λ. At $N = 10^{-4}$ V (horizontal dashed line), which is the N_{th} at $\lambda = 10^{-1}$, the P_i at i = 7–10 would be below the noise, and thus corrupted. The corresponding C_7–C_{10} would be affected. At $\lambda = 10^{-1}$ damping just reaches $i = 13$ (C_{13} is 5% smaller than its value at $\lambda = 10^{-6}$), and as a result the corresponding C_7–C_{10} remain undamped. Thus, the image would be perturbed. This example illustrates what is meant in the literature that at a certain noise level, the number of singular values that can be employed by the reconstruction is limited.

At the highest noise levels, differences in the largest P_i lead to differences in noise performance, as expected from E($|\boldsymbol{\Delta}|$) (figure 6.7). Differences in N_{th} among these I–M spectra, which all have the same rank, appear at large λ where, as shown in chapter 5, behavior becomes increasingly dominated by loss of sensitivity to conductivity changes at the center of the sensor.

The comparison of the I–M patterns at the same λ in figure 6.11(b) is not entirely 'apples to apples'. As shown in chapter 5, raising λ had a greater effect on 1–1 than on 7–1: the slope $\mathrm{d}i/\mathrm{d}\lambda$ at which $\mathbf{v}_i$ at index i were dampened as λ increased, was higher for 1–1. Thus for large λ, 1–1 had smaller contributions than 7–1 from the $\mathbf{v}_i$ eigen-images and larger contributions from prior information. One would hence need to employ a smaller λ with 1–1 to obtain a similar resolution to that of 7–1. In addition, in figure 6.11(a) at large λ the pattern 7–1 had a greater number of coefficients above a given noise level than 1–1. The number of P_i above N_{th} is plotted versus N_{th} in figure 6.12(a). Not only were the N_{th} on the x-axis higher for 7–1 than 1–1, but so were their positions on the y-axis. Thus, not only was 7–1 more noise immune, but it also had a larger number of contributing $\mathbf{v}_i$ at the λ needed for its N_{th}, resulting in finer resolution. Upward shifts of the Picard spectra are thus doubly beneficial.

Cross-sections are shown in figure 6.12(b) to demonstrate this difference in resolution. At $\lambda = 10^{-1}$ the peak for 7–1 (black) was more focused than the peak for 1–1 (red), which was true in the absence and in the presence of the same amount of noise. Thus, while the performance of 1–1 and 7–1 were similar at small λ, at large λ 7–1 was both less susceptible to noise and less affected by the deleterious effects of regularization.

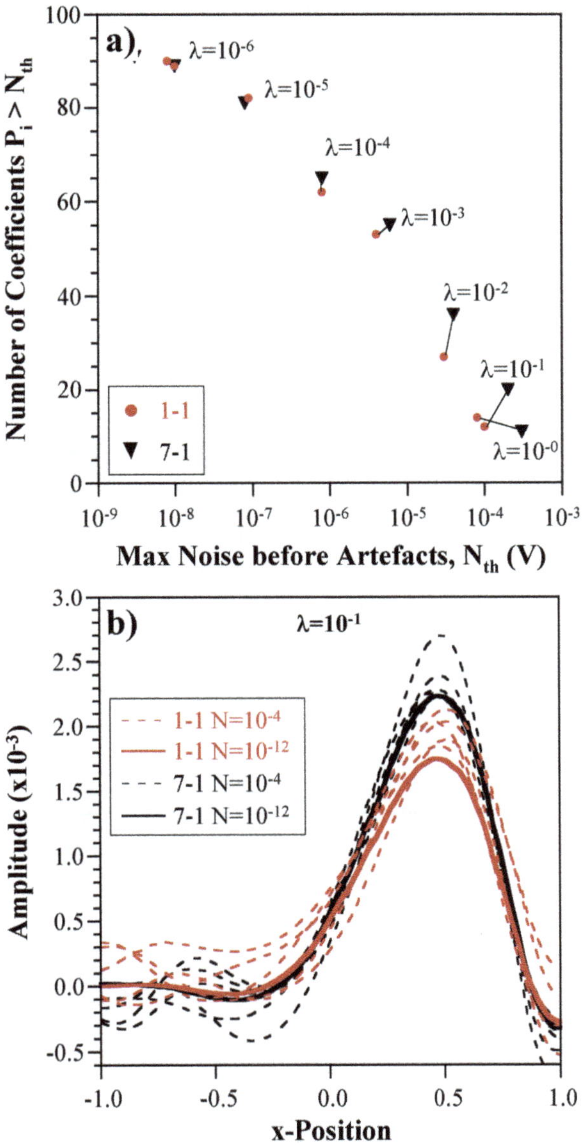

Figure 6.12. (a) The number of Picard coefficients above N_{th} as a function of N_{th} at various hyperparameters for I–M = 1–1 and 7–1 with a triangular target at $x = 0.5$. (b) Cross-sections (at $y = 0$) for $\lambda = 10^{-1}$ with noise (dashed lines, 4 replicates) and with negligible noise (solid lines). (16 electrodes, $\sigma_0 = 10^{-2}$, $\sigma_T = 0.6\sigma_0$, $I = 1 \times 10^{-3}$, $r_T = 0.2$)

6.2.2 Number of electrodes

Most tactile sensor work has used 16 electrodes (chapter 2). A larger number of electrodes incurs considerable increases in measurement and reconstruct times. Under low noise when a small λ can be employed, a larger number of electrodes around the perimeter allows higher resolution since more measurements yield more independent terms in **J**. However, when a large hyperparameter is employed additional electrodes are not useful [30] (see section 5.4).

In this section we compare the noise susceptibility of 8, 12, 16, and 32 electrode systems, which require 32, 96, 192, and 896 measurements, respectively, for the pseudo-polar, or 'nearly opposite', I–M pattern, which is 3–1 for 8 electrodes, 5–1 for 12, 7–1 for 16, and 15–1 for 32. Simulations were otherwise identical. Figure 6.13(a) shows the $|\mathbf{U}^{\mathrm{T}}\boldsymbol{\Delta}|$ in size-sorted order, with horizontal lines indicating the noise levels at which artefacts appeared for each system using $\lambda = 10^{-5}$ and $\lambda = 10^{-2}$.

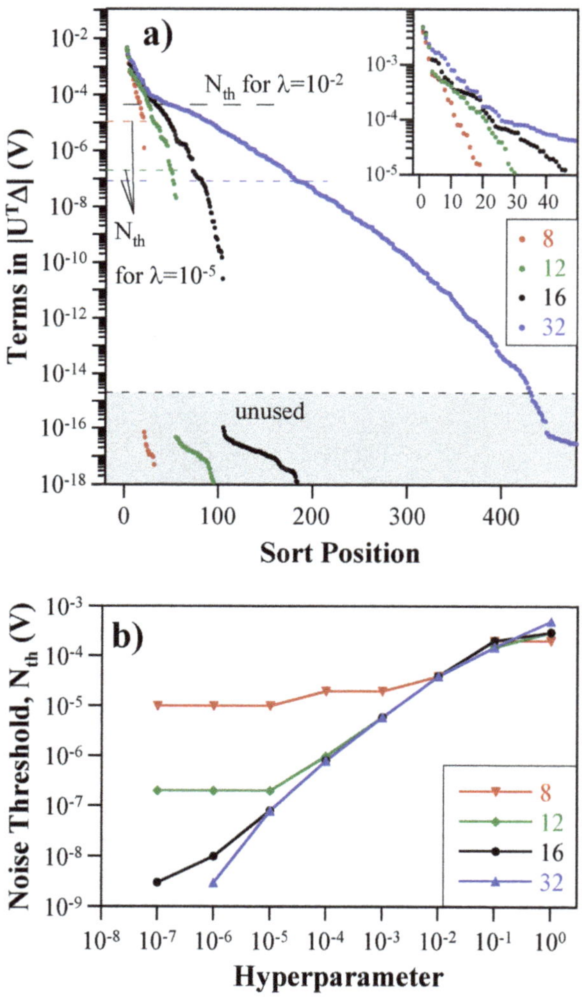

Figure 6.13. (a) The coefficients $|\mathbf{U}^{\mathrm{T}}\boldsymbol{\Delta}|$ in size-sorted order for systems with 8, 12, 16, and 32 electrodes employing nearly-opposite I–M configurations (3–1, 5–1, 7–1, and 15–1, respectively). Noise thresholds at two hyperparameters are indicated. The inset shows a close-up of the upper left. (b) N_{th} as a function of λ for varying numbers of electrodes. ($\sigma_0 = 10^{-2}$, $\sigma_{\mathrm{T}} = 0.6\sigma_0$, $I = 10^{-3}$, triangular target, $x = 0.5$, $r_{\mathrm{T}} = 0.2$) (Below $\lambda = 10^{-7}$ reconstructions failed for 32 electrodes.)

At $\lambda = 10^{-5}$, for 8 electrodes the noise threshold $N_{th} = 1 \times 10^{-5}$ V (dashed red line) was orders of magnitude higher than the $N_{th} = 2 \times 10^{-7}$ V for 12 electrodes (green line) and the 8×10^{-8} V for 16 and 32 electrodes (blue line). This strong noise performance was related to the low rank, $r = 20$. (N_{th} was just below the 19th coefficient. Additional noise that resulted in the loss of the 18th P_i lead to artefacts.) For $\lambda = 10^{-2}$, on the other hand, N_{th} was the same for all four systems.

The noise thresholds as a function of λ are shown in figure 6.13(b). The 8-electrode system was immune to noise below $N = 10^{-5}$ V and there was no dependence of N_{th} on λ up to $\lambda = 10^{-2}$ because all the P but one were larger than 10^{-5} V. Similarly, the 12-electrode system was immune to noise below 2×10^{-7} V, below which were the five smallest P_i.

The curve for 16 electrodes joined the one for 32 at $\lambda = 10^{-5}$ in figure 6.13(b). Thus, the dependence of N_{th} on λ for 16 and 32 electrodes was the same over most of the range, following the same power law. The curve for 12 electrodes joined them at $\lambda = 10^{-4}$, and finally the one for 8 electrodes joined at $\lambda = 10^{-2}$ so that all four systems had the same N_{th}. The information in figure 6.13(a) and (b) corresponded completely. Above $\lambda = 10^{-2}$ the N_{th} order reversed, with 32 having a somewhat better immunity to noise and 8 somewhat worse. Thus, the question of the best number of electrodes for susceptibility to noise depended on λ, as well as on the level of the noise in relation to the smallest P_i.

The EIT images and HM threshold images for $\lambda = 10^{-2}$, at which the four systems had the same $N_{th} = 2 \times 10^{-5}$, are shown in figure 6.14 to allow visual comparison of the peak amplitude and resolution at that point. At N_{th} (top row of images) the resolution was finer for 32 electrodes than for 16, with a greater concentration of energy in the peak, and both were finer than for 8 electrodes. (Amplitude and resolution dependence on λ were quantified in chapter 5.) The better performance is due to the larger number of $\mathbf{v}_i$ above N_{th} contributing to the image.

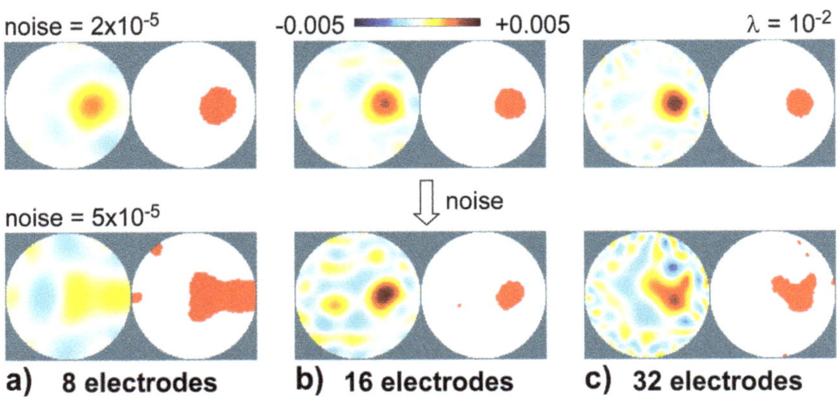

Figure 6.14. EIT and threshold images at (top row) and above (bottom row) N_{th} for (a) 8, (b) 16, and (c) 32 electrodes for $\lambda = 10^{-2}$, at which N_{th} is the same for all three systems. (I–M = nearly opposite, $\sigma_0 = 10^{-2}$, $\sigma_T = 0.6\sigma_0$, $I = 10^{-3}$, triangular target, $r_T = 0.2$, $x = 0.5$)

An important result of this section is that, for a given I–M pattern, the noise threshold N_{th} was the same regardless of the number of electrodes, once the noise was large enough to affect more than the smallest several P_i. However, the resolution at N_{th} improved with the number of electrodes, since that depends on the number of P_i used in the reconstruction, although the resolution improvement from 16 to 32 electrodes is small, as shown in chapter 5.

6.2.3 Effect of target position

Figure 6.6(a) showed that the average voltage was smaller for targets in the center of the sensor than at the perimeter, yet figure 6.6(b,c) showed that the noise performance only depended on target position at large λ. To understand this apparent contradiction, the P_i at five target positions are shown in figure 6.15 together with vertical lines indicating the index at which the given hyperparameter starts to dampen the image $\mathbf{v}_i$ (from chapter 5), and thus to remove noise (smaller C_i, figure 6.10). Horizontal lines indicate the N_{th} from figure 6.6(b,c). No noise was included in these $\mathbf{\Delta}$. (The negligibly small coefficients below 10^{-12} above $i = 104$ are due to numerical rounding errors and are not shown because the associated $\mathbf{v}_i$ are not used in the reconstruction.)

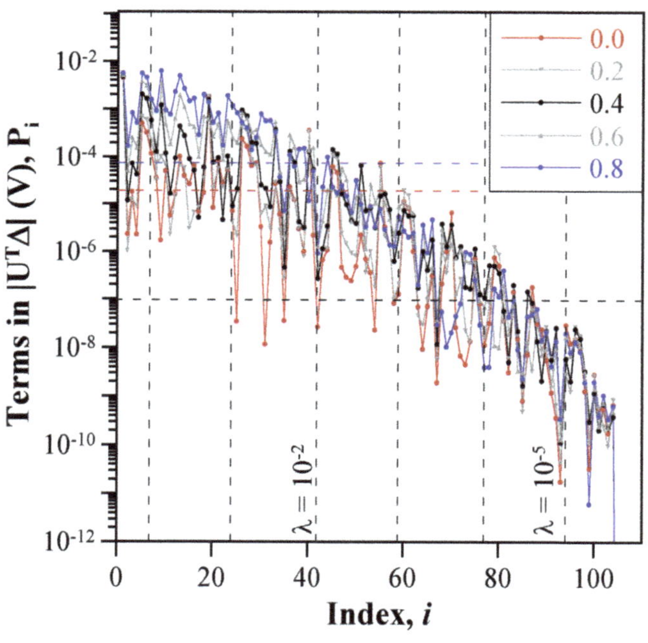

Figure 6.15. (a) The Picard coefficients P_i as a function of singular value index i for targets at positions between $x = 0$ and 0.8. Dashed vertical lines indicate where various values of λ begin to dampen the eigen-images $\mathbf{v}_i$, with λ increasing by factors of 10 from right to left. Dashed horizontal lines indicate N_{th} from figure 6.6(b), 1×10^{-7}, and figure 6.6(c), 2×10^{-5} and 7×10^{-5}. (16 electrodes, I–M = 7–1, $\sigma_0 = 0.01$, $\sigma_T = 0.6\sigma_0$, $I = 10^{-3}$, triangular target, $r_T = 0.2$, $N = 1 \times 10^{-12}$)

At large index i, associated with small hyperparameters, the P_i for targets at different positions were comparable. However, as i decreased the spectra separated, with the P_i becoming lowest at the center of the sensor and the highest at the perimeter. The points for $x = 0$ split from the others below $i = 80$, below the index corresponding to $\lambda = 10^{-2}$, followed by those for $x = 0.2$, and ending with the separation of those for $x = 0.6$ at $i = 40$, corresponding to $\lambda = 10^{-2}$. Thus, at the smallest noise levels, N_{th} at all positions would be expected to be similar, but for higher noise N_{th} would be expected to be smaller at the center. This result is consistent with those of figure 6.6(b,c).

The differences in the $|\mathbf{U}^T\mathbf{\Delta}|$ spectra in figure 6.15 were due only to differences in $\mathbf{\Delta}$, since $\mathbf{U}$ is fixed by the sensor configuration (see section 4.3), which was the same for all five target positions. Nevertheless, greater information can be obtained by displaying this spectrum, or fingerprint, than from a plot of $\mathbf{\Delta}$ alone (figure 6.1). For example, one can see that the P_i for $x = 0$ are relatively large at $i = 1, 19, 40, 55, 70, 87$, which correspond to the circularly symmetric $\mathbf{v}_i$, and these P_i can be directly compared to the noise level to determine when each $\mathbf{v}_i$ would be lost. These spectra are ordered by i, or decreasing order of importance to the sensitivity matrix $\mathbf{J}$. They thus reflect the information in the sensitivity map: the target at $x = 0$ had negligible contributions from 3 of the first 4 eigen-Δ, whereas the target at $x = 0.8$ employed all of them. The fingerprints thereby show that for the nearly-opposite pattern 7–1, the sensitivity at the center of the sensor is smaller than at the edge.

6.2.4 Size and number of targets

The previous sections used a single target of one size, but tactile targets will vary in size and number [31, 32]. Given that smaller targets generate a smaller $\mathbf{\Delta}$, their noise susceptibility would be expected to be higher, but it is unclear by how much. This section examines the relationship between target size and N_{th}, and it also looks at an issue arising from the solution of the inverse problem.

6.2.4.1 Target size

Figure 6.16(a) shows $|\mathbf{U}^T\mathbf{\Delta}|$ for circular targets of increasing size, sorted from largest to smallest (as opposed to sorted by index as in figure 6.9, figure 6.11, figure 6.15). The spectra had similar dependence on sort number, but at low sort positions they were vertically offset. The downward shifts were greatest for the smallest target radii r_T. However, the offsets were not uniform with sort position; with increasing position number, the spectra increasingly overlapped.

The N_{th} for these targets at $\lambda = 10^{-2}$ is indicated by the horizontal lines in figure 6.16(a). The N_{th} intercepted the coefficient curves in corresponding locations: the number of P_i above N_{th} was the same for all the r_T. In contrast, as shown in appendix F.9, $E(|\mathbf{\Delta})|$ increased with the square of the radius (as does signal strength defined as $||\mathbf{\Delta}||_2$ [7]), rather than tapering off at larger r_T, so it did not correlate with N_{th} for large targets.

Figure 6.16(b) shows the noise thresholds for these target sizes as a function of hyperparameter. The amplitudes of N_{th} were shifted strongly downward for radii

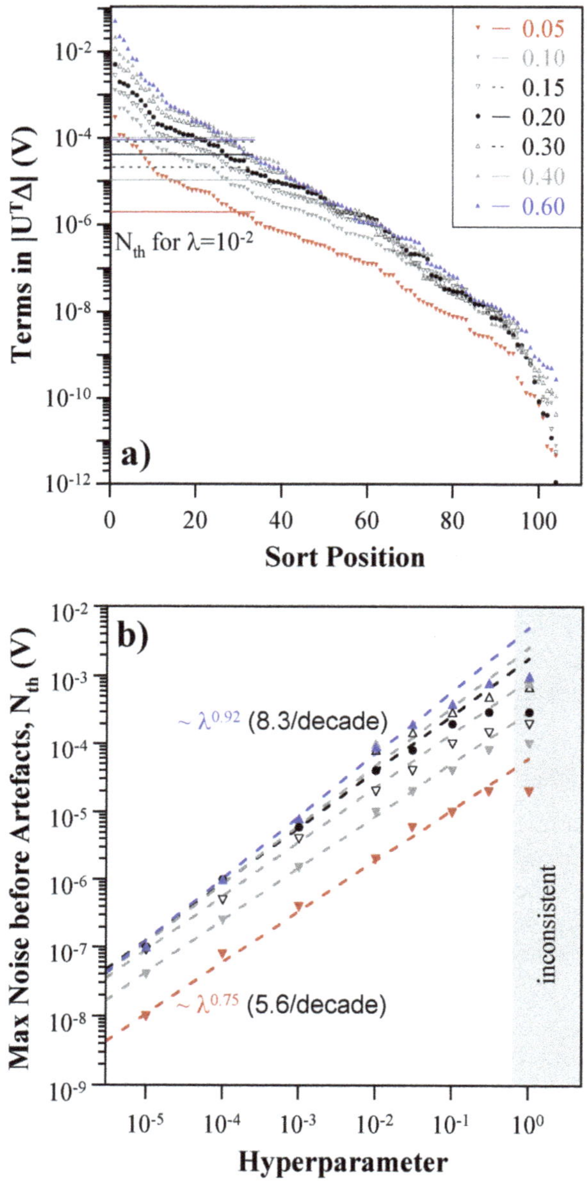

Figure 6.16. (a) The coefficients in $|\mathbf{U}^T\mathbf{\Delta}|$, in size-sorted order, for circular targets of varying radius r_T, indicated in the legend. Noise thresholds at $\lambda = 10^{-2}$ are indicated. (b) Noise thresholds as a function of λ for these targets (points) and curve fits (dashed lines). (16 electrodes, I–M = 7–1, $\sigma_0 = 10^{-2}$, $\sigma_T = 0.6\sigma_0$, $I = 10^{-3}$, $N = 10^{-12}$, $r_T = 0.2$, $x = 0.3$)

below $r_T = 0.2$, as would be expected: smaller features produce smaller changes in the measured voltages, and so are more easily lost to noise. For a given λ, the N_{th} scaled with the feature area for radii below $r_T = 0.3$ (see appendix F.9). Above that, however, the N_{th} plateaued, becoming the same for $r_T = 0.4$ and 0.6.

For $\lambda < 0.1$, the data in figure 7.8(b) could be fit to a power law, $N_{th} = a\lambda^b$, as shown by the dashed lines. At the larger hyperparameters, at which the feature began to occupy a substantial fraction of the sensor area (figure 6.2), N_{th} plateaued; the larger the target, the lower the λ at which the deviation from the model occurred since they filled the sensor area earlier. The exponent b depended on the target radius, increasing with r_T up to 0.4: $b = 0.49r_T + 0.73$ ($R^2 = 0.997$). Thus, the noise threshold increased with λ by a factor of 5.6/decade for the smallest target $r_T = 0.05$, but it increased more strongly for the largest targets $r_T = 0.4$ and 0.6, by a factor of 8.3/decade. So, larger targets were not only more impervious to noise, but they also became increasingly relatively more impervious as λ was raised.

6.2.4.2 Number of targets

To explore the noise susceptibility of a multi-contact target, such as arising from finger touches on a sensor [31, 33–37] a target was employed consisting of three circles, each of $r_T = 0.2$, located at (0,0.4), (0.4,0), and (0.8, 0.4) (figure 6.17(a)). For a contrast of 0.4, used in the previous sections, reconstructions with even negligible noise showed errors (figure 6.17(b)). The apparent artefact between the outmost target circles using $\lambda = 10^{-5}$ was not due to noise, but to a failure of the algorithm to represent circles that were close together: this fourth peak appeared in every simulation. When λ was raised to 10^{-4} the fourth feature became a merger of two of the circles. In general, the algorithm struggled with large-area, large-amplitude targets (chapter 5), particularly near the perimeter. Under these conditions the linear approximations made in the solution become increasingly invalid. Lowering the contrast (figure 6.17(c)) took care of the problem: the three distinct peaks were correctly represented at $\lambda = 10^{-5}$ and 10^{-2} without noise. The lower contrast of course resulted in smaller-amplitude peaks (the EIT images are shown using the same scale in the figure), but the images still improved. (Recall that N_{th} scales linearly with the contrast, as shown in figure 6.5, so lower contrast will result in greater noise susceptibility.)

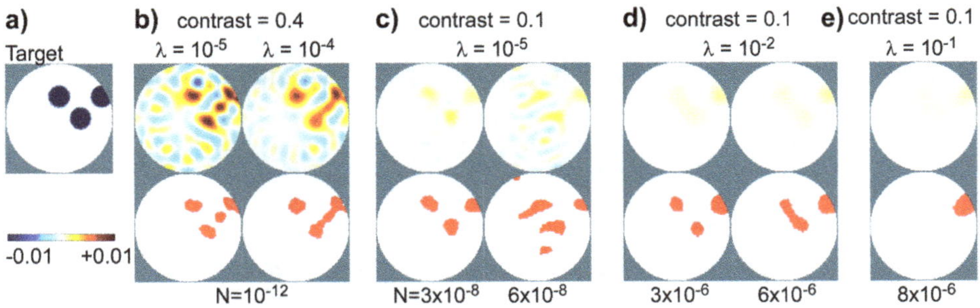

Figure 6.17. EIT reconstructions and threshold images for (a) a three-circle target. (b) At a contrast of 0.4, reconstructions with negligible noise at hyperparameters $\lambda = 10^{-5}$ and $\lambda = 10^{-4}$. At a contrast of 0.1, images below and above N_{th} at (c) $\lambda = 10^{-5}$, (d) $\lambda = 10^{-2}$. (e) At a contrast of 0.1, images below N_{th} at $\lambda = 10^{-1}$. (16 electrodes, I–M = 7–1, $\sigma_0 = 10^{-2}$, $I = 10^{-3}$, 3 circles, $r_T = 0.2$)

The addition of noise at small hyperparameters resulted in artefacts (figure 6.17(c)), while at larger hyperparameters it typically resulted in feature merging (figure 6.17(d)). The spatial dependence of the hyperparameter was evident when λ was raised to 10^{-1}; the peaks at the center sank below the $A/2$ threshold. (See chapter 5 for further information about masking at large λ.)

The noise thresholds for the three-circle target were lower than those of a one-circle target having the same radius $r_T = 0.2$; they were comparable to those of a single circle having $r_T = 0.1$ (see appendix F.9). The additional features rendered the image more sensitive to perturbations, since a larger number of terms is required to represent them correctly.

The above results show that, as a practical matter, the hyperparameter needs to be chosen for the smallest expected target size and the greatest number of targets, as well as the smallest expected change in conductivity (lightest touch). The former two are more sensitive to noise and thus require a larger λ, while the latter needs a small λ for the peak to emerge, so these requirements conflict with each other. The difference in noise thresholds based on size can be as large as two orders of magnitude, meaning a required increase in λ by over one order of magnitude. Experimentalists must therefore reduce noise in the system as much as possible to allow a smaller λ to be employed to be able to visualize light touches and touches at the center. In addition, signals that are too large can produce image artefacts, so the dynamic range of contacts must be considered and managed.

6.3 Summary and conclusions

This chapter has quantitatively examined the issue of noise in EIT for tactile imaging. Given the importance of identifying the correct number, locations, and strengths of highly variable touches, this entailed using the onset of artifacts as a metric. It also involved showing how signal components are degraded by noise by examining the Picard coefficients. While the handling of noise is intimately related to the effects of the hyperparameter, noise susceptibility was here considered separately from the defocusing caused by increasing λ.

Although in practical applications the hyperparameter can simply be raised until the images appear by eye to be reasonable, it is of interest to understand the relationship between noise and the hyperparameter, and how noise susceptibility is affected by changes in system and target parameters. This allows the development of protocols for improving images in a particular application so that they better represent the input, as illustrated by figure 6.17.

6.3.1 Evaluating noisiness

Measures of noisiness define when a reconstruction has been significantly degraded by perturbation errors. A method of evaluating noisiness was introduced in this work, the noise threshold N_{th}, based on when artefacts begin to appear in the image, as opposed to using detectability or resolution criteria, because the absence of non-target features is essential for tactile imaging. N_{th} at a given hyperparameter was found to be an efficient metric, as shown in chapter 7, requiring only a handful of replicate images for repeatable determination of the onset of instability to guide decisions on system configurations and the required regularization.

There has been much discussion of the best way to select the hyperparameter [18, 22], which essentially involves finding a good compromise between feature defocusing and image break-up. The noise threshold approach is most closely related to the BestRes [18] and f-slope [22, 38] methods for objectively choosing a hyperparameter as discussed in chapter 7.

6.3.2 Signal and SNR

The terms signal and SNR have been used in various ways in the EIT literature. The most frequently employed definitions of signal involve some average of $\mathbf{\Delta}$; also utilized are the dynamic range of $\mathbf{\Delta}$ or the maximum values. These are relevant, and of course expedient on the spot, for a given experiment to improve its SNR by increasing data collection times, changing current settings, and the like. However, measures based on $\mathbf{\Delta}$ alone were not found to correlate well with image noisiness when comparing different systems or different targets.

For an experimentalist coming from another field, the necessity of obsessively excluding noise that is orders of magnitude smaller than the measured voltage differences may be surprising. Target-induced voltage changes may be 1000 times greater than the noise on a given channel—a far cry from the SNR = 2 rule of thumb often employed in other systems—yet preventing image break-up may still require a large hyperparameter, to the detriment of resolution, amplitude, and uniformity. Moreover, it makes no difference whether the noise is on the smallest or the largest measurements: it is equally destructive anywhere in the measurement frame. The images are so noise sensitive because $\mathbf{\Delta}$ behaves as a sum of patterns, or 'eigen-Δs' $\mathbf{u}_i$, the coefficients of most of which are orders of magnitude smaller than the values in $\mathbf{\Delta}$. Overwhelming these tiny so-called Picard coefficients with noise results in artefacts, which renders the image useless without sufficient regularization.

The challenge of comparing performance across systems and targets motivated the development of measures such as the noise factor [12] and distinguishability [11]. Distinguishability contains information from both the system and the voltage differences $\mathbf{\Delta}$. It has the advantage of providing a single number that can be used as an SNR for a given measurement scenario.

The alternate approach advocated here of using the $|\mathbf{U}^T\mathbf{\Delta}|$ spectrum of Picard coefficients P_i as an indication of SNR dates back to using SVD for solving inverse problems and regularizing ill-conditioned matrices [25]. The P_i incorporate all the forward problem information (not reconstruction information such as λ). The inclusion of measurement system information via $\mathbf{U}$ permits comparisons across systems. Target information is included via $\mathbf{\Delta}$. Using $|\mathbf{U}^T\mathbf{\Delta}|$ spectra offers two advantages. First, the P_i have units of volts, allowing direct comparison with the amount of noise. Second, the spectra provide insight. For example, they reveal why differences in noise susceptibility depend on the hyperparameter, under what conditions one system may outperform another, and how different variables, such as target size, affect N_{th}.

While the $|\mathbf{U}^{\mathrm{T}}\boldsymbol{\Delta}|$ spectra allow comparison of different scenarios, they do not provide a single value to be used as an SNR ratio. They instead offer an overview of the noise relative to the amplitudes of the various signal components for a particular scenario.

Signal components $\mathbf{u}_i$ with coefficients P_i that are larger than the noise have corresponding image components $\mathbf{v}_i$ that are meaningful. The intrinsic resolution of the image is given by the number of meaningful $\mathbf{v}_i$ [7]. Those $\mathbf{v}_i$ associated with smaller P_i must be eliminated by an appropriately set λ. The hyperparameter is adjusted to replace noise-corrupted $\mathbf{v}_i$ with prior information, allowing the most reasonable approximate solution to be obtained. The required λ can be obtained from the linear relationship between $\log(N_{\mathrm{th}})$ and $\log(\lambda)$ for a given I–M pattern.

$|\mathbf{U}^{\mathrm{T}}\boldsymbol{\Delta}|$ spectra alone cannot predicting the exact point at which noise overwhelms an image since they are derived only from the forward problem. Factors that come into play in the inverse problem, such as the 'prior' employed, also affect the image, which is why distinguishability has been an attractive metric.

6.3.3 Some relationships

Tolerable maximum noise in the image, given by N_{th}, increased as λ^b. For I–M = 7–1 and a single triangular target under these simulation conditions, $N_{\mathrm{th}} \sim \lambda^{0.87}$, a factor of 7.4 for each factor of 10 increase in λ, up to $\lambda = 10^{-2}$; above that the N_{th} leveled off. The exponent b depended on target characteristics, but it did not depend on the number of electrodes.

Differences in N_{th} among the three full-rank I–M patterns studied here were noise-level-dependent. For example, differences between 7–1 and 1–1 were negligible at low noise but increased at higher noise, reflecting an increasing separation of their $\mathbf{U}^{\mathrm{T}}\boldsymbol{\Delta}$ spectra at low singular value index i. Thus, a determination of the best I–M pattern regarding noise performance is more nuanced than has been generally recognized.

In tactile imaging, for some applications it may be important to detect and accurately represent multiple targets of varying size. Unfortunately, small radius targets ($r_{\mathrm{T}} = 0.05$) tolerate 50x less noise than those with large radii ($r_{\mathrm{T}} = 0.4$). Other applications, such as human–machine tactile interactions based on finger-touches, will have similar-size targets. However, the number of those contacts will vary, and as the number of targets increases, so does noise susceptibility. In addition, matrix inversion issues may manifest themselves, such as artefacts appearing between closely spaced targets. Lowering the contrast can help alleviate the latter problem, as can increasing λ, but at large λ spatial non-uniformity becomes pronounced, so light touches at the center of the sensor accompanied by heavier touches near the perimeter become particularly challenging. Thus, it is essential to have a low noise to obtain a useful image.

At small λ, systems with 8 and 12 electrodes were more immune to noise than those with 16 or 32: because of their low rank the former had fewer small Picard coefficients P_i. Of course, they also had lower resolution. Above $\lambda = 10^{-2}$, N_{th} did not depend appreciably on the number of electrodes: 8, 12, 16, and 32 electrode set-ups were equally susceptible to noise. Furthermore, as shown in other chapters, in the presence of so much noise that $\lambda > 10^{-2}$ is required, it may improve the image if 12 electrodes are used instead of 16 or 32.

6.3.4 Noise, increasing $\boldsymbol{\Delta}$

It is clear that to obtain images of reasonable resolution, to have sensitivity to small and to light touches, and to reduce amplitude non-uniformity over the sensor, every effort must be made to reduce noise so that a smaller λ can be employed. For the smallest targets, given the relationship between N_{th} and target size, noise may need to be reduced by additional orders of magnitude. Standard measures include electromagnetic shielding and employing low-noise circuit components and ADCs. They also include averaging a larger number of voltage readings, although the latter may be infeasible if contacts with the sensor are short-lasting, and although noise only decreases as the square root of the number of measurements. A noise-free reference image based on a large number of readings on each channel should certainly be obtained prior to using the sensor.

Of course the other way to increase SNR is to boost the signal. This can be done by using a sensor with greater resistivity or increasing the injected current, provided that the noise is *independent* of the current, for example because it is dominated by noise in the data acquisition system [6]. Both result in linear improvements in N_{th} through linear increases in $\boldsymbol{\Delta}$ following Ohm's law, but they also increase power consumption. The best approach is to use a sensor with a higher gauge factor (sensitivity to strain) or to mechanically amplify tactile contacts. Unfortunately, obtaining sensors with high and isotropic gauge factors along with other desired characteristics can be challenging, and mechanical amplification increases system complexity. The problem of boosting the signal too high must also be borne in mind, since that can result in artefacts when there are multiple touches.

References

[1] Seagar A D, Barber D C and Brown B H 1987 Theoretical limits to sensitivity and resolution in impedance imaging *Clin. Phys. Physiol. Meas.* **8** 13

[2] Vauhkonen M, Lionheart W R, Heikkinen L M, Vauhkonen P J and Kaipio J P 2001 A MATLAB package for the EIDORS project to reconstruct two-dimensional EIT images *Physiol. Meas.* **22** 107–11

[3] Polydorides N and Lionheart W R B 2002 A Matlab toolkit for three-dimensional electrical impedance tomography: a contribution to the Electrical Impedance and Diffuse Optical Reconstruction Software project *Meas. Sci. Technol.* **13** 1871–83

[4] Adler A and Lionheart W R B 2006 Uses and abuses of EIDORS: an extensible software base for EIT *Physiol. Meas.* **27** S25–42

[5] Dai T 2008 Image reconstruction in EIT using advanced regularization frameworks *PhD thesis* Department of Systems and Computer Engineering Carleton University

[6] Shi X T, Dong X Z, Shuai W J, You F S, Fu F and Liu R G 2006 Pseudo-polar drive patterns for brain electrical impedance tomography *Physiol. Meas.* **27** 1071–80

[7] Gaggero P O 2011 Miniaturization and distinguishability limits of electrical impedance tomography for biomedical application *PhD thesis* University of Neuchâtel, Landquart,

Switzerland Nanomedecine Division, Centre Suisse d'Electronique et de Microtechnique (CSEM)
[8] Russo S, Nefti-Meziani S, Carbonaro N and Tognetti A 2017 A quantitative evaluation of drive pattern selection for optimizing EIT-based stretchable sensors *Sensors* **17** ARTN 1999
[9] Adler A, Dai T and Lionheart W R B 2007 Temporal image reconstruction in electrical impedance tomography *Physiol. Meas.* **28** S1–S11
[10] Yasin M, Bohm S, Gaggero P O and Adler A 2011 Evaluation of EIT system performance *Physiol. Meas.* **32** 851
[11] Adler A, Gaggero P O and Maimaitijiang Y 2011 Adjacent stimulation and measurement patterns considered harmful *Physiol. Meas.* **32** 731–44
[12] Braun F, Proença M, Solà J, Thiran J-P and Adler A 2017 A versatile noise performance metric for electrical impedance tomography algorithms *IEEE Trans. Biomed. Eng.* **64** 2321–30
[13] Adler A and Guardo R 1996 Electrical impedance tomography: regularized imaging and contrast detection *IEEE Trans. Med. Imag.* **15** 170–9
[14] Lionheart W, Polydorides N and Borsic A 2005 Chapter 1. The reconstruction problem *Electrical Impedance Tomography: Methods, History and Applications, Series in Medical Physics and Biomedical Engineering* ed C G Orton, J H Nagel and J G Webster (Bristol: IOP Publishing)
[15] Breckon W R and Pidcock M K (ed) 1988 *Some mathematical aspects of electrical impedance tomography* vol 39 (Berlin, Heidelberg: Springer)
[16] Chen Y 2018 Tactile sensing with compliant structures for human–robot interaction *PhD thesis* Department of Mechanical Engineering, University of Maryland
[17] Tawil D S, Rye D and Velonaki M 2011 Improved image reconstruction for an EIT-based sensitive skin with multiple internal electrodes *IEEE Trans. Robot.* **27** 425–35
[18] Graham B M and Adler A 2006 Objective selection of hyperparameter for EIT *Physiol. Meas.* **27** S65–79
[19] Zhang L, Wang H and Zhang L 2010 Single source current drive patterns for electrical impedance tomography *IEEE Instrumentation & Measurement Technology Conf. Proc (Austin, TX, 3–6 May)* pp 1477–80
[20] Adler A *et al* 2009 GREIT: a unified approach to 2D linear EIT reconstruction of lung images *Physiol. Meas.* **30** S35–55
[21] Adler A and Boyle A 2017 Electrical impedance tomography: tissue properties to image measures *IEEE Trans. Biomed. Eng.* **64** 2494–504
[22] Correia T, Gibson A, Schweiger M and Hebden J 2009 Selection of regularization parameter for optical topography *J. Biomed. Opt.* **14** 034044
[23] Hansen P C 2010 *Discrete Inverse Problems: Insight and Algorithms, Fundamentals of Algorithms* (Philadelphia, PA: Society for Industrial and Applied Mathematics (SIAM)
[24] Kantartzis P, Abdi M and Liatsis P 2013 Stimulation and measurement patterns versus prior information for fast 3D EIT: A breast screening case study *Sig. Process* **93** 2838–50
[25] Hansen P C 1990 The discrete Picard condition for discrete ill-posed problems *BIT Numer. Math* **30** 658–72
[26] Hansen P C 2010 *DIAS 006—Discrete Inverse Problems—Day 1, slides based on Discrete Inverse Problems: Insight and Algorithms vol 2020, Fundamentals of Algorithms* (Philadelphia: Society for Industrial and Applied Mathematics (SIAM))

[27] Grychtol B and Adler A 2013 Uniform background assumption produces misleading lung EIT images *Physiol. Meas.* **34** 579–93

[28] Grychtol B and Adler A 2014 Choice of reconstructed tissue properties affects interpretation of lung EIT images *Physiol. Meas.* **35** 1035–50

[29] Polydorides N and McCann H 2002 Electrode configurations for improved spatial resolution in electrical impedance tomography *Meas. Sci. Technol.* **13** 1862–70

[30] Newell J 2005 Chapter 13: The Rensselaer experience *Electrical Impedance Tomography: Methods, History and Applications, Series in Medical Physics and Biomedical Engineering* ed C G Orton, J H Nagel and J G Webster (Bristol: IOP Publishing)

[31] Tawil D S, Rye D and Velonaki M 2012 Interpretation of the modality of touch on an artificial arm covered with an EIT-based sensitive skin *Int. J. Robot. Res.* **31** 1627–41

[32] Visentin F, Fiorini P and Suzuki K 2016 A deformable smart skin for continuous sensing based on electrical impedance tomography *Sensors* **16** ARTN 1928

[33] Kato Y, Mukai T, Hayakawa T and Shibata T 2007 Tactile sensor without wire and sensing element in the tactile region based on EIT method *IEEE Sensors, 2007 (Atlanta, GA, Oct. 28-31)* pp 792–5

[34] Nagakubo A, Alirezaei H and Kuniyoshi Y 2007 A deformable and deformation sensitive tactile distribution sensor *IEEE Int. Conf. Robot. Biomimetics (ROBIO) (Sanya, China, Dec. 15–18)* pp 1301–8

[35] Lee H, Kwon D, Cho H, Park I and Kim J 2017 Soft nanocomposite based multi-point, multi-directional strain mapping sensor using anisotropic electrical impedance tomography *Sci. Rep.* **7** 39837

[36] Russo S, Nefti-Meziani S, Carbonaro N and Tognetti A 2017 Development of a high-speed current injection and voltage measurement system for electrical impedance tomography-based stretchable sensors *Technologies* **5** 48

[37] Chen Y, Yu M, Bruck H A and Smela E 2018 Compliant multi-layer tactile sensing for enhanced identification of human touch *Smart Mater. Struct.* **27** 125009

[38] Wu L M 2003 A parameter choice method for Tikhonov regularization *Electron Trans. Numer. Anal.* **16** 107–28

Chapter 7

Experimental decisions

Given the prior discussions of the workings of electrical impedance tomography (EIT), regularization, and noise, the practitioner will ask, what conditions should I use for my work? The following sections discuss hyperparameter selection and I–M patterns. While these topics have been touched upon previously, they require further study in order to answer this question. The number of electrodes to use also becomes clear in the latter discussion.

As detailed in prior chapters, noise destabilizes EIT images, and the onset of instability is associated with the appearance of artefacts, which are spurious image features that are not associated with sensor responses to contacts. Artefacts are detrimental because the essential features of contacts, or targets, must be correctly represented, including how many there are and their approximate shapes and locations, yet their presence has not previously been used as a performance measure. Regularization, the extent of which is determined by the hyperparameter λ, is used to manage the destabilization, but it results in spatially non-uniform defocusing of image features. We therefore introduced an efficient criterion for evaluating tactile sensor image quality based on the onset of artefacts. In this chapter, using simulated data and the one-step Gauss–Newton reconstruction algorithm with the Laplace prior, the noise level at which artefacts first appear at a given hyperparameter, or noise threshold $N_{th}(\lambda)$, are found. How the relationship depends on target characteristics and other factors is shown, and N_{th} can vary by orders of magnitude. The conceptually similar BestRes method and the classical L-curve and generalized cross-validation (GCV) methods for determining an optimal hyperparameter are evaluated using the criterion of artefact-free images. The L-curve generates hyperparameters that are well matched to the onset of artefacts, except at high noise; the other two result in artefacts. For high dynamic range tactile inputs, setting the threshold at a fixed value using a method such as N_{th} is not advisable, and automatic regularization tailored to the input may be needed using a method such as the L-curve or GCV, provided that the computational overhead is tolerable.

doi:10.1088/978-0-7503-5402-8ch7

The current injection and voltage measurement (I–M) patterns that are most frequently used in EIT for tactile sensing are bipolar. In this chapter, the total set of 36 unique combinations for 16-electrode systems is investigated using simulations. Performance is evaluated on a circular sensor as a function of hyperparameter and target position with respect to critical performance measures for tactile sensing; these include not only peak amplitude and resolution, but also susceptibility to noise and, importantly, the uniformity of performance over the sensor area. The determination of which pattern to employ can therefore be based on the needs of the particular application. The relative performance of the I–M patterns is determined at small hyperparameters by electrode placement symmetry, but at large hyperparameters by sensitivity at the center of the sensor. Patterns with high spatial symmetry should be avoided; these include electrode pairs on opposite sides of the sensor. Patterns with electrodes in adjacent positions, which have been the norm for tactile sensing, should also not generally be used. If performance on all metrics across a wide range of hyperparameters is needed, then placing both the injection and measurement electrodes three spaces apart (the 3–3 pattern) can be a good strategy. The use of 13 electrodes instead of 16 is also examined. The absence of symmetry provides greater flexibility in the choice of I–M pattern, and the loss in performance may be small; furthermore, the reduction in data collection time may be advantageous. Beyond avoiding the worst I–M patterns, the most important measure to take is decreasing noise on the signal to permit the use of a smaller hyperparameter; this is of greater importance than selecting from among the remaining I–M patterns.

7.1 Considering artefacts in hyperparameter selection

The material in this section is from the paper Smela E 2022 EIT for tactile sensing: considering artefacts in hyperparameter selection *Eng. Res. Expr.* **4** 035057 [22].

Here we consider noise in EIT from the perspective of tactile imaging, performed for example using a piezoresistive ‘smart skin’. Even small amounts of noise can be surprisingly detrimental to EIT images, but at what point does it become so severe that the image is no longer useful for correctly detecting the ‘target’ stimulus, or spatial pattern of induced impedance changes? For tactile imaging [1–12], as reviewed in [13, 14], the goal of EIT is generally to provide ‘actionable intelligence’ from the sensing system. This may be the interpretation of a human touch or knowledge about physical contacts made by a robot with its environment. This can be challenging because the timing, number, locations, sizes, and strengths of contacts are unknown and in some applications can be highly variable. The signal may be relatively small, arising, for example, from a human finger gently pressing on a sensor, or relatively large, as from a robot with a sensing skin bumping into an object. Furthermore, the reconstruction of each image must be sufficiently reliable for real-time inferences and decision-making, for example to understand gestures [2, 5, 12], so averaging many images is infeasible.

Noise arises from numerous sources, as reviewed in [15], and it can make the image unusable for determining how many touches, where, when, what size, and how strong because, in addition to other image distortions, noise introduces *artefacts*, which are peaks that do not correspond to the target touches, as shown below. In fact, artefacts have been found to be the main reason for image degradation, including position errors, in tactile imaging [4]. At even higher noise levels, the image breaks up completely.

The level of noise dictates the extent of regularization, which is controlled by the hyperparameter λ, required during image reconstruction to remove artefacts [16] (see appendix G.4). The effective strength of the hyperparameter depends on measurement parameters such as the current and sensor conductivity (as discussed in section 4.4.4 and shown in appendices E.1 and E.2), and it will therefore differ among studies. The onset of stability has been defined, for a single target, as the point at which spatially disjoint elements are removed from the image by regularization, leaving only one set of adjacent elements [17]. Unfortunately raising λ also results in image distortions, primarily 'defocusing,' or broadening of features (loss of resolution and amplitude), which is spatially non-uniform. This non-uniformity can result in the masking of contacts at the center of the sensor by contacts at the perimeter. Thus, much attention has been given to the optimal choice of hyperparameter, as reviewed in [16–18]. However, the question has not yet been examined from the perspective of tactile imaging experimentalists.

In this section we examine the onset of artefacts as a performance metric and a criterion for choosing the hyperparameter, based on the need for accurately determining the most essential information about contacts. Determining the presence of artefacts is efficient even at low signal-to-noise ratios (SNRs), and this metric of image quality can be used to compare different systems. We also examine the practical question of hyperparameter selection when the dynamic range of expected SNRs is large, and recommend, in this case, optimization of the hyperparameter for each image, within preset limits.

7.1.1 Image artefacts and the noise threshold

As discussed previously, in tactile imaging touches can occur anywhere on the sensor at any time. Since knowing whether touches have occurred and their number and locations is paramount, in this work the onset of the occurrence of artefacts [19] was used as an estimate of the onset of instability. Artefacts are features that do not correspond to targets from the forward model but that appear in the reconstructed image due to noise, as shown in figure 7.1 (previously introduced in figure 3.2). Since the number, amplitudes, sizes, and shapes of touches are typically unknown, artefacts cannot readily be distinguished from contacts. (Artefacts can also be introduced by strains at the electrodes [4] or from electrode motion, but these are not addressed here.)

Although given in section 3.2, we repeat some definitions here. Following convention, the maximum amplitude $\Delta\sigma_R$ in the reconstruction, or peak height, was found. Image elements with values greater than $\Delta\sigma_R/2$ were used to identify targets and artefacts. Those elements are referred to as being in the half max (HM) amplitude set and the binary image of these elements is the HM image. Then,

$$\text{Num. Artefacts} = (\text{Num. Features with Peak Amplitude} > \Delta\sigma_R/2) - (\text{Num. Targets}) \quad (7.1)$$

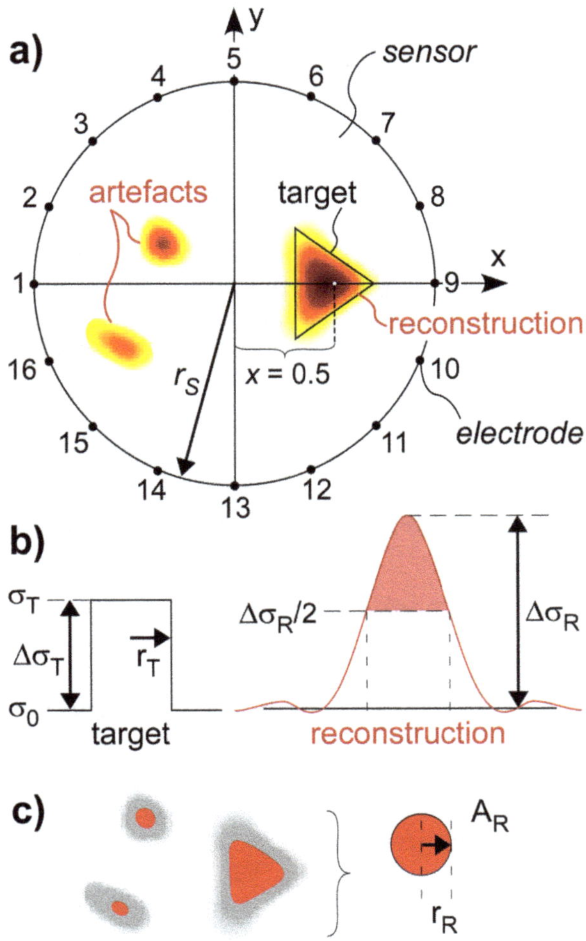

Figure 7.1. (a) Example EIT reconstruction on a circular sensor with constant conductivity σ_0 and 16 electrodes at the boundary. (Conductivity changes of opposite sign, such as due to ringing, are not shown in this example image.) Here the target at position $x = 0.5$ has a triangular shape, (b) size $r_T = 0.2$, and fixed amplitude conductivity change $\Delta\sigma_T$. The half amplitude set consists of points with amplitudes greater than half of the reconstructed peak amplitude. Here the reconstructed image of the target is accompanied by two artefacts. Although the figure indicates a positive amplitude, $\Delta\sigma_T$ actually decreases in this work, corresponding to an increase in resistance. (c) Resolution r_R is defined as the square root of the area A_R, a circle with equivalent area to the half-amplitude set (red).

(The number of artefacts was obtained using the Matlab function *regionprops* on the HM image.)

A noise threshold $N_{th}(\lambda)$ was defined as the highest level of noise at a given hyperparameter at which there were no artefacts in the EIT images in five replicate trials.

$$(N_{th} \in \text{Noise}) | \text{ Num. Artefacts } |_{5\text{ trials}} = 0 \tag{7.2}$$

While the total number of artefacts could be used instead, that metric is inefficient, requiring a large number of replicates due to a high variability; N_{th} is more consistent (see appendix G.1). Equivalently, a minimum hyperparameter $\lambda_{th}(N)$ was found at a given level of noise N at which there were no artefacts in the EIT images in five replicate trials:

$$(\lambda_{N_{th}} \in \text{Hyperparameters})| \text{ Num. Artefacts } |_{5\text{ trials}} = 0 \tag{7.3}$$

The resolution of the reconstructed features determines the ability to distinguish adjacent touches. Peak widths are used in numerous fields to define resolution or resolvability: two peaks of equal size separated by a distance equal to their widths at half of their height (full width at half max, FWHM) can be readily resolved, having a dip between them of roughly half their heights, while peaks separated by half that width can just be resolved, having a small dip between them. Figure 3.2(c) illustrates the points in the half amplitude set, which includes the areas from artefacts, and which occupy a total area A_R. An equivalent circle of area A_R has a radius r_R, specified as a fraction of r_S. Thus, in EIT resolution is often defined as the square root of the normalized area:

$$\begin{aligned}\text{Resolution} &= \sqrt{A_R/A_S} = r_R/r_S \\ &= r_R \text{ } if \text{ } r_S = 1\end{aligned} \tag{7.4}$$

By this definition, smaller numbers are preferable since they show finer resolution. (EIDORS 3.10 calculates resolution using a threshold of $\Delta\sigma_R/4$ by default; this threshold can be changed in eval_GREIT_fig_merit.m.) Feature radii increases with the hyperparameter. For a point target, the resolution is the blur radius, the additional radius added to targets of any size.

7.1.2 Overview: noise and blurring in tactile images of a single target

We begin by reviewing the deleterious effects of noise on a tactile image, although this has been shown in previous chapters. We emphasize that these simulations employed the Gauss–Newton one-step inversion, the most commonly used for tactile imaging, with the Laplace prior, the associated default in EIDORS, which influence how noise affects the image (for examples of the effects of other algorithms see e.g. [20, 21]). Figure 7.2 shows how, for a given set of simulation parameters, an image first loses fidelity and eventually breaks up completely as the noise amplitude increases. (These are so-called perturbation errors.) The noise level at which this occurs depends on the hyperparameter λ. Considered in reverse, increasing the hyperparameter at a given level of noise results in an onset of stability [17].

Figure 7.2(a) employed a small hyperparameter, $\lambda = 10^{-5}$; the top row shows the EIT images and the second row shows the corresponding threshold or HM images. (Even at the tiny amount of noise in the first image, it is difficult to discern the triangular target shape at this λ.) The onset of artefacts occurred over a narrow noise range; for this case between $N = 1 \times 10^{-7}$ and 2×10^{-7} V. N_{th} was thus 1×10^{-7} at this λ. Above N_{th} the images varied substantially from one simulation run to the next.

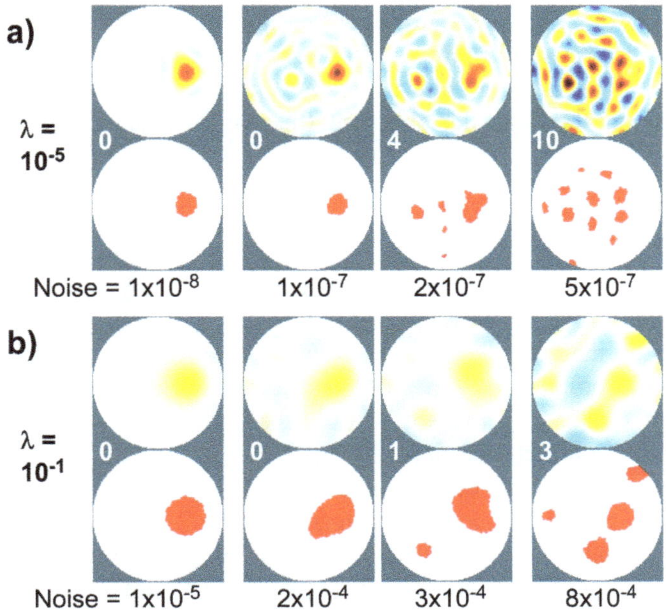

Figure 7.2. EIT images (top rows) and the corresponding HM threshold images (bottom rows) for two hyperparameters: (a) $\lambda = 10^{-5}$, for which $N_{\mathrm{th}} = 1 \times 10^{-7}$ V, and (b) $\lambda = 10^{-1}$, for which $N_{\mathrm{th}} = 2 \times 10^{-4}$ V. The noise amplitude increases from left to right; the center two images have noise levels just below and above the onset of artefacts, the number of which is indicated by the white text. Decreases in conductivity are shown as red, increases as blue. (Identical color bars used for all the EIT images.) (16 electrodes, I–M = 7–1, $\sigma_0 = 10^{-2}$, $\sigma_{\mathrm{T}} = 0.6\sigma_0$, $I = 10^{-3}$, triangular target, $r_{\mathrm{T}} = 0.2$, $x = 0.5$)

At and just below N_{th} the shape of the target was distorted, but its size and location were approximately correct. Near but above N_{th}, shortly after the onset of artefacts, the target remained technically 'detectable' in the sense that there was still a peak at the target location. Nonetheless, since in tactile imaging there is no *a priori* knowledge of target numbers and locations, the images may become essentially unusable for interpretation of tactile information, without further information or processing, above N_{th}. For example, in figure 7.2(a) just above N_{th} there appear to be at least two targets. Increasing the noise even further, the images broke up into many small peaks, all of which were artefacts.

Figure 7.2(b) employed, using the same target, the much larger hyperparameter $\lambda = 10^{-1}$, and N_{th} was thus orders of magnitude higher. Larger λ results in a loss of concentration of the image energy, meaning the feature broadens and reduces in amplitude, which is evident when comparing figures 7.2(a) and (b). (These are so-called regularization errors.) This 'defocusing' occurs because increasing λ eliminates higher spatial frequency image modes in the reconstruction [22]. The areas of the artefacts were thus also larger at the greater λ. Again there was a narrow range, relative to the greater noise amplitude, over which artefacts began to appear. Again the target was identifiable although distorted at N_{th}, but above N_{th} it was unclear how many targets there were. In figure 7.2(a), it was apparent that the final

EIT image had broken up due to noise, but in figure 7.2(b), there appear to be 3 or 4 touches. In applications with known minimum target radii or strengths, additional image processing based on the blur radius at a given λ could eliminate some of the artefacts based on their smaller size, but this will not generally be the case (see section 5.5.2).

7.1.3 Hyperparameter versus N_{th}

To handle smaller SNRs in voltage difference data, **Δ**, the hyperparameter λ must be increased. There is an expected relationship between λ and N_{th}, which will depend on the reconstruction method among other things. For example, an approach based on minimizing the resolution showed a linear relationship between log(λ) and noise at high noise levels [17]. The present work utilized a one-step inverse that defines λ = average noise/conductivity change [23].

The relationship between the required hyperparameter and the noise level was found for the sensor and target parameters of figure 7.2 by fixing λ and gradually increasing the noise level N. Five trials were run at each condition and the number of trials without artefacts was determined, as shown in figure 7.3(a). (Corresponding EIT images are shown in appendix G.2.) The range of noise studied was larger than would be encountered in practice, but was used to understand trends.

The highest noise level that resulted in no artefacts (100% runs without artefacts from figure 7.3(a)), N_{th}, is shown as a function of hyperparameter in figure 7.3(b). The relationship between them followed a power law between $\lambda = 10^{-6}$ and 10^{-1}: N_{th} went as $\lambda^{0.87}$ for the triangular target, for two levels of current. Thus, for each increase in λ by a factor of 10, the tolerable noise increased by a factor of 7.4. The noise thresholds were the same for an equivalent positive contrast $\sigma_T = 1.67\sigma_0$. For a circular target the relationship was similar, with N_{th} increasing by 6.8 for each increase in λ by a decade. At higher noise and λ, N_{th} plateaued: once the feature reached a certain broadened size, further regularization offered less improvement in noise immunity. N_{th} was the same for both $I = 1 \times 10^{-3}$ and 3×10^{-3} at the same values of λ in figure 7.3(b), which was expected based on the scaling to be applied when forward problem conditions are varied (section 4.4.4).

The results of varying the forward and inverse mesh sizes are shown in appendix G.3. Keeping the forward mesh fixed at the finest level of j2d4c, N_{th} was unaffected by the inverse mesh until the mesh elements were no longer small compared to the smallest EIT feature size (which, decreasing from h2d4c, first occurred at mesh d2d4c). Likewise, keeping the inverse mesh fixed at a coarse e2d4c (the mesh still fine enough not to affect N_{th}), N_{th} was unaffected by the forward mesh, which was kept finer (varying from j2d4c to f2d4c) than the inverse mesh.

As shown above, just above N_{th} artefacts often have smaller amplitudes than the feature associated with the target. Thus, raising the image threshold level above $\Delta\sigma_R/2$, for example to $3\Delta\sigma_R/4$, could slightly increase tolerance to noise, allowing a target to be correctly identified. This change is readily implemented in the EIDORS code. However, given the steepness of the curves in figure 7.3(a), the benefit would only be slight. More importantly, this approach would also eliminate lighter touches.

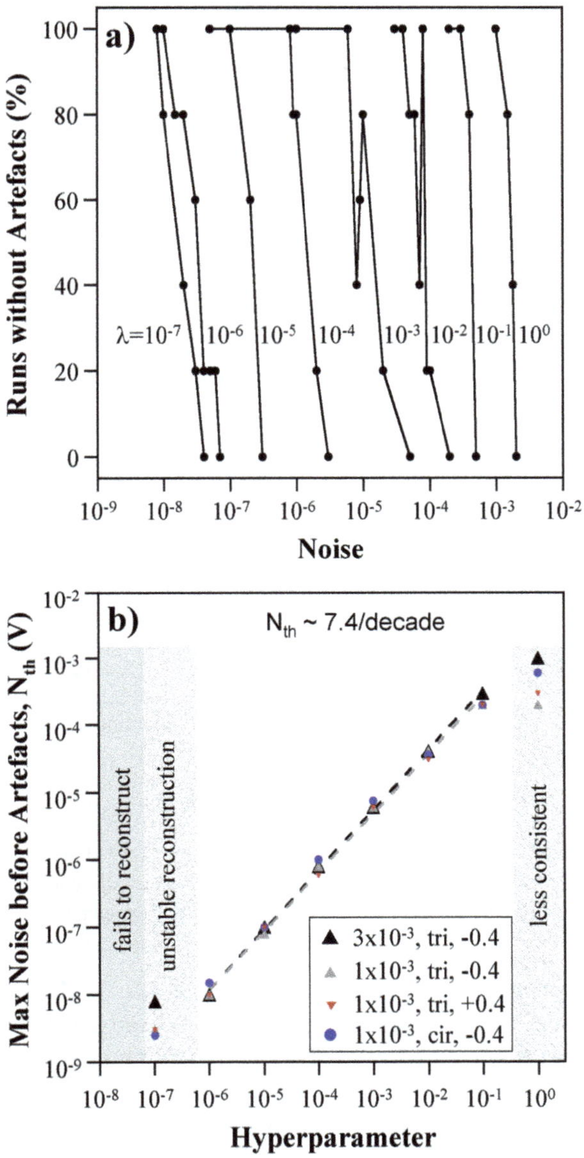

Figure 7.3. (a) The fraction of five trials with no artefacts as a function of noise at different values of the hyperparameter (triangular target, $I = 1 \times 10^{-3}$, $\sigma_T = 0.6\sigma_0$). (b) The maximum noise N_{th} before artefacts appear as a function of hyperparameter for triangular and circular targets at two currents ($I = 1 \times 10^{-3}$ and 3×10^{-3}) for both positive and negative contrasts of 40% (16 electrodes, I–M = 7–1, $\sigma_0 = 10^{-2}$, $\sigma_T = 0.6\sigma_0$ and $1.67\sigma_0$, $r_T = 0.2$, $x = 0.5$).

The artefact-based approach can readily be used to compare not only experimental parameters (see appendices G.13, G.14 and G.16) but also different systems, unlike metrics such as the noise figure [24]. For example, as shown in figure 7.4(a), noise thresholds for injection–measurement patterns I–M = 1–1 and 7–1 are identical up to $\lambda = 10^{-4}$, but 1–1 becomes more susceptible to noise at larger λ. (Note that the effective

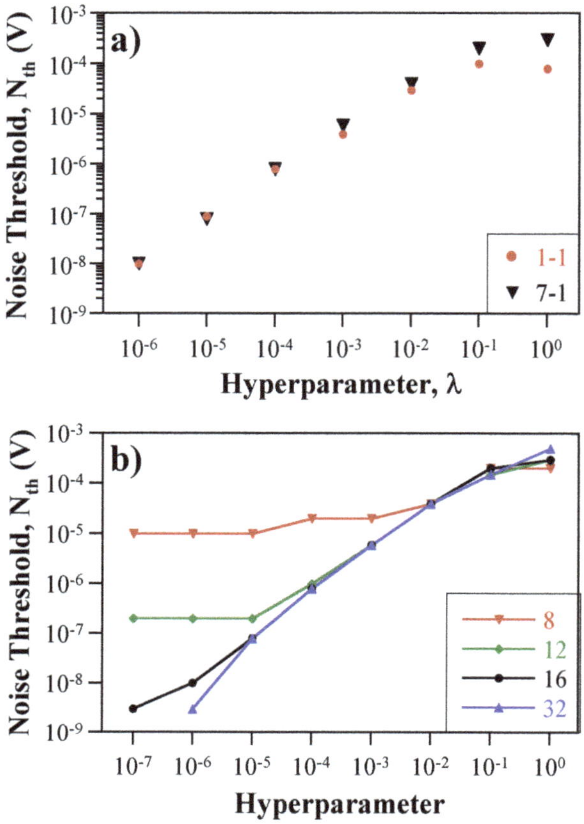

Figure 7.4. (a) Noise thresholds as a function of hyperparameter for I–M = 1–1 and 7–1 (16 electrodes). (b) N_{th} as a function of λ for varying numbers of electrodes (I–M = pseudo-polar-adjacent: 15–1 for 32 electrodes, 7–1 for 16, 5–1 for 12, and 3–1 for 8). ($\sigma_0 = 10^{-2}$, $\sigma_{\text{T}} = 0.6\sigma_0$, $I = 10^{-3}$, triangular target, $x = 0.5$, $r_{\text{T}} = 0.2$)

strength of the hyperparameter also differs for these two I–M patterns as shown in chapters 5 and appendix G.15: for large λ, at which behavior becomes increasingly dominated by loss of sensitivity to conductivity changes at the center of the sensor, 1–1 experiences greater defocusing.) As another example (figure 7.4(b)), above $\lambda = 10^{-5}$, $N_{\text{th}}(\lambda)$ is identical for 16 and 32 electrode systems having equivalent I–M patterns. In fact, even for fewer electrodes N_{th} becomes equivalent once the noise reaches the level of the smallest Picard coefficients for the system. Stated differently, systems with fewer electrodes, which have lower resolution, lack the high spatial frequency image components that are corrupted at smaller levels of noise, but the lower spatial frequency components are similarly affected by noise.

7.1.4 Comparison of hyperparameters obtained from L-Curve, GCV, and BestRes considering N_{th}

Notwithstanding the prior work on this issue, the optimal method for hyper-parameter selection still requires further consideration [25] for tactile sensing.

Numerous approaches have been developed to optimize the image for use in various fields based on different criteria. For example, in prior work for optical topography, 11 different methods for choosing the hyperparameter were reviewed [18] with the conclusion that the classical L-curve was the best. For medical imaging, the BestRes method [17], to which our approach is conceptually similar, was favorably compared to five other methods including generalized cross-validation (GCV) [26, 27], another frequently used technique (although under the conditions in [17], GCV resulted in severely under-regularized solutions and was found to be unreliable). Therefore, here we compare the hyperparameter at the onset of artefacts to hyperparameters selected using BestRes, the L-curve, and GCV.

The L-curve compares the 'size', given by the L2 norm (variously written as $||x||_2$, $||L(x_\lambda - x_0)||_2$, etc), of the 'regularized solution', which in our case is the EIT image $\boldsymbol{\sigma}$, with the size of the 'residual,' which is the difference between what the regularized solution would predict for the input voltage difference data and the actual input data (written as $||Ax_\lambda - b||_2$, etc) [28]. In EIT this residual is the difference $\mathbf{J}_{\text{reg}}\boldsymbol{\sigma}-\boldsymbol{\Delta}$, where $\mathbf{J}$ is the Jacobian or sensitivity matrix and $\mathbf{J}_{\text{reg}}$ is the regularized $\mathbf{J}$ [22]. The size of the image is larger when there are more features. For example in figure 7.2(a) the image size is larger for $N = 2 \times 10^{-7}$ than for $N = 1 \times 10^{-7}$ because of the artefacts (see appendix G.4). On the other hand, the size of the residual increases as the feature becomes increasingly smoothed (see appendix G.5). L-curves can be generated in EIDORS using the *l_curve* function in the add-on *regtools* toolbox [29–31]. This function takes $\mathbf{U}$ and $\mathbf{S}$ from the singular value decomposition (SVD) of $\mathbf{J}$ [22], as well as the voltage difference data $\boldsymbol{\Delta}$ (with noise) as inputs, which are all from the forward problem. (Note that *l_curve* requires running *csvd*, or compact SVD, on $\mathbf{J}$. For some notes on the calculation, see appendix G.6.) This code dampens the image coefficients by $s_i^2/(s_i^2 + \lambda^2)$, where i is the index of the coefficient and the s_i are the singular values in $\mathbf{S}$; this differs from the actual dampening resulting from the Laplace prior (section 5.1.3 and appendix G.7). The L-curve for a given $\boldsymbol{\Delta}$ is generated automatically for 200 values of λ, providing an approximate optimal hyperparameter. Since the curve is found for a particular $\boldsymbol{\Delta}$, which contains noise, the hyperparameter varies somewhat from run to run. L-curve minima have been considered to be over-regularized based on visual inspection of the resulting images, although the size of the target may have played a role [32]; the role of target size is further examined below.

GCV is another method for calculating the optimal λ for a frame of data; it is based on a statistical approach, as well described in [16], and has been successfully validated and used in other fields. Conceptually, one element of the dataset is omitted and the remaining points are used to calculate a solution, which is then used to predict the missing element. The λ that minimizes the prediction error for all the data points is then found. For Tikhonov regularization, in practice the minimum of a function $G(\lambda)$ is found. $G(\lambda)$ can be generated in EIDORS using the *gcv.m* and *gcvfun.m* functions in the add-on *regtools* toolbox [29–31]. Like the L-curve calculation, this function takes $\mathbf{U}$, $\mathbf{S}$, and $\boldsymbol{\Delta}$ from *csvd* as inputs. This code uses the filter $f = \lambda^2/(\mathbf{S}^2 + \lambda^2)$. G is calculated as the ratio of the norm of the square of the product of f with $\mathbf{U}^{\mathrm{T}}\boldsymbol{\Delta}$ and the sum of the square of the terms in f. (For details, see appendix G.8.) The *G* curve is also generated automatically for 200 values of λ, and its minimum is at the optimal hyperparameter. This λ is optimal, in the sense of predicting omitted points, for the particular dataset $\mathbf{\Delta}$. Under some conditions, like other methods, GCV can fail [16].

The BestRes method of obtaining the hyperparameter is based on the resolution of the images [17], since resolution has been considered to be the primary metric of image quality [25]. BestRes obtains the minimum area occupied by the half amplitude set: that area increases due to the presence of artifacts when λ is too small and it increases again due to feature broadening when λ is too large. The procedure involves, for a fixed level of noise, reconstructing a number of images, with 50 being recommended, as a function of λ (see appendix G.11 for plots of some resolution data.). Resolution is found in EIDORS using *eval_GREIT_fig_merit.m*, and it is defined as r_R (equation (4), figure 7.1), which includes artefacts. The minimum in r_R versus λ is then located. As opposed to the L-curve and GCV, BestRes is used to set a fixed λ for subsequent imaging. A method based on BestRes was used to set the hyperparameter for a tactile sensing system, employing 150–200 replicates at every mesh element [13, 33].

The BestRes method employs an impulse contrast at a single mesh element located at $x = 0.5$. To compare the outcomes of these methods, a circular target with a small radius, $r_T = 0.05$, was therefore used: in our system, below this radius the amplitude of the reconstructed feature decreases but its resolution does not. In fact, its resolution is only somewhat smaller than that of a target with $r_T = 0.2$, although its amplitude is much smaller.

Four L-curves at different noise levels *N* are shown in figure 7.5(a), together with the located corner points and the values of the hyperparameters there (orange). The standard deviations of the hyperparameters over five trials were 6%–8%. One of the criticisms of the L-curve method is that there are cases when the curve does not have a clear corner so that it fails, which occurs when the solution is very ill-posed [18]. Such a failure can be seen at $N = 10^{-5}$ (green). The lack of a corner resulted in a completely incorrect identification of λ. This happened whenever the SNR was low. A corner developed at $N = 10^{-5}$ when the size of the target was increased from $r_T = 0.05$ to 0.2, improving the SNR.

The $G(\lambda)$ curves obtained with GCV are shown in appendix G.9 at the same four noise levels, and the corresponding EIT and threshold images are shown in appendix G.10 and in figure 7.7 at $N = 3 \times 10^{-6}$. The optimal hyperparameters were smaller than for the L-curve approach, and the images had artefacts at noise levels of $N = 10^{-6}$ and above.

The outcome of the BestRes approach is shown in figure 7.5(b), employing the recommended 50 trials at each point. The optimal hyperparameter is the one that gives the minimum resolution, as indicated (pink). Using five trials (open circles) is insufficient, as shown for $N = 3 \times 10^{-6}$ V (blue curves). The standard deviations of the resolutions for 50 trials, shown for two of the noise levels, are substantial, increasing both at smaller λ for a given noise and at higher noise for a given λ. The BestRes method, like the L-curve and GCV, failed at high noise (green).

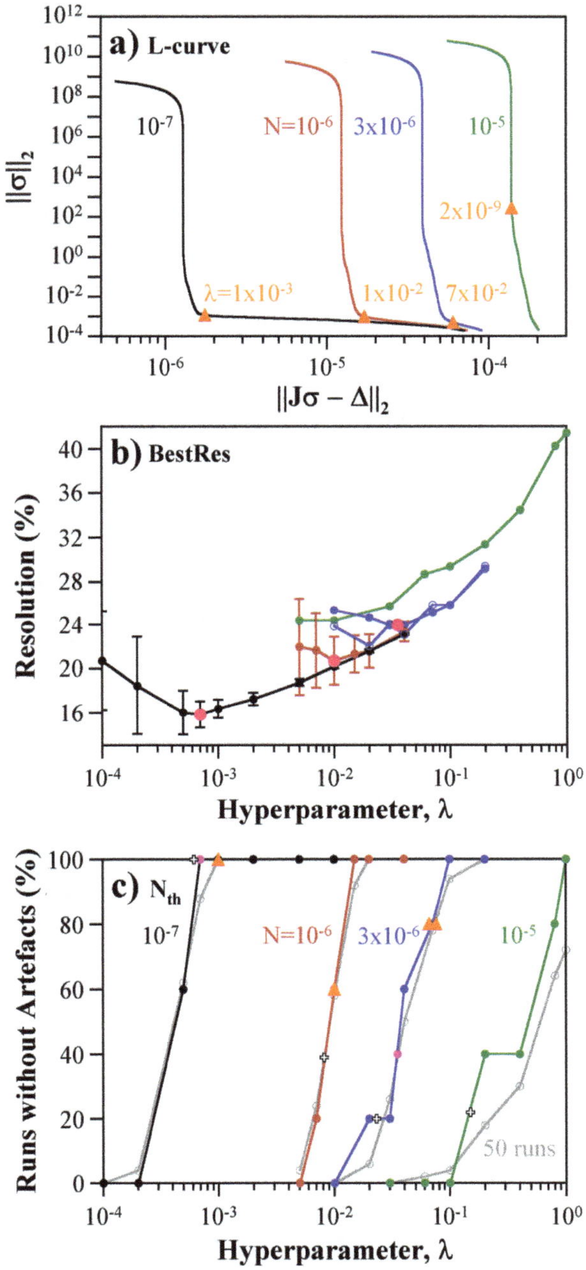

Figure 7.5. (a) L-curves at four noise levels and the associated corners (orange symbols); a single run is shown. (b) At the same noise levels, average resolution over 50 trials as a function of λ and the associated minima (pink). Also shown are standard deviations for two of the noise levels and the results of only five trials at $N = 3 \times 10^{-6}$ (open symbols). (c) Fraction of trials without artefacts in five trials (color) and 50 trials (open gray). For comparison, the optimal λs found in (a) and (b) are also shown (y-axis positions placed on the curve), with the minimum and maximum of five trials for the L-curve method at $N = 3 \times 10^{-6}$. The optimal λs found using GCV are shown as open '+' signs. (16 electrodes, I–M = 7–1, $\sigma_0 = 10^{-2}$, $\sigma_T = 0.9\ \sigma_0$, $i = 10^{-3}$, circular target, $r_T = 0.05$, $x = 0.5$)

The fraction of runs without artefacts is shown in figure 7.5(c) as a function of λ. (Note the x-axis change from figure 7.3(a), since in this case the noise was fixed and λ was varied.) Five trials is sufficient, as shown by comparison with the 50-trial curves. The optimal hyperparameters from the L-curve, λ_L (orange triangles), from GCV, λ_{CV} (black '+' signs), and from BestRes, λ_{BR} (pink circles), are also indicated on the figure, with their y-axis positions set to lie them on the N_{th} curves. (These L-curve values came from a single trial, with the exception of the points at $N = 3 \times 10^{-6}$, which show the minimum and maximum from five trials. The GCV hyperparameters are the average of five trials.) At $N = 1 \times 10^{-7}$, the hyperparameter obtained from using 100% of five trials without artefacts, λ_{th}, was the same as λ_{CV} and λ_{BR}, while λ_L and the 50-run artefact count agreed and were somewhat higher than the first three. With increasing noise, however, λ_{CV} and λ_{BR} became smaller than the other two, allowing a greater number of artefacts.

The heuristic method of choosing images involves looking at them to determine the best choice of λ. Example threshold images for $N = 3 \times 10^{-6}$ are shown in figure 7.6 at (a) $\lambda_{BR} = 3 \times 10^{-2}$ and (b) $\lambda_L = 7 \times 10^{-2}$. Although the resolution was on average slightly lower at λ_{BR} (23.95%) than the resolution at λ_L (24.66%, a size increase of 3%) (see also figure 7.5(b)), the artefacts with the former were significant. It could be argued that just below λ_{th}, at 80% artefact-free trials, corresponding to figure 7.6(b), the artefacts are sufficiently small and few to live with, and that this

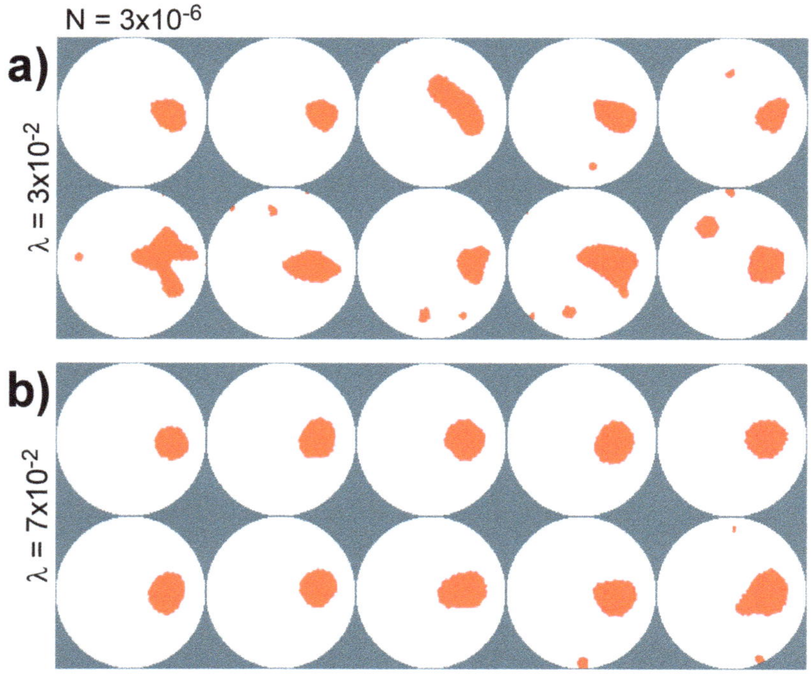

Figure 7.6. Representative half-max threshold images at a noise level of $N = 3 \times 10^{-6}$ at (a) $\lambda = 3 \times 10^{-2}$, the BestRes minimum, and (b) $\lambda = 7 \times 10^{-2}$, the L-curve corner. (16 electrodes, I–M = 7–1, $\sigma_0 = 10^{-2}$, $\sigma_T = 0.9\sigma_0$, $I = 10^{-3}$, circular target, $r_T = 0.05$, $x = 0.5$)

would be a better threshold than 100% artefact-free. The 'sufficiently small' criterion is based on the fact that the blur radius at a given hyperparameter is known, so features that are substantially smaller than that could be safely ignored; this would be the case if the dynamic range of expected contacts was small and that λ was small; otherwise a light contact simultaneous with a heavy one, or a contact at the center simultaneous with one at the edge, will appear to be small (section 5.5.2). Even at 60% artefact-free, the images were reasonable (not shown), with artefacts being much smaller than the feature and features having no gross distortions. However, down at 20% trials without artefacts (figure 7.6(a)), several of the images were sufficiently distorted, and the size of the artefacts sufficiently large, to lead to problems if a machine was relying on such images to make decisions. For example, in the 3rd, 6th, and 9th images, the shape of the contact is completely incorrect (the 3rd image suggests a sliding touch modality), and in the final image there appear to be two contacts, neglecting the smallest artefacts. At low noise (see appendix G.12 for images), $N = 1 \times 10^{-7}$, images had no artefacts at λ_{th} ($\lambda = 7 \times 10^{-4}$), but at the smaller $\lambda = 5 \times 10^{-4}$ (60% without artefacts) occasional images had artefacts of size comparable to the feature. Thus, 70%–100% artefact-free would appear to be a good working limit. If there are multiple contacts, some of which are considerably smaller or lighter, or some of which are closer to the center of the sensor, the higher limit may be preferred.

Figure 7.7 shows the EIT and corresponding threshold images produced by setting a fixed λ using N_{th} versus using optimal λs determined by the L-curve and GCV on the same five data frames ($N = 3 \times 10^{-6}$). (Images at other noise levels are shown in appendix G.10.) The λ_{L} were close to, but a little smaller than, λ_{th}, thereby giving a slightly better resolution, but the λ_{CV} were up to an order of magnitude smaller, and thus showed artefacts.

The answer to the question of which approach is 'better' depends on the needs of the application. A set-and-forget approach, like N_{th} or BestRes, can work well if the SNR does not vary much for a given application. Methods that optimize λ for a particular dataset, such as L-curve and GCV, are desirable if the sensor may experience multiple contacts, particularly transient contacts. (While code could be readily be written to automate the counting of artefacts, reducing λ until only a single region remained, that would not work for tactile sensing applications with the possibility of more than one touch at the same time.) Since under-regularization is detrimental, the L-curve may be a good option. This question is further examined below.

We can conclude that for tactile sensing, resolution is not an ideal criterion for hyperparameter selection. Furthermore, it is inefficient, requiring a large number of replicates because of the high variability of resolution among images, and it fails at high noise. It may be argued that the need for determining λ at high noise is questionable, since it would be far better to increase the SNR. However, there may be cases when this cannot be done. The more conservative L-curve estimates result in images with a little more blur than BestRes, but with more consistently correct representations of target characteristics. With even a single run, the L-curve provided a good estimate of a hyperparameter that could be used for set-and-forget, although at low SNR the method also failed.

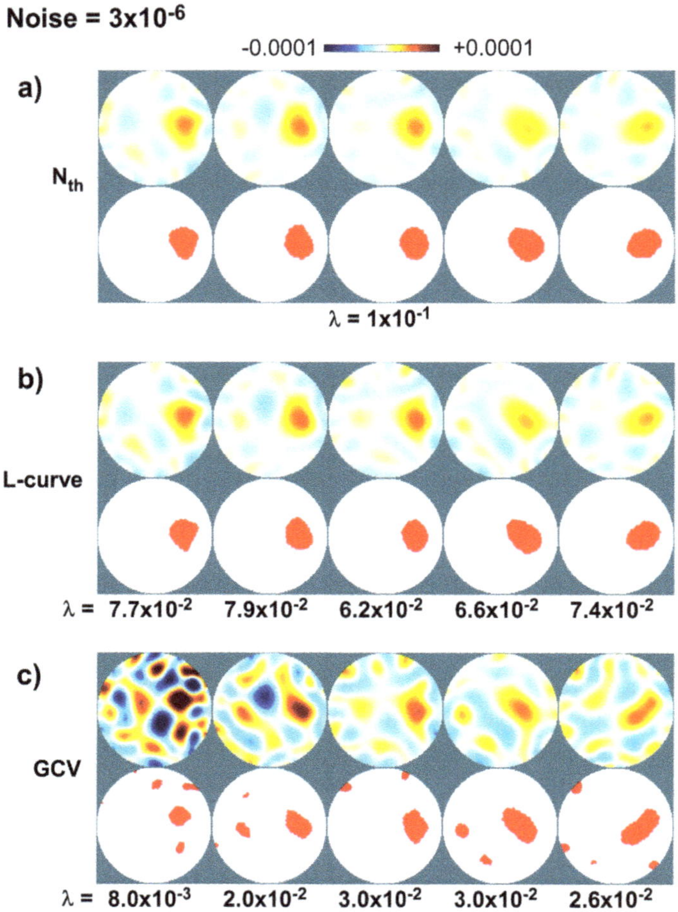

Figure 7.7. EIT and half-max threshold images produced for the same five trials at a noise level of N using the fixed (a) N_{th} hyperparameter and the optimal (b) L-curve and (c) GCV hyperparameters. (16 electrodes, I–M = 7–1, $\sigma_O = 10^{-2}$, $\sigma_T = 0.9\sigma_O$, $i = 10^{-3}$, circular target, $r_{\text{T}} = 0.05$, $x = 0.5$)

7.1.5 Practical implications

We turn to the issue of handling variability of contacts with a tactile sensor. For some applications, such as interpreting finger touches on an artificial skin [3, 10, 11, 34, 35], the dynamic range of the expected signals may not be large, allowing a hyperparameter to be set in advance. The dynamic range for other applications may, however, be large. The SNR, and thus the required λ, depends directly on the strength of the touch, which may be a light contact from one finger (1–2 N) or it may be a strong blow from a fist (1600 N) [36] or from an accidental bump into a large protrusion; some applications experience a wide range of pressure [37]. An examination of noise thresholds as a function of target size (figure 7.8) shows that the required hyperparameter at a given noise level can vary by two orders of

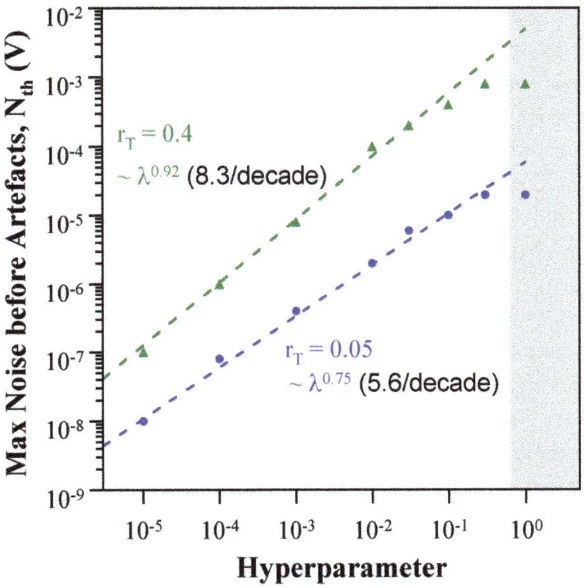

Figure 7.8. Noise thresholds as a function of λ for circular targets of small and large radius r_T (points) and curve fits (dashed lines) (16 electrodes, I–M = 7–1, $\sigma_0 = 10^{-2}$, $\sigma_T = 0.6\sigma_0$, $I = 10^{-3}$, $x = 0.3$).

magnitude for a target of $r_T = 0.05$ versus one of $r_T = 0.4$. Furthermore, the dependence of N_{th} on λ differs for the two radii, becoming steeper for larger targets.

Regarding the accuracy of the representation of different-sized targets, the effect of a large λ on amplitude is even more severe than its effects on resolution. Smaller targets, $r_T < 0.2$, have reduced amplitudes even at the smallest λ because of the minimum resolution with which they can be represented (since the volumes of features are maintained, amplitude drops with r_T), and their amplitudes are further reduced by increases in λ. In contrast, large targets, $r_T \geqslant 0.4$, are little affected by λ. In addition, the optimal hyperparameter depends on target position at low SNRs (not shown). Thus, setting λ in advance based on the worst-case SNR scenario of a small, light target at the center of the sensor would result in potentially greatly and unnecessarily over-blurred images for other targets, rendering pointless the exercise of obtaining an optimal hyperparameter.

To handle a large dynamic range in SNR, the hyperparameter should ideally be dynamically and automatically set. This is contrary to the conventional wisdom of choosing λ in advance for a range of data based on the view that it is impractical to set λ for each measurement [24]. The artefact-based approach presented here is unsuitable for dynamically determining λ because the number of touches is *a priori* unknown. Methods such as those based on image SNR also require knowledge of the targets [24]. However, the L-curve and GCV are run on one frame of data and require no prior information about the contacts. A concern is the additional computational time and capability required. The SVD for the system, to obtain **U** and **S** from **J**, only needs to be done once, and setting the range of λ in advance would allow some pre-computation; it may also be possible to reduce the number of tested hyperparameters. Another concern arises from the fact that most of the time the sensor will not experience a touch, so the measurement frames contain only noise. Under these conditions the L-curve and GCV fail, yielding a tiny hyper-parameter (figure 7.5(a)) and generating an image overwhelmed by noise. A minimum λ may therefore be required. This could be set in advance, for example using a calibration contact representing the maximum expected SNR. As an aside, to avoid visual confusion the image color scale may also need to be selected automatically, employing a minimum and maximum, since a fixed color scale can struggle with dynamic range (e.g. figure 7.2(a) versus (b)). A third concern is that the L-curve may over-regularize the images, and the GCV under-regularize it. A multiplier on λ_L orλ_{CV} could be employed to adjust it, and such a multiplier could be set to apply to different ranges or circumstances. A recommendation for future work is therefore an investigation of a 'light weight' method of choosing the hyperparameter that can be run quickly (to allow low latency for decision-making) and on a platform such as a mobile phone. The use of available prior information, such as from a sliding contact or a longer touch, could also be employed to guide the selection of λ.

Given the minimalism of the system, data being in principle obtained from periphery voltage measurements on a simple continuous resistor, and given that simulations of potential drops at the perimeter due to conductivity variations within the sensor area (the forward problem) are straightforward and unambiguous, simulations and experiments would be expected to give the same results, provided that the assumptions in the model are valid. However, in actual experiments these assumptions may not hold: the initial resistance over the sensor may not be known or uniform, the noise on the electrodes may not be white, and the electrical connections may not be ideal points, as assumed in this work. Without understanding these non-idealities and their effects, discrepancies between experimental and simulation results can be challenging to interpret. In future work, therefore, several topics need to be studied. One is the effect of non-uniform sensor conductivity. The spray-coating of piezoresistive films, for example, may result in thickness variations across the surface, and differences in drying rates may result in stratification of conductive phases, both producing variations in conductivity. Accurately mapping the initial conductivity distribution $\sigma_0(x,y)$ is time consuming, but an incorrect $\sigma_0(x,y)$ entered into the algorithms results in inaccurate predictions. An acceptable tolerance for non-uniformity has not been established based on EIT performance metrics such as amplitude, shape, and position accuracy. Another related issue is anisotropic conductivity, which is significant in fabric-based sensors. Because of the many advantages of forming smart skins from conductive fabrics, understanding how to incorporate anisotropies due to different weaves into EIT forward models is a priority. A second area for examination is the nature of the noise arising from tactile sensors. In particular, does the noise depend on the distance of the measurement electrodes from the injection electrode or ground, or on the distance between the two measurement electrodes? On a given electrode, is the noise Gaussian? In this work, the noise was assumed to be the zero-mean, normally distributed and the same on every channel, but that would only be the case if the dominant source of noise was a common analog-to-digital converter or the power supply. Other sources of noise in a particular experiment [15], such as arising from the current flowing in the sensing material, could invalidate this assumption. The nature of the noise may be highly system-specific. A third important topic concerns the electrical connections. Electrode size is known to affect the reconstruction, as does contact impedance. Even more significant can be sensor strain concentrated at the electrodes, which is sensitive to the location and strength of any tactile contacts and depends on the mechanical clamping conditions. Such strains can dominate the EIT image since they occur at the perimeter, where sensitivity to changes in conductivity is greatest.

7.2 Considerations regarding the injection–measurement pattern

Much of the material in this section is from the paper Smela E 2022 EIT for tactile sensing: considerations regarding the injection–measurement pattern *Eng. Res. Expr.* **4** 045041 [59], but there is additional text here, most of which was in the Supporting Information of the article.

In order to understand the strengths and weaknesses of the I–M patterns for use in tactile imaging, we begin with negligible noise added to the simulations. In an overview we show EIT images for two targets. Then we look at reconstructed feature size metrics—amplitude, resolution, and volume—and position error. The noise susceptibility of the patterns is next examined. Lastly, a system with 13 electrodes is studied. Based on the totality of the data, recommendations are made.

7.2.1 Introduction

EIT [38] is attractive for tactile sensing [35] because it can be used to create an image of conductivity changes due to a contact within a continuous sensing area using electrodes placed only at the perimeter. Some of those electrodes inject current while others measure the resulting voltages. There has been considerable research concerning the choice of current injection and voltage measurement (I–M) electrode placements for EIT; see for example [35, 39]. While there are advantages to using patterns that involve multiple current sources, much of the focus has been on *bipolar* configurations (also called pairwise or differential), which involve one pair of electrodes for current injection and another pair for voltage measurement. In particular, the adjacent (ADJ), polar (POL or opposite), and pseudo-polar (PP) electrode placements have received the most attention.

To elucidate these electrode placement designations, in a bipolar configuration a sequence or *frame* of measurements is made, with the current-injecting electrode pair and the voltage-measuring pair rotating systematically around the perimeter (for further information see section 4.2). The current-injecting electrodes are typically not used for voltage measurement, so the frame consists of between 192 and 208 measurements for a 16-electrode system, depending on the I–M pattern. Figure 7.9 illustrates examples of two positions during a single

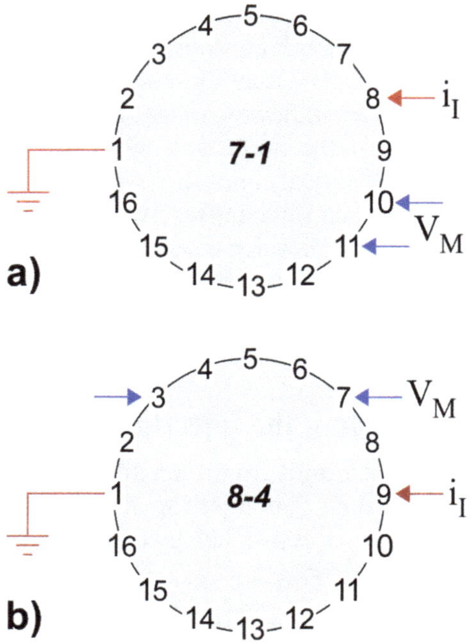

Figure 7.9. I–M electrode patterns are designated by the relative positions of the electrodes in each pair. (a) In I–M = 7–1, the current injecting electrode (indicated by i_I) is offset seven positions away from ground, while the voltage is measured between adjacent electrodes (indicated by V_M). (b) In 8–4, the current injecting electrode is eight positions away from ground, and the voltage is measured between electrodes four spaces apart. Reproduced from [59].

measurement of the frame. The names used in this work for the injection and measurement electrode pairs are based on the number of positions between the electrodes, or the *offset*, which is maintained fixedly during their rotations. Thus, adjacent electrodes have an offset of 1 and electrodes on opposite sides of the sensor have an offset of 8 in the 16-electrode system, as shown in table 7.1. (This differs from the skip-*m* convention, in which adjacent electrodes are indicated by 0.) The angle between the electrodes has also been used in the literature to designate relative positions.

The susceptibility to uniform noise is quantified using the noise threshold metric N_{th} of section 7.1. This study does not address experimental issues that affect implementation, such as quantization errors or noise that depends on electrode positions or separations.

As discussed in chapter 4, the conductivity change image, $\boldsymbol{\sigma}$, and the changes in perimeter voltages, $\boldsymbol{\Delta}$, are related by $\sigma = \mathbf{J}_{\mathbf{reg}}^{-1}\Delta$, where $\mathbf{J}$ is the sensitivity matrix, or Jacobian, and $\mathbf{J}_{\mathbf{reg}}$ is the regularized $\mathbf{J}$. (The extent of regularization is controlled by the hyperparameter, λ.) $\mathbf{J}$ for a given I–M pattern has a rank r equal to the number of independent measurements, which is smaller than the total number of

Table 7.1. Nomenclatures for specifying bipolar electrode positions.

Offset			Angle	Name
Number of electrodes				
16	8	32		
1		2	22.5	Adjacent (ADJ)
2	1	4	45.0	
3		6	67.5	
4	2	8	90.0	
5		10	112.5	
6	3	12	135.0	
7		14	157.5	Pseudo-polar (PP)
8	4	16	180.0	Polar, Opposite (POL)

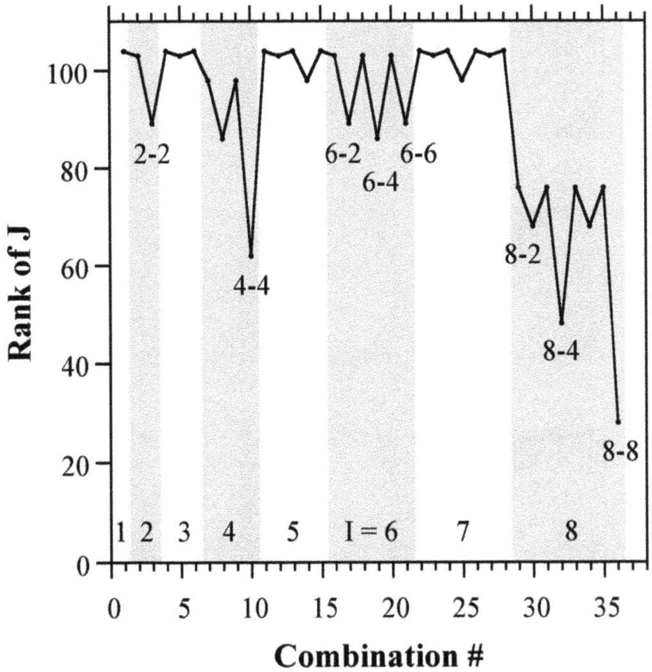

Figure 7.10. Rank r of the Jacobian, which is equal to the number of independent measurements, for the 36 unique I–M combinations for 16 electrodes. Labels are included for some of the I–M patterns. Reproduced from [59]. Copyright IOP Publishing Ltd. All rights reserved.

measurements due to various electrode position symmetries. Figure 7.10 shows the ranks of **J** for all 36 unique bipolar configurations for a sensor with 16 electrodes. (By reciprocity, driving the current between pair A and measuring the voltage between pair B is equivalent to driving between pair B and measuring between pair A [53] (e.g. reconstructions for 7–1 and 1–7 are identical), so only half of all the numerical possibilities require examination, yielding 36 patterns.) The I–M patterns in figure 7.10 are ordered by a combination number determined by the first offset value for I, grouped into shaded areas, and then by the second offset value for M, which goes from 1 to I. The highest symmetry patterns have the lowest rank. Low-rank patterns have poor resolution even at low levels of regularization, e.g. at small hyperparameters (λ), for reasons discussed in section 7.1. The results below show that rank determines I–M performance at small hyperparameters. The set of patterns with a rank of at least 80 are designated here as the 'I–M_{80+}'.

The rows of **J** show the sensitivity of the voltages to conductivity changes on the sensor surface for given positions of the injection and measurement pairs in the measurement frame. Figure 7.11 shows the 1st, 3rd, and 7th rows of **J**, or the

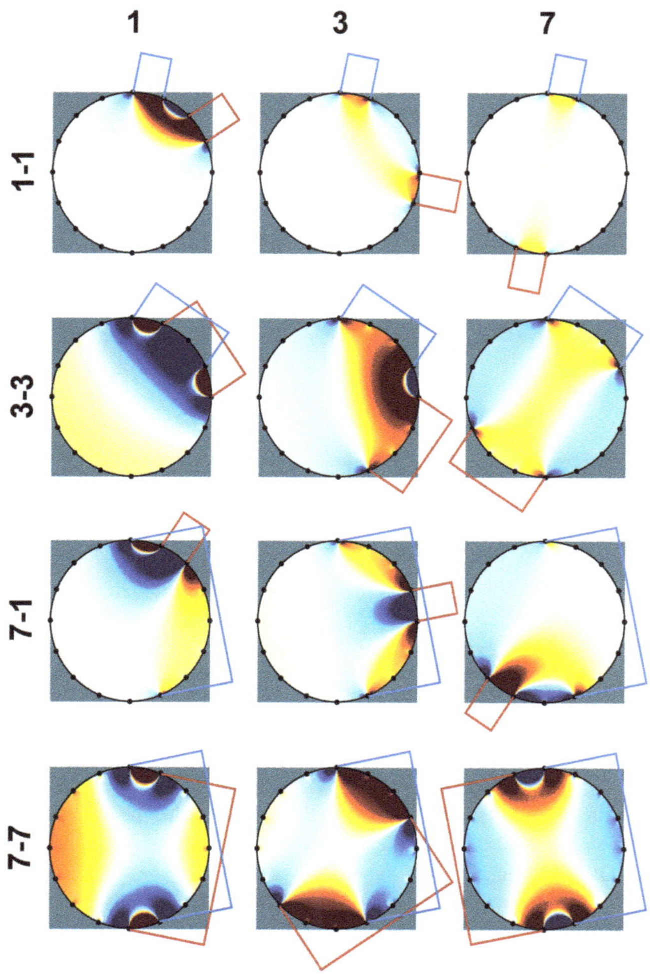

Figure 7.11. Sensitivity maps resulting from visualization of rows 1, 3, and 7 of the Jacobian **J** for four of the I–M patterns. Colored lines indicate the connection points for current injection and voltage measurement; by reciprocity exchanging them gives the same outcome. Reproduced from [59]. Copyright IOP Publishing Ltd. All rights reserved.

sensitivity maps, for four of the I–M patterns. (The first seven rows are shown in appendix C for all of the I–M patterns; by symmetry, the rest are known from those.) For I–M = 1–1, when the injection and measurement pair are next to each other (offset 1), there is high positive sensitivity, indicated by the dark red color, near the edge. As the electrode pair separation increases, the sensitivity decreases until, at the point in the data collection sequence when the pairs are opposite each other (I and M are offset by 7), there is very little sensitivity anywhere, as indicated by the white color. Thus, I–M = 1–1 is sensitive primarily to targets, or conductivity contrasts, at the periphery. Looking at I–M = 3–3, there is strong negative sensitivity when the electrode pairs are offset by 1 position, which changes to strong positive sensitivity for offset 3. When the pairs are on opposite sides of the sensor, there is still significant sensitivity in the center, and the sensitivity is fairly uniform between them. Thus, I–M = 3–3 covers the entire area reasonably well. I–M = 7–1, like 1–1, has sensitivity primarily at the edge, whereas 7–7 has good coverage in the center for offsets 1 and 7 and also high sensitivity at the edge for offset 3. The results presented below show how sensitivity determines I–M performance at large hyperparameters. (For a discussion of the relative degradation of images for different I–M patterns due to regularization, see figure 5.2 and section 5.3.)

Not explicitly shown on the sensitivity maps are the magnitudes of the potential drops. Since the resistance between electrodes is proportional to their separation, for a fixed injection current, greater electrode separation results in larger potential differences. Because the electrodes for I or M = 1 are closer together than for other positions, the maximum values in the measurement frame are smaller, and this lowers the SNR, necessitating the use of larger hyperparameters [22].

Unless otherwise specified, other model parameters are given in table 5.1. Noise was uncorrelated zero-mean Gaussian. A single circular target of radius $r_T = 0.2$ with a uniform conductivity decrease was used. Because reconstructions have previously been shown to have circular symmetry [19, 33, 34], only target positions along the x-axis were studied.

Recommendations regarding the best bipolar pattern have varied [13, 15, 25, 33, 39–52], as summarized in table 7.2, because outcomes depend on factors such as the extent of regularization, the performance measures employed, the method of adding noise (e.g. fixed versus percentage), the inverse algorithm and prior that were used, and the target characteristics, not all of which have always been specified. The ADJ pattern was frequently used in the early years, although other work recommended POL. More recently, in publications on this topic PP has emerged as a consensus among these three. PP has been reported to produce greater detectability of conductivity changes, allowing the use of smaller injection currents [47], and to be have better noise performance [34, 43, 44]. Another study on the angle between the current injecting and ground electrodes found that the range from 60° to 150° (table 7.1) was best [15]. Still others have advised choosing a pattern with a high sensitivity to conductivity changes in the region of interest [39], employing different patterns for detecting changes at the center and edge of the sensed area [52]. Despite those studies, however, the tactile sensing community has converged on the use of I–M = ADJ–ADJ (1–1).

Table 7.2. Summary of some conclusions from prior work on the choice of bipolar I–M patterns.

Recommendations	Basis and additional observations	References
Use POL instead of ADJ for moderate-high regularization.	Simulations with TSVD. Based on singular value spectra, resolution at different truncation points (e.g. regularization), noise performance. Noise was highest near the perimeter.	[40]
Choose pattern with high sensitivity to region of interest.	Review.	[39]
Use ADJ.	Simulations. Based on rate of convergence of iterative reconstruction with noise. No regularization employed.	[41]
No pattern is preferred; can combine multiple patterns.	Simulations. Based on sensitivity maps. ADJ was least sensitive in the center but had best proportional selectivity for seeking location of change.	[42]
PP is optimal. Avoid ADJ.	Equivalent circuit model. Based on boundary voltage change & dynamic range, # independent measurements, anti-noise performance, singular value spectra.	[43, 44]
Use PP–PP.	Theory Based on sensitivity distribution, rank.	[45]
Place an electrode(s) in the interior of the sensor. Avoid ADJ.	Simulations & tactile sensor experiments. Based on resolution, position error, and resolution with noise.	[13, 33]
Use PP.	Simulations. Based on iso-potential lines, number of measurements, voltage dynamic range, voltage change, conductivity error.	[46]
Use PP–PP. Avoid symmetric patterns. Avoid ADJ.	Simulations. Based on distinguishability (probability of detection) of all I–M bipolar pairs. Saline tank experiments. Based on eight I-positions; M-position was ADJ.	[47]
Use offsets from 4 to 14 at high noise ($>10^{-4}s_1$), optimally 12 (123°).[a] Use large offsets to reduce dependence on target position. Use POL for best distinguishability.	Simulations, 32 electrode system. Based on singular value spectra, Jacobian correlation, number of independent measurements, $\|\|\mathbf{\Delta}\|\|_2$.[b]	[15]

(*Continued*)

Table 7.2. (*Continued*)

Recommendations	Basis and additional observations	References
Minimize symmetry by using a prime number of electrodes. Use 32 electrodes instead of 16. Avoid even-number electrode spacings, particularly POL and others of high symmetry. Avoid offsets >12.		
Use an offset of 4 for most visually reliable images. Avoid small offsets (0–3) to minimize shape distortions. Avoid intermediate offsets (5–12) to minimize ringing and blurring. Avoid large offsets (13–15) to minimize autocorrelation (e.g. mirroring).	Saline tank experiments, 32 electrodes. Based on EIT images.	[15]
Use POL.	Experiments with chicken tissue. Based on boundary voltages, image quality, noise.	[48]
Use large angles between injection electrodes.	Simulations. Based on distinguishability, correlation coefficient, relative error.	[49]
Use ADJ rather than POL.	Simulations. Based on electric fields, EIT images.	[50]
Use a prime number of electrodes. Avoid 90° and 180° separations.	Simulations, 32 electrode system. Based on rank, singular values, and global uncertainty.	[51]
Dynamically change pattern depending on target location. Use PP–PP for multiple touches.	Tactile sensor experiments. Based on image quality metrics, $\|\|\boldsymbol{\Delta}\|\|_2$[b], SNR.	[52]
Use either ADJ or POL.	Simulations. Based on norm of conductivity difference.	[25]

Notes:

[a] is the largest singular value.

[b] Signal strength = boundary voltage change = $\|\boldsymbol{\Delta}\|_2 = \sqrt{\sum(\Delta_i)^2}$, where $\boldsymbol{\Delta} = \mathbf{V}_{\text{touch}} - \mathbf{V}_{\text{ref}}$ is the vector of voltage differences with and without a target, respectively.

An in-depth comparison of the performance of different bipolar I–M patterns on criteria important for in tactile sensing has not yet been presented. This chapter describes comprehensive simulations of all the patterns for a circular sensor with 16 electrodes. The extent of regularization, here controlled by the hyperparameter λ, and the position of the target are varied, and the resulting performance on a number of measures, or metrics, is quantified to elucidate the conditions under which some patterns perform well or poorly. The metrics that are of most interest for tactile imaging were introduced previously, in chapter 3, namely (a) resolution, amplitude, and volume; (b) uniformity of resolution, amplitude, and volume over the sensing area; (c) position error; and (d) noise susceptibility.

This study shows how the choice of I–M pattern depends on the hyperparameter and the relative importance of the metrics. Plots present the performance of all the patterns, and these can be used to guide decisions if the hyperparameter will remain within a narrow range and certain performance criteria dominate the choice. There are some bipolar patterns that should not be used, including those with ADJ and POL positions, among others. While there are differences in performance across the acceptable I–M patterns, those are small in comparison with differences brought about by changes in λ, so every effort should be made to reduce noise. For tactile encounters requiring a hyperparameter that might vary greatly and that need good performance across all metrics, for the 16-electrode system I–M = 3–3 provides a good compromise, as does 2–2 under low noise conditions. The results also show that reducing the number of electrodes from 16 to 13 can be advantageous.

This simulation study examines outcomes under the best conditions for a two-dimensional circular sensor, a step change in conductivity for a circular target of a particular radius ($r_T = 0.2$), and identical Gaussian noise on every channel. These forward model parameters result in a set of simulated electrode voltage differences, $\mathbf{\Delta}$, that reflect an ideal tactile experimental set-up. The study does not address experimental actualities that affect real-world outcomes, such as non-uniform and anisotropic sensor conductivity, fluctuations in injected current, electrode motion and impedance, hysteresis and other memory effects, stress concentrations at the electrodes due to contact, Joule heating, or noise that depends on electrode positions or separations. These issues will perturb the voltages going into the inverse problem that creates the image of conductivity changes, $\boldsymbol{\sigma}$. Furthermore, the simulations employ a particular inverse algorithm and prior. Other inversion techniques might give somewhat different outcomes.

Full details of the simulations were given in chapter 3. Briefly, EIDORS (version 3.10, Matlab version R2018b) [54–56] was employed with the Gauss–Newton one-step algorithm and the Laplace prior. The mesh size used for the forward problem was the finest j2d4c, and for the inverse it was h2d4c. Prior work showed that results were mesh invariant [22]. The threshold $f = 2$ was used for the $1/f$ max amplitude set (e.g. the half amplitude set, consisting of image

Table 7.3. Simulation parameters for the baseline case.

Forward model parameter	Symbol	Value	Target parameter	Symbol	Value
# Electrodes	$N_{\text{electrodes}}$	16	# Targets	–	1
Injected current	I	1×10^{-3}	Target position	x	0.1
				y	0.0
Noise	N	1×10^{-12}	Target radius	r_{T}	0.2
Sensor shape	Circle		Target shape	Circle	—
Sensor conductivity	σ_0	1×10^{-2}	Target conductivity	σ_{T}	$0.9\ \sigma_0$ (Contrast = −10%)

elements $\Delta\sigma_i > \Delta\sigma_{\mathrm{R}}/2$, where $\Delta\sigma_{\mathrm{R}}$ is the largest amplitude in the image, was the region of interest, ROI). Unless otherwise specified, other model parameters are given in table 7.3. Noise was uncorrelated zero-mean Gaussian. A single circular target of radius $r_T = 0.2$ with a uniform conductivity decrease was used. Because reconstructions have previously been shown, both in simulation and experimentally, to be substantially circularly symmetric [19, 33, 34, 57], only target positions along the x-axis were studied.

The hyperparameter values specified in this work are specific to the current and sensor baseline conductivity used in these simulations, and values of λ need to be scaled to account for changes in those parameters for λ to have the same level of influence on the final image (see section 4.4.4). As discussed in prior chapters, the hyperparameter values given here are specific to the current and conductivity used in these simulations, and values of λ need to be scaled to account for changes in those parameters for λ to have the same level of influence on the final image. The higher the current I, the larger λ must be to have the same effect, with a linear relationship: for each 2x increase in current, the size of λ must be increased by 2x. On the other hand, the larger the sensor conductivity σ_0, the smaller λ must be have the same relative strength, and this effect goes as the square: for each 2x increase in conductivity, the size of λ must be decreased by 4x. Changing the contrast, defined as the conductivity change $\Delta\sigma$ relative to the baseline sensor conductivity σ_0, does not change the width of the feature and therefore requires no scaling of λ. (A scaled hyperparameter λ_s that allows comparison across experimental conditions is $\lambda_s = \lambda\sigma_0^2/i$, which here would be $\lambda_s = 0.1\lambda$.) (table 7.3)

7.2.2 Overview

EIT images resulting from different I–M patterns provide some context for the quantitative metrics presented below. In figure 7.12 images with negligible noise are shown using two different targets: a cross-shaped target and a three-circle target. The current injection pair is given on the vertical axis and the measurement pair on the horizontal axis, increasing in opposite directions for the two targets.

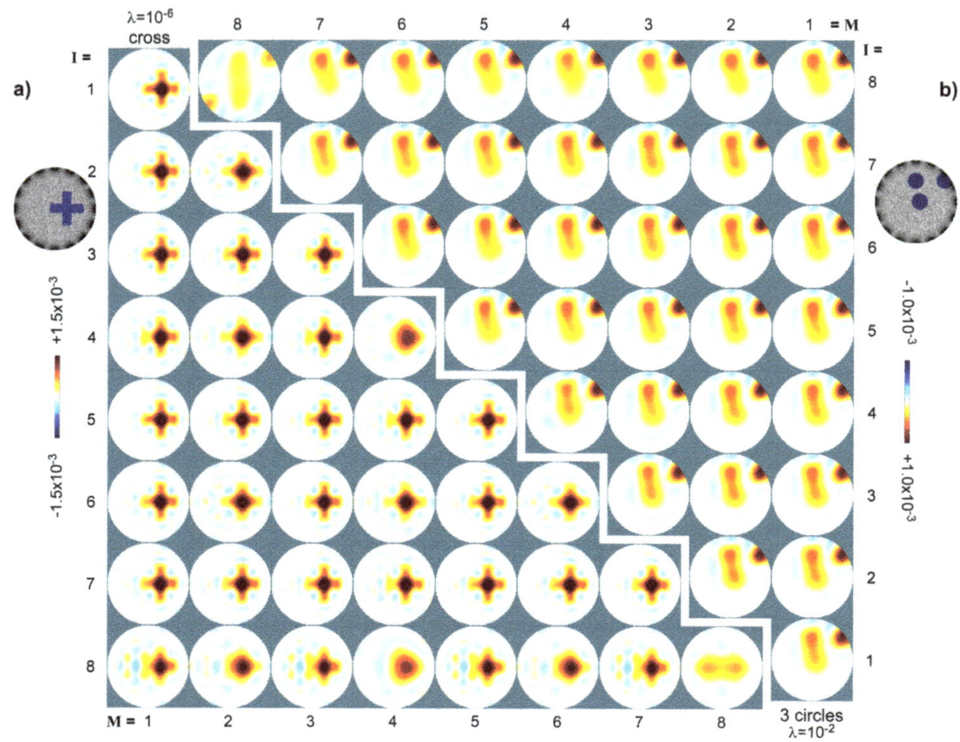

Figure 7.12. The effect of I–M pattern on reconstructions, organized by I-position up-down and M-position left-right. (a) A cross-shaped target centered at $x = 0.3$ using $\lambda = 10^{-6}$. (b) A three-circle target, each circle of $r_T = 0.2$, using $\lambda = 10^{-2}$. Decreases in conductivity are shown as red, increases in conductivity as blue, reversed from the convention used in medical imaging. (Targets and color bars are shown.) (16 electrodes, $I = 10^{-3}$, $\sigma_0 = 10^{-2}$, $\Delta\sigma = 0.9\sigma_0$, negligible noise $N = 10^{-12}$.) Reproduced from [59].

Figure 7.12(a) shows images made with little regularization, here at $\lambda = 10^{-6}$ (which scales with experimental parameters as shown in section 4.4.4), and thus illustrates the best that each I–M pattern can achieve. Reconstructions for the full-rank, or nearly full rank, I–M patterns (figure 7.10) were virtually identical. However, those of lower rank lacked detail, resulting in missing arms. For the strongly rank-deficient I–M patterns, 4–4 and several of the 8-# family (designating 8–1, 8–2, …, 8–8), the reconstructions were missing any indication of the arms. Furthermore, the high symmetry of 8–8 resulted in a mirror image; several other low-rank patterns also showed some positive or negative mirroring. (Mirroring is more clear in additional images for different targets shown in appendix G.17.) Much has been made of the number of independent measurements (equal to the rank r) that results from particular I–M patterns [15]. As figure 7.12(a) illustrates, rank is important at small hyperparameters, where it limits the resolution.

As discussed in section 4.3, the EIT image can be considered to be a sum of eigen-images or modes, denoted $\mathbf{v}_i$, where i goes from 1 to r. With increasing i, the spatial frequency of the modes increases, so the resolution and detail that can be produced in the final EIT image likewise increases with r. The coefficients of the $\mathbf{v}_i$ in the sum depend on the I–M pattern, as well as on the target characteristics, hyperparameter, and number of electrodes.

The medium to high range of regularization is of greater relevance experimentally, so it is given more attention in this chapter. Increasing the hyperparameter λ results in preferential defocusing (broader, shorter features) at the center of the sensor. (The effects of λ were described in detail in chapter 5.) Thus, while differences among I–M patterns at small λ are due to rank, differences at large λ are due instead to varying sensitivities to conductivity changes at the center of the sensed area (figure 7.11). Lower sensitivity at a given location, encoded in $\mathbf{J}$, occurs due to electric fields being weaker at the perimeter or to more weakly interacting fields, and it results in greater defocusing.

Figure 7.12(b) shows a three-circle target reconstructed with a larger hyperparameter, $\lambda = 10^{-2}$. Among the full-rank I–M patterns, differences in performance appeared due to differences in sensitivity. For example, I–M = 3–3 better represented the center target than 5–1 did. For all the patterns, while the target circle at the perimeter was represented as a tall, narrow (focused) peak, the target circle at the center was represented as a short, broad (defocused) peak. This target illustrates a problem for tactile imaging: due to the spatially non-uniform effects of regularization, targets nearer the center can be 'masked' by simultaneous touches elsewhere, meaning that larger amplitude peaks overwhelm the image so that smaller amplitude peaks are not seen. It should be emphasized that differences among the I–M_{80+} (the patterns that were not strongly rank deficient) were smaller than changes wrought by increasing regularization. Increasing the hyperparameter further to $\lambda = 10^{-1}$, the images were uniformly poor, and by $\lambda = 1$ they became unusable for distinguishing multiple touches.

The question of choosing a best I–M pattern is one of subtle distinctions, after putting aside the highly rank deficient patterns 4–4 and 8–#. The question addressed in the remainder of this chapter is, is there an overall best compromise?

7.2.3 Performance metrics

This section examines differences in image metrics quantitatively for a single circular target of radius $r_{\mathrm{T}} = 0.2$. (The effect of target radius were investigated in chapter 5.) Performance on any metric depends on both target position and hyperparameter, as shown above (figure 7.12). Because performance is worst at the center of the sensor, later sections focus on targets at $x = 0.1$.

7.2.3.1 Peak amplitude

The peak amplitude of the reconstructed feature, $\Delta\sigma_R$, is the maximum value in the image,

$$\text{Peak amplitude} = \Delta\sigma_R = \max(\Delta\sigma_i)\big|_{\text{image}} \tag{7.5}$$

obtained in this work by averaging the 10 largest image values. Amplitude uniformity is given by the ratio of the minimum to maximum peak amplitudes across target positions from the center to the periphery along the x-axis.

$$\text{Amplitude uniformity} = (\Delta\sigma_{R,\ \min}/\Delta\sigma_{R,\ \max})|_x \tag{7.6}$$

Peak amplitudes are shown in figure 7.13(a) and (b) as a function of position x for medium and large hyperparameters. Each curve was created by placing the target at a series of 10 positions from 0.0 to 0.9. Note that for $x = 0.9$, the target extended beyond the sensor perimeter; this is indicated by gray shading in the figures. Corresponding EIT images are shown for several of the I–M patterns in figure 7.14(a) and (b).

At the medium value of $\lambda = 10^{-3}$, the low-rank I–M patterns (gray lines) had smaller peak amplitudes, particularly near the center of the sensor, than those of full

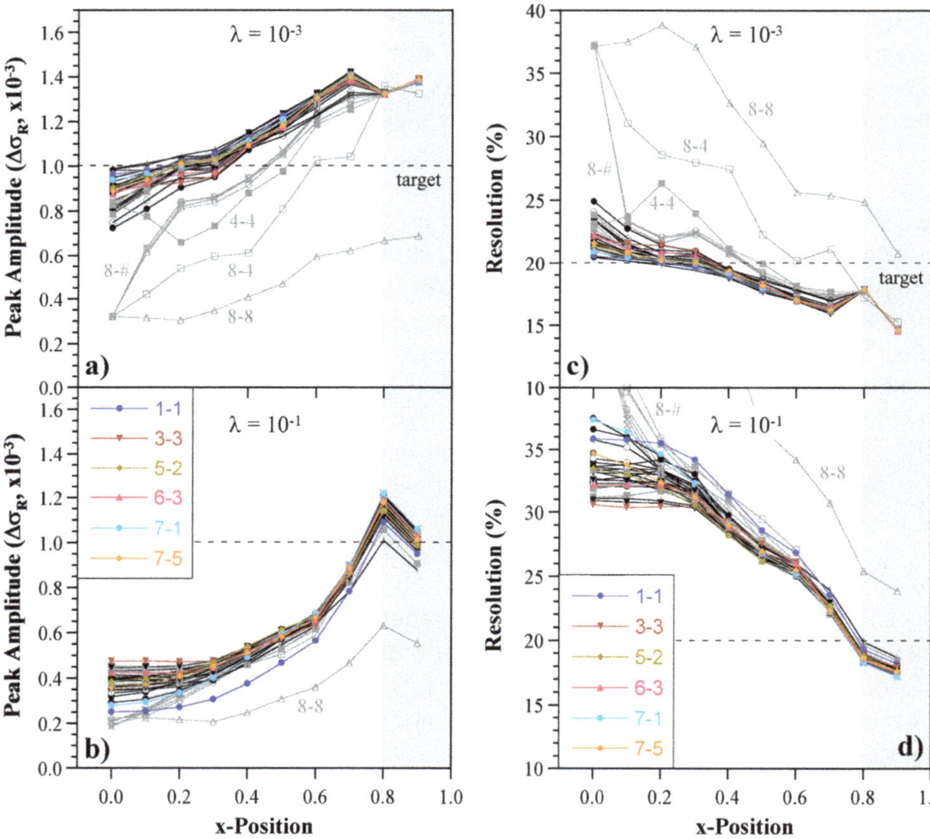

Figure 7.13. (a), (b) Peak amplitude and (c), (d) resolution for a circular target for the 36 I–M patterns as a function of x-position at (a), (c) $\lambda = 10^{-3}$ and (b), (d) $\lambda = 10^{-1}$. Aside from the I–M patterns in the legend, 4–4 and 8–# are shown in gray and the others in black. The gray regions on the right indicate where the target extends beyond the sensor perimeter. The horizontal dashed lines indicate the target values. (The y-axis scales for (c) and (d) are the same, but they do not go to zero) (16 electrodes, $I = 10^{-3}$, $\sigma_0 = 10^{-2}$, $\Delta\sigma = 0.9\sigma_0$, $r_T = 0.2$, negligible noise $N = 10^{-12}$). Reproduced from [59].

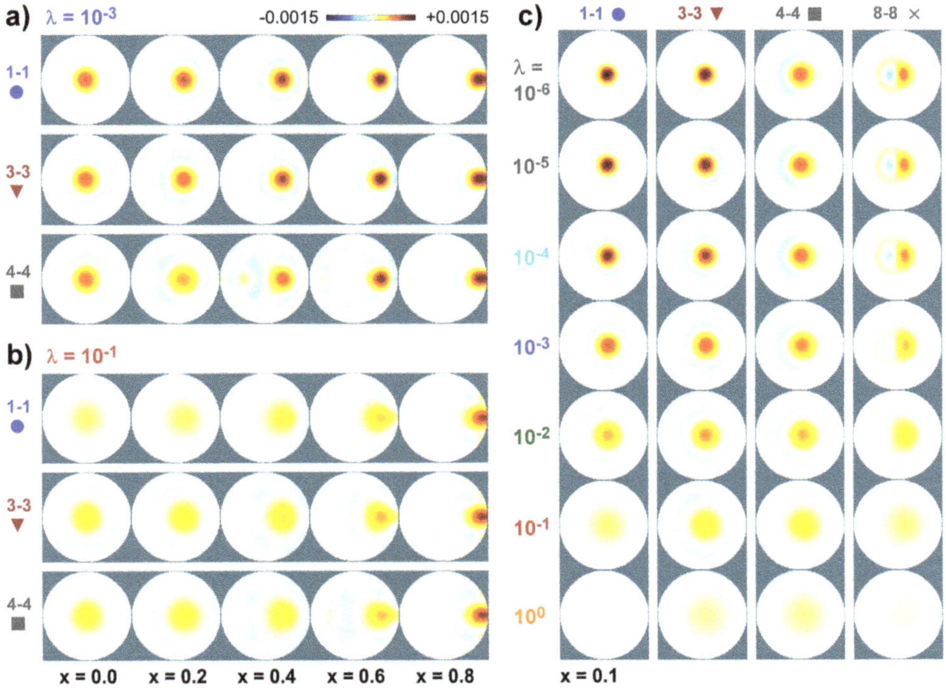

Figure 7.14. EIT images corresponding to several of the I–M patterns in figure 7.13, figure 7.15, and subsequent plots, with matching symbols and colors. EIT images at different x-positions, increasing left to right, for (a) $\lambda = 10^{-3}$ and (b) $\lambda = 10^{-1}$. (c) EIT images at $x = 0.1$ as λ increases top to bottom. (The color scales are the same for all the images.) (16 electrodes, $i = 10^{-3}$, $\sigma_0 = 10^{-2}$, $\Delta\sigma = 0.9\sigma_0$, $r_T = 0.2$, negligible noise $N = 10^{-12}$.) Reproduced from [59].

or nearly full rank, the I–M$_{80+}$ (black and color lines), because the former have fewer $\mathbf{v}_i$ contributing to the final EIT images. For the I–M$_{80+}$ this value of the hyperparameter introduced some spatial non-uniformity, with peak heights near 1.3 at $x = 0.8$ but near 0.9 at $x = 0.0$. At the even higher $\lambda = 10^{-1}$, peak heights were diminished at every position for all the patterns, but they were more reduced at the center of the sensor, the hyperparameter having most strongly dampened the high frequency image components there. Spatial uniformity was even lower: amplitudes were near 1.1 at $x = 0.8$ but dropped steeply to near 0.4 at $x = 0.0$. The relative positions of individual I–M patterns within the group changed with λ. For example, at $x = 0$, 1–1 went from having one of the largest amplitudes at $\lambda = 10^{-3}$ to one of the smallest at $\lambda = 10^{-1}$.

Note that the peaks of all the I–M$_{80+}$ were similar in being highest at the perimeter and lowest at the center. (Among the low-rank patterns, 4–4 at $\lambda = 10^{-3}$ was lowest at $x = 0.2$ due to mirroring, as shown in figure 7.14(a).) Chapter 5 showed that for some of the I–M, the peak amplitude could be described as $-ax^2\log(\lambda)$ while for others there was less dependence on x at the center. Figure 7.13(b) shows that some of the I–M$_{80+}$ patterns flattened at higher levels and larger x than others. The set of 3–1, 3–2, and 3–3—collectively 3–#—were among the least diminished at the center. The pattern 3–3 had a flat plateau from $x = 0$ out to $x = 0.3$. (Resolution, also shown in figure 7.13, is discussed in the next section.)

Figure 7.15 shows the peak amplitude data as a function of hyperparameter for a target position near the center of the sensor at $x = 0.1$. (Data are shown for $x = 0.5$ in appendix G.19.) EIT images corresponding to some of the I–M patterns are shown in figure 7.14(c). The position $x = 0.1$ was used instead of $x = 0.0$ because the latter is a special case for a circular target, reconstructed solely from the circularly symmetric $\mathbf{v}_i$. The shape and amplitudes of the low-rank I–M curves in figure 7.15 (gray lines) are a

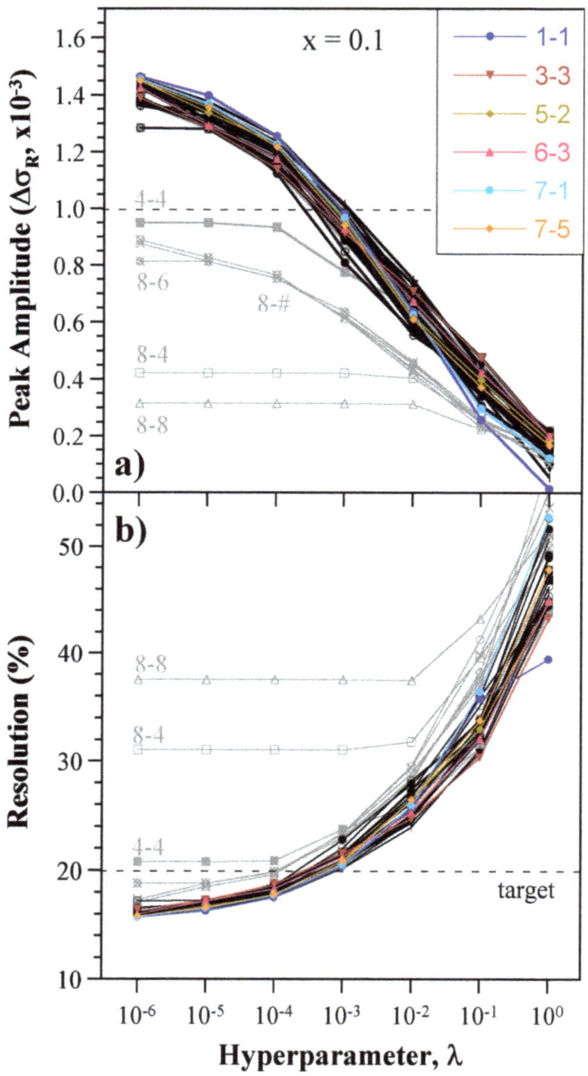

Figure 7.15. (a) Peak amplitude and (b) resolution for a circular target at $x = 0.1$ for the 36 I–M patterns as a function of hyperparameter. Aside from the I–M patterns in the legend, 4–4 and 8–# are shown in gray and the others in black. (16 electrodes, $I = 10^{-3}$, $\sigma_0 = 10^{-2}$, $\Delta\sigma = 0.9\sigma_0$, $r_T = 0.2$, $N = 10^{-12}$.) Reproduced from [59]. Copyright IOP Publishing Ltd. All rights reserved.

result of the lack of high spatial frequency contributions to the EIT images, as well as information lost due to symmetry, as discussed in chapter 5. Briefly, λ is akin to a low-pass filter that, in essence, reduces the amplitudes of the modes, the reduction starting with the highest spatial frequency $\mathbf{v}_i$ at small λ and moving to lower spatial-frequency $\mathbf{v}_i$ as λ increases. Since there are no high spatial frequency $\mathbf{v}_i$ contributing to the EIT images of the low-rank I–M, the reconstructed features were short and broad, even at small λ, and the low-pass filtering did not affect them until λ became large enough. For example, the curve for 4–4 joined those for the I–M_{80+} above $\lambda = 10^{-3}$. Note from figure 7.15 that the performance of 1–1 deteriorated relative to the other I–M_{80+} only above $\lambda = 10^{-2}$.

Figure 7.15 again illustrates the reason for differences in performance among the I–M at low versus high λ. Small amplitude and poor resolution due to low rank were most pronounced at small λ. On the other hand, defocusing for the I–M_{80+} increased with λ, and above $\lambda = 10^{-4}$ the amplitude dropped as $-\log(\lambda)$. These results go some way toward explaining the divergent recommendations in table 7.2. The extent of regularization must be taken into account.

Figures 7.13 and 7.15 emphasize the similarities among the I–M patterns. To more clearly show the differences, figure 7.16 presents the peak amplitude as a function of I–M combination at the target position $x = 0.1$, where the effects of λ are severe. The gray and white regions alternate between sets of increasing I, as in figure 7.10. The differences in low and high λ behaviors are again clear. Also evident

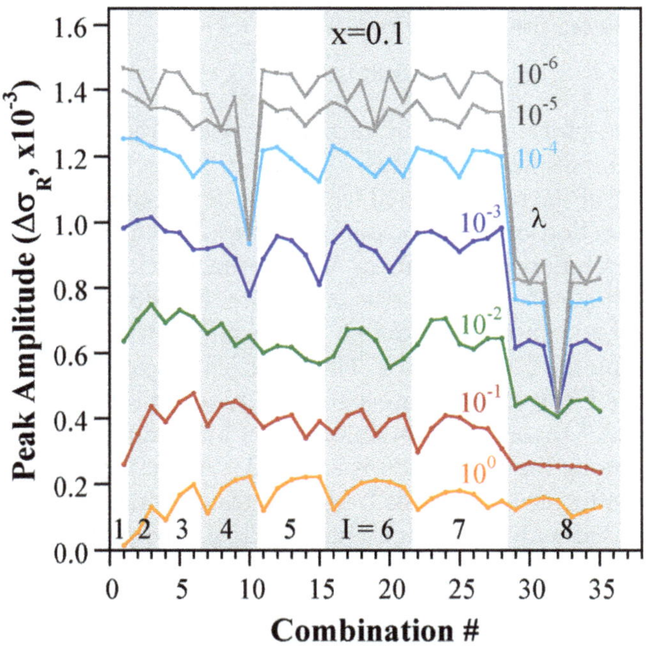

Figure 7.16. Peak amplitude for a circular target at $x = 0.1$ for the 36 I–M patterns at different hyper-parameters (indicated on the plot). (16 electrodes, $I = 10^{-3}$, $\sigma_0 = 10^{-2}$, $\Delta\sigma = 0.9\sigma_0$, $r_T = 0.2$, $N = 10^{-12}$.) Reproduced from [59].

are cycles that repeat with I. For example one that becomes apparent is that at large λ (orange, red) there is a local dip in amplitude for all of the #–1 patterns. However, at the intermediate λ (light and dark blue) there are dips at all the #–4 positions. The dips due to low rank at small λ, for 4–4 and 8–#, lessen as λ increases. This figure also illustrates that differences among the I–M_{80+} are smaller than differences caused by changing λ by a factor of 10.

Peak amplitudes were also examined at two different target sizes at one hyper-parameter, $\lambda = 10^{-2}$ (plots are shown in appendix G.20). For a point target of $r_T = 0.02$, the relative amplitudes were largely unchanged from those in figure 7.16, although they were reduced by a factor of 100. For a target of $r_T = 0.4$ the differences among the I–M patterns were reduced, since regularization affects large targets less strongly.

Given the detrimental effect of masking of one target by another for tactile imaging applications, as illustrated in figure 7.12(b), amplitude uniformity over the sensor is a critical consideration. Figure 7.17(a) presents the peak amplitude uniformity across target positions between $x = 0$ and 0.8. The same trends are visible as in figure 7.16, since uniformity is dominated by what occurs in the center of the sensor and since the behavior at the edge is similar for all the I–M.

7.2.3.2 Resolution

To distinguish two or more features for tactile imaging, not only must the representation of their peak amplitudes not be too different to avoid masking, but also the resolution must be fine enough that the peaks can be differentiated. Resolution is defined, for a sensor radius of $r_s = 1$, as

$$\text{Resolution} = r_r. \tag{7.7}$$

Smaller values of r_r mean finer resolution. Resolution uniformity is defined analogously to amplitude uniformity.

The resolution of the reconstructed features, as a percentage of the sensor radius, is shown as a function of target position in figure 7.13(c) and (d) for the 36 I–M patterns. The resolution decreased, or became finer, with x, in tandem with the increase in amplitude of the reconstructed feature. Resolution was found in section 4.5 to be linked to amplitude through a constant feature volume, which is an advantage of using the Laplace prior. Thus, 1–1 had one of the finest resolutions at $\lambda = 10^{-3}$ (figure 7.13(c)) reflecting its high amplitude (figure 7.13(a)), but one of the coarsest at $\lambda = 10^{-1}$ (figure 7.13(d)) reflecting its low amplitude (figure 7.13(b)).

The spread among the I–M patterns at $x = 0$ was small compared to differences due to x and λ. Difference among the I–M_{80+} were even smaller for $x \geqslant 0.5$, although the spread increased with λ (see also figure 7.15(b)). The pattern 3–3 had the finest resolution at the center of the sensor at $\lambda = 10^{-1}$.

Figure 7.15(b) shows that the I–M_{80+} had the same resolution at small hyper-parameters, consistent with the findings in [34]. The resolution coarsened as λ increased; chapter 5 showed that the resolution rose as $[\log(\lambda)]^{-0.5}$. (Resolution is shown as a function of I–M pattern for different λ in appendix G.18.)

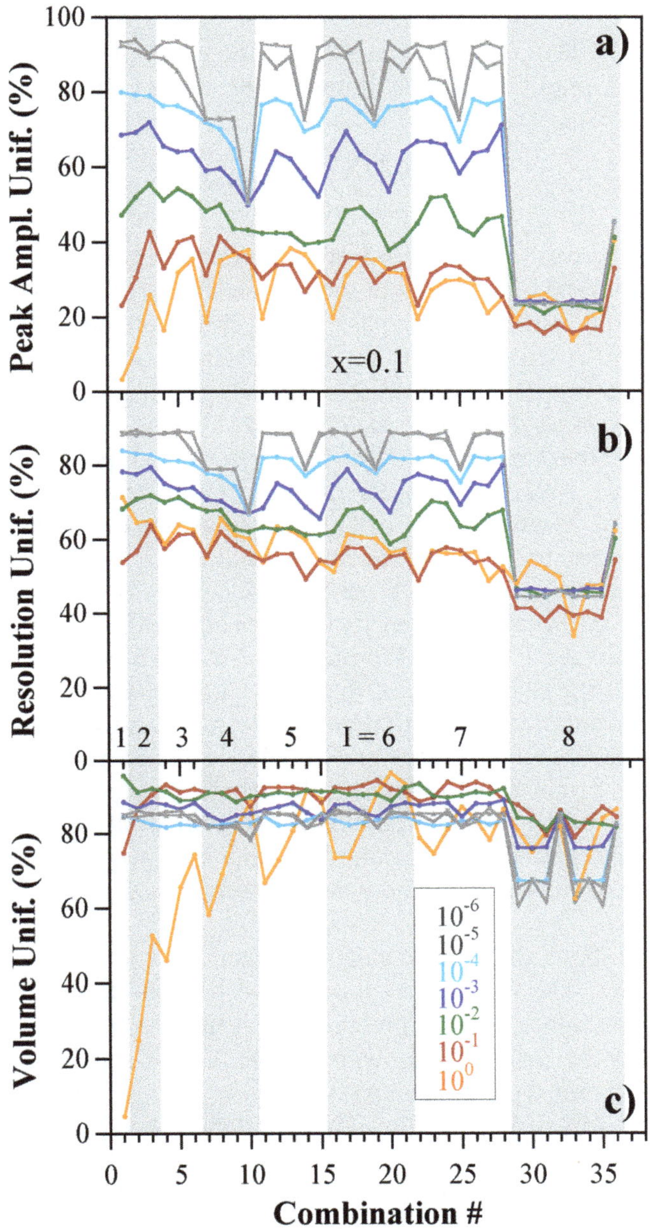

Figure 7.17. Uniformity of (a) peak amplitude, (b) resolution, and (c) volume for a circular target for the 36 I–M patterns at different hyperparameters. (16 electrodes, $I = 10^{-3}$, $\sigma_0 = 10^{-2}$, $\Delta\sigma = 0.9\sigma_0$, $r_T = 0.2$, $N = 10^{-12}$.) Reproduced from [59].

The resolution uniformity (figure 7.17(b)) closely resembled the peak amplitude uniformity. However, uniformity was higher overall since resolution depended less strongly on λ than amplitude did. Also, the uniformity was anomalously high at $\lambda = 10^{-1}$.

7.2.3.3 Volume

The volume of the feature, also referred to as its energy [17], takes into account both its area and amplitude. It was found as the sum of elements $\Delta\sigma_i$ in the half amplitude set:

$$\text{Volume} = \sum_{\text{elements}} \Delta\sigma_i|_{\Delta\sigma_i > \Delta\sigma_R/2} \tag{7.8}$$

The feature volume was found to be constant over a large range of λ in chapter 5 for several of the I–M: the total energy of the feature was largely conserved during the reconstruction process using the Laplace prior. High volume uniformity indicates good coverage of the sensor area by the I–M pattern. Loss of energy, on the other hand, represents a loss of information.

Figure 7.18(a) shows the reconstructed feature volume as a function of position at the large hyperparameter $\lambda = 0.1$. The pattern 1−1 performed particularly poorly with regards to the preservation of energy in the peak: a target at the center was represented as having only ¾ of the volume as one at the edge. This loss of volume reflects a greater relative lack of information about conductivity changes near the center, arising physically from the low current there, requiring a higher reliance on prior information. Other #–1 targets also suffered from loss of energy at the center as did some of the 7–# patterns—7–2, 7–6, and 7–7. The 8–# targets had full energy at the exact center of the sensor, at $x = 0.0$, but just off center, at $x = 0.1$, they also suffered substantial volume loss. One pattern, 5–5, experienced a unique loss near $x = 0.4$; others had smaller losses at $x = 0.5$. The losses at various positions might be considered to be 'blind spots' for the pattern, due to either small fields or symmetry. Three of the low-rank patterns, specifically 4–4, 8–4, and 8–8, experienced an inflation of volume near $x = 0.4$. The two patterns with the flattest curves were 3–3 and 6–3, followed by 4–3 and 5–3, and then 5–2, 6–2, and 7–5.

Figure 7.18(b) shows the volume data as a function of λ at a single position near the center, $x = 0.1$. The volume loss for the 8–# patterns was not a problem that manifested only at high λ, but was present even at the smallest $\lambda = 10^{-6}$. In fact, for some of the 8–# the problem was worst at small λ. The I–M$_{80+}$ generally had volumes that increased slightly with log(λ) up to $\lambda = 10^{-2}$; the slopes were similar for all of them (0.010 to 0.015). The lowest slope and most linear change were found in 3–3. The #−1 patterns had linear changes in this range, whereas the most irregular increases in volume with hyperparameter were found in 2–2,4–3,4–4, 5–4, 6–2, 6–4, and 6–6. In general the volume decreased with regularization above $\lambda = 10^{-2}$. A particularly noticeable trend was that this volume loss was greatest for the #−1, as well as for 4–4. In contrast to the position dependence, the patterns that were the flattest were 4–4, 8–4, and 8–8. The pattern 3–3 emerged from both plots as favored from a conservation of energy perspective. (Volume is shown as a function of I–M pattern for different λ in appendix G.18.)

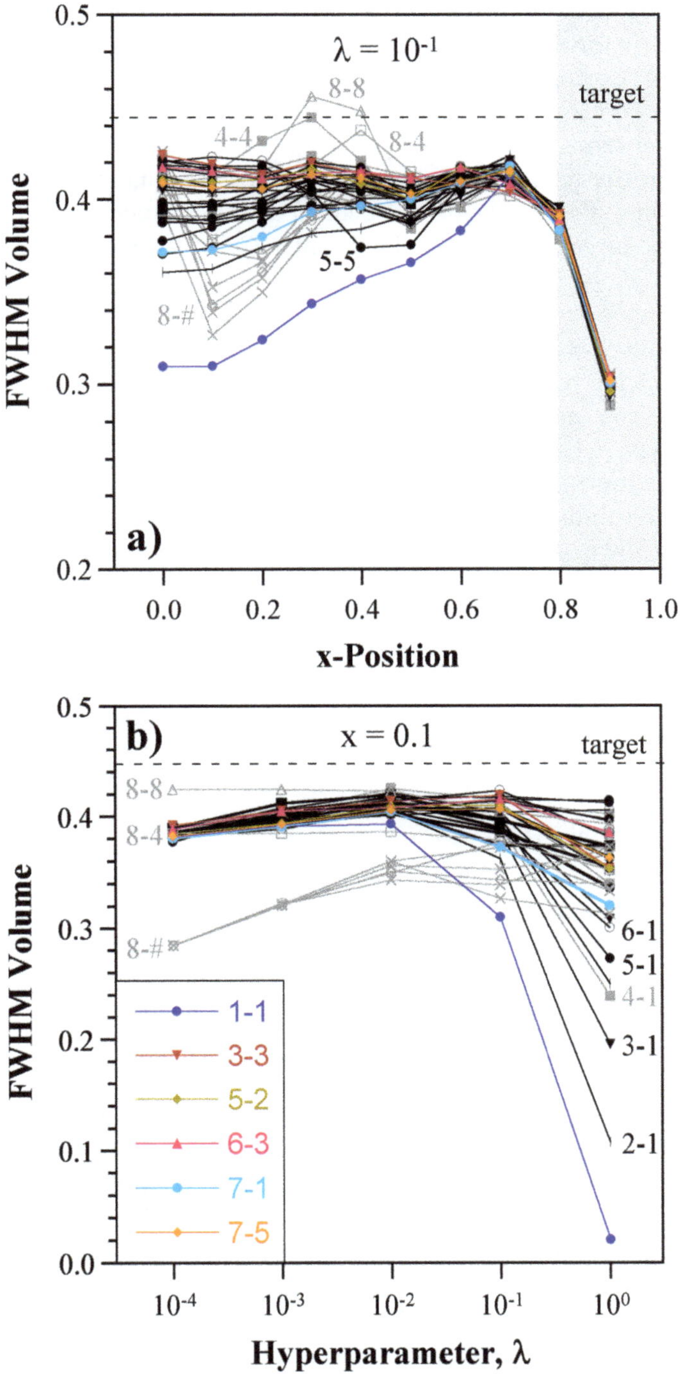

Figure 7.18. Volume for a circular target for the 36 I–M patterns as a function of (a) position at $\lambda = 10^{-1}$ and (b) hyperparameter at $x = 0.1$. Note that y-axis scales differ and the y-axis scale for (a) does not go to zero. Aside from the I–M patterns in the legend, 4–4 and 8–# are shown in gray and the others in black. The gray regions indicates where the target touches, or extends beyond, the sensor perimeter (16 electrodes, $I = 10^{-3}$, $\sigma_0 = 10^{-2}$, $\Delta\sigma = 0.9\sigma_0$, $r_T = 0.2$, $N = 10^{-12}$). Reproduced from [59]. Copyright IOP Publishing Ltd. All rights reserved.

Volume uniformity is shown in figure 7.17(c). It became strongly compromised at $\lambda = 1$, particularly for the low-angle patterns, meaning offsets of 1 to 4 in either I or M. For the 8–#, except 8–5, volume uniformity was low only at small λ.

7.2.3.4 Position error

Among the non-size-related metrics, position error is arguably the most important for tactile imaging. Position error was defined as the distance between the weighted center C_T of the target and the weighted center C_R of the reconstructed feature:

$$\text{Position error} = C_R - C_T. \tag{7.9}$$

Position errors at $x = 0.1$, where they were greatest, are shown in figure 7.19 as a function of λ, with positive values indicating positions closer to the perimeter. Position errors were near zero for the I–M_{80+}, increasing for a few of them up to ±5% at the largest hyperparameter. For the low-rank patterns, this error was larger: +10% for 8–8 across all λ, and for 8–5 at $\lambda = 1$, 16%. The same data are shown as a function of pattern number in figure 7.19(b). For most of the I–M_{80+}, the position error was small and negative. For 4–4, the error was positive at all λ. The errors were also generally positive for the 5–# and 6–# patterns at large λ. Position errors decreased with x, and beyond $x = 0.5$ were small and almost the same for all the patterns, with 8–8 excepted. At $x = 0$, position errors were zero for all the I–M patterns for this circular target.

Shape errors are also included in appendix G.21. For the I–M_{80+}, shape errors were near 2% for large λ and up to 4% for medium and small λ.

7.2.4 Noise susceptibility

The I–M patterns were next challenged by adding noise. A useful metric for evaluating the effects of noise on tactile images is the onset of artefacts (chapter 6, section 7.1). Susceptibility to noise was determined by finding the noise level at which artifacts just started to appear for a given λ. The noise threshold $N_{th}(\lambda)$ was defined as the highest level of noise for which a series of five trials contained no artefacts:

$$N_{th} = \max(\text{N})\,|_{\lambda}\ \ \varepsilon\ \text{Artefacts} = 0 \text{ in five trials}. \tag{7.10}$$

Higher values of N_{th} signify greater stability in the presence of noise. For noise above N_{th} the images become unusable for tactile imaging because of artefacts and severe distortions. In these simulations, at $\lambda = 10^{-3}$ the N_{th} were on the order of 10^{-6} V.

Figure 7.20(a) plots N_{th} as a function of λ and figure 7.20(b) as a function of the I–M combination for the circular target at $x = 0.1$. Among the I–M_{80+}, target position did not significantly affect N_{th}: the values at $x = 0.1$ and 0.5 were similar. (The latter is shown in appendix G.25). There were large differences in N_{th} among the I–M_{80+} for $\lambda \geqslant 10^{-1}$, greater than a factor of 10 at $\lambda = 1$, with the #–1 patterns being the most susceptible to noise; 7–6 and 8–5 were also particularly susceptible. This result is consistent with prior work [34, 40]. The practical implication of a small N_{th} is that an even larger λ is needed to suppress the noise. For $\lambda < 10^{-1}$, however, the patterns behaved similarly. At the very low $\lambda = 10^{-6}$ and 10^{-5}, among

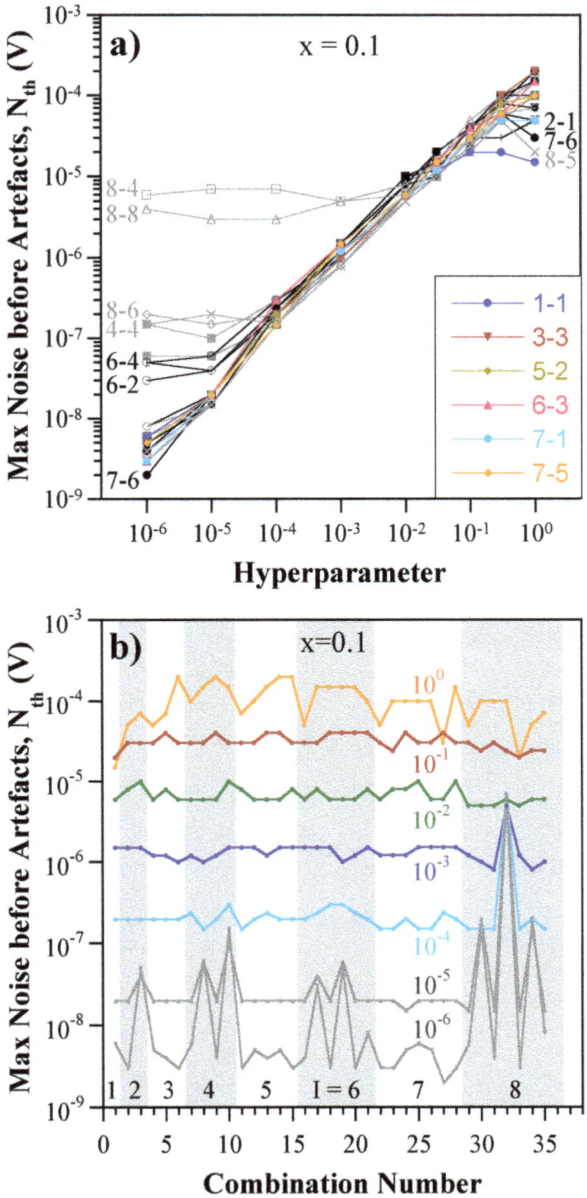

Figure 7.19. Position error as a function of (a) hyperparameter and (b) I–M pattern for a circular target at $x = 0.1$. (16 electrodes, $I = 10^{-3}$, $\sigma_0 = 10^{-2}$, $\Delta\sigma = 0.9\sigma_0$, $r_T = 0.2$, $N = 10^{-12}$.) Reproduced from [59]. Copyright IOP Publishing Ltd. All rights reserved.

the I–M$_{80+}$, 2–2,4–2, 6–2, and 6–4 had the highest N_{th}. The low rank patterns had greater noise stability, as expected and as discussed in chapter 6.

The noise level can be compared to $|\mathbf{U}^T\mathbf{\Delta}|$ spectra [58], where $\mathbf{\Delta}$ is the vector of voltage differences in the measurement frame and the $\mathbf{u}_i$ in $\mathbf{U}$ are a set of orthogonal basis vectors, or 'eigen-Δs', with which $\mathbf{\Delta}$ can be expressed. The absolute values of

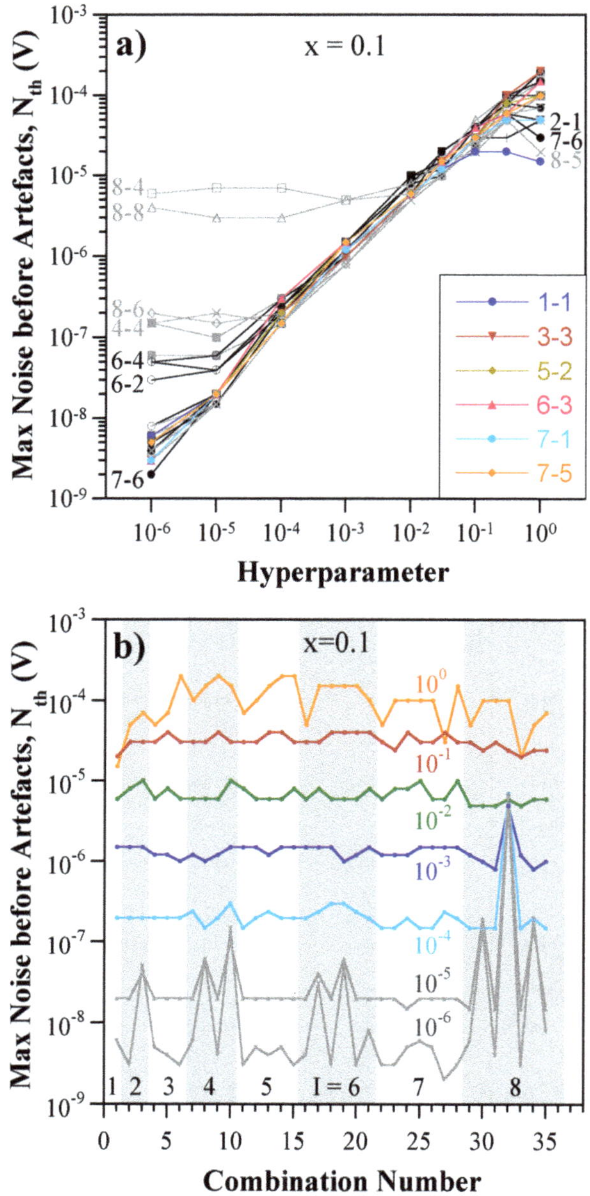

Figure 7.20. Noise threshold as a function of (a) hyperparameter and (b) I–M combination for a circular target at $x = 0.1$. (16 electrodes, $I = 10^{-3}$, $N = 10^{-12}$, $\sigma_0 = 10^{-2}$, $\Delta\sigma = 0.9\sigma_0$, $r_T = 0.2$.) Reproduced from [59].

the amplitudes of the coefficients in this expansion of $\mathbf{\Delta}$ into $\mathbf{u}_i$, the Picard coefficients, are shown in appendix G.22 for all 36 I–M patterns.

The question arises whether the presence of noise would confound the selection of an I–M pattern based on data from the previous sections. To explore the effect of noise on the metrics, the peak amplitude and resolution were collected at the N_{th} for

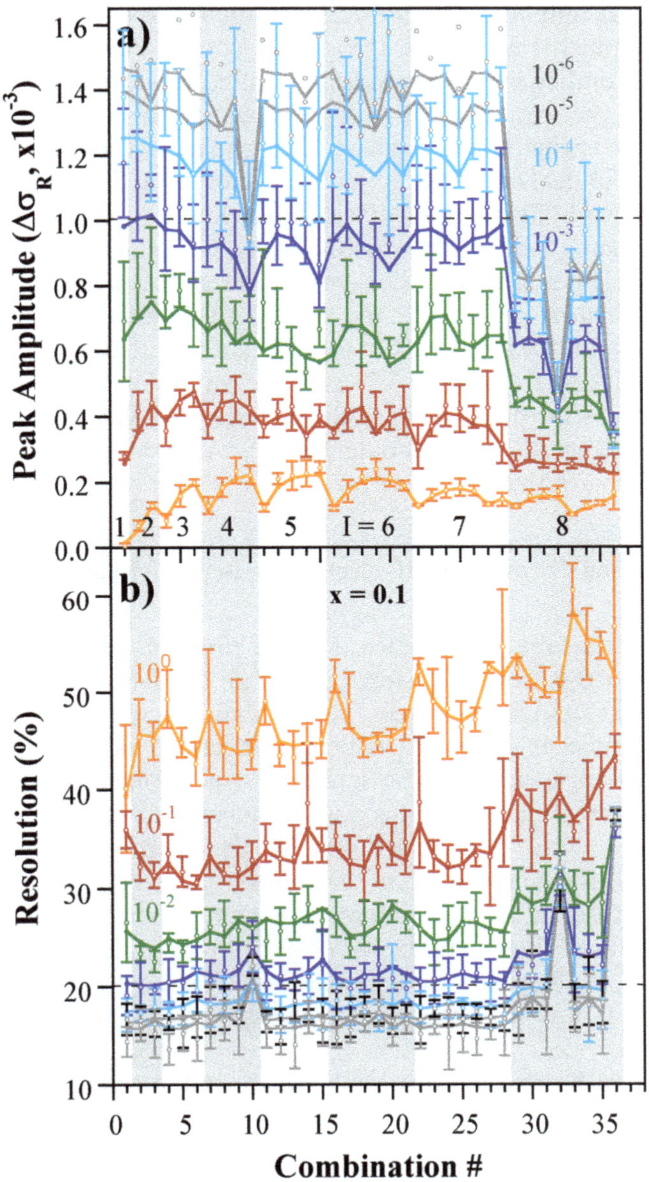

Figure 7.21. (a) Peak amplitude and (b) resolution as a function of I–M pattern for different values of λ for a circular target at $x = 0.1$. Solid points and lines show values at negligible noise ($N = 10^{-12}$). Open circles show the average values of 5 replicate trials with noise of N_{th}, which differs for each pattern, and the error bars show the standard deviations of the replicates. (16 electrodes, $I = 10^{-3}$, $\sigma_0 = 10^{-2}$, $\Delta\sigma = 0.9\sigma_0$, $r_T = 0.2$.) Reproduced from [59]. Copyright IOP Publishing Ltd. All rights reserved.

each pattern (the values in figure 7.20) for a circular target at $x = 0.1$. They are shown in figure 7.21 for various hyperparameters, with open circles and error bars showing the average and standard deviation of 5 replicates and lines showing the negligible-noise values. For medium and large hyperparameters, $\lambda \geqslant 10^{-3}$, the differences in peak amplitudes (figure 7.21(a)) among the I–M patterns were largely maintained. Despite the deviations, the average points were reasonably close to the noise-free values or they slightly magnified the differences. However, with decreasing hyperparameter, the scatter in the data grew, and the average values increasingly deviated from the negligible-noise values. The standard deviations increased tenfold, from an average of 0.02 at $\lambda = 10^0$ to an average of 0.2 at $\lambda = 10^{-6}$. Thus, the error bars are not shown in figure 7.21(a) for points below $\lambda = 10^{-4}$.

Turning to figure 7.21(b), the resolution at N_{th} followed the negligible-noise values at all λ. The scatter was, conversely, lower at small and medium hyperparameter and higher for large λ: the standard deviations of the five replicates jumped from 1.7–2.0 for $\lambda \leqslant 3 \times 10^{-2}$ to 2.7–3.2 above that.

The key conclusion from figure 7.21 is that even in the presence of noise that is high, but still below the point at which the EIT images break up, one can select the I–M pattern based on the previous data. Thus, we are now prepared to perform an overall comparison of the I–M patterns.

7.2.5 Summary and discussion of 16-electrode system I–M pattern performance at $x = 0.1$

Table 7.4 summarizes the performance of the 36 bipolar I–M patterns for a target at $x = 0.1$, near $x = 0$ where the performance of all the I–M_{80+} patterns was worst, starting at the smallest realistic level of regularization, $\lambda = 10^{-4}$. Filled, downward-facing triangles indicate the several worst performers (a 'bad' rating), while empty, upward-facing triangles indicate the several best performers ('good'). Blue text is used to present the results of the two largest hyperparameters, $\lambda = 10^0$ and 10^{-1}, purple text for $\lambda = 10^{-2}$, and black text for the intermediate hyperparameters, $\lambda = 10^{-3}$ and 10^{-4}. Summary counts of the number of good and bad ratings are given at the bottom of the table. Red columns highlight patterns with 10 or more bad ratings, gray columns show patterns with 5–9 bad ratings, and white columns have 2–4 bad ratings. Light yellow columns are used to show patterns with 0–1 bad ratings. Finally, dark yellow shows patterns with 0 bad ratings and 9 or more good ratings.

It should be emphasized that for some metrics and hyperparameters, differences among the I–M_{80+} patterns were slight, while for others they were substantial, so the table entries are not all 'apples to apples'. Furthermore, the summary counts give all metrics equal weight. The plots in the previous sections thus serve as better guides. Nevertheless, it can be useful to see all the relative performances in one place.

The patterns with no especially poor performance on any of the metrics studied here were 3–3, 5–2, 5–3, 6–2, 6–3, and 7–3. By far the best among these, based on the number of categories in which it was consistently among the top, was 3–3. This was due to its exceptionally flat curves at the center of the sensor (figure 7.13) at large λ.

One pattern that should also be mentioned is 2–2, which performed well with 16 good ratings, but it was among the worst on amplitude and volume conservation at

Table 7.4. Performance of the bipolar I–M patterns (circular target at $x = 0.1$, 16 electrodes). Shading: red = 10+ bad ratings, gray = 5–9 bad, white = 2–4 bad, light yellow = 0–1 bad, dark yellow = 0 bad ratings and 10+ good.

	comb.	1	2	3	4	5	6	7	8	9	10	11	12	13	14	15	16	17	18	19	20	21	22	23	24	25	26	27	28	29	30	31	32	33	34	35	36
	I-M	1-1	2-1	2-2	3-1	3-2	3-3	4-1	4-2	4-3	4-4	5-1	5-2	5-3	5-4	5-5	6-1	6-2	6-3	6-4	6-5	6-6	7-1	7-2	7-3	7-4	7-5	7-6	7-7	8-1	8-2	8-3	8-4	8-5	8-6	8-7	8-8
rank		104	103	89	104	103	104	98	86	98	62	104	103	104	98	104	103	89	103	86	103	89	104	103	104	98	104	103	104	76	68	76	48	76	68	76	28
peak amplitude	$\lambda = 10^{0}$	▼	▼	▼	▼			▼			△	▼			△	△	▼						▼					▼		▼				▼	▼	▼	
	$\lambda = 10^{-1}$	▼				△	△			△					▼					▼			▼						▼	▼	▼	▼	▼	▼	▼	▼	▼
	$\lambda = 10^{-2}$		△	△		△	△								▼	▼	▼				▼	▼		△	△					▼	▼	▼	▼	▼	▼	▼	▼
	$\lambda = 10^{-3}$	△	△	△							▼					▼		△			▼								△	▼	▼	▼	▼	▼	▼	▼	▼
	$\lambda = 10^{-4}$	△	△	△							▼						△													▼	▼	▼	▼	▼	▼	▼	▼
amplitude uniformity	$\lambda = 10^{0}$	▼	▼		▼		△	▼	△	△	△	▼		△	△		▼		△	△			▼							▼				▼	▼		△
	$\lambda = 10^{-1}$	▼		△		△	△		△						▼								▼						▼	▼	▼	▼	▼	▼	▼	▼	
	$\lambda = 10^{-2}$		△	△		△	△								▼	▼	▼				▼	▼			△					▼	▼	▼	▼	▼	▼	▼	
	$\lambda = 10^{-3}$		△	△							▼					▼		△			▼								△	▼	▼	▼	▼	▼	▼	▼	▼
	$\lambda = 10^{-4}$	△	△	△						▼	▼				▼									△		▼				▼	▼	▼	▼	▼	▼	▼	▼
resolution	$\lambda = 10^{0}$	△			▼		△	▼		△	△	▼					▼						▼	▼	▼		▼	▼	▼	▼	▼	▼	▼	▼	▼	▼	▼
	$\lambda = 10^{-1}$	▼		△		△	△		△	△					▼					▼			▼						▼	▼	▼	▼	▼	▼	▼	▼	▼
	$\lambda = 10^{-2}$		△	△	△	△	△														▼			△	△					▼	▼	▼	▼	▼	▼	▼	▼
	$\lambda = 10^{-3}$										▼					▼														▼	▼	▼	▼	▼	▼	▼	▼
	$\lambda = 10^{-4}$										▼																			▼	▼	▼	▼	▼	▼	▼	▼
resolution uniformity	$\lambda = 10^{0}$	△	△	△					△								▼						▼					▼		▼			▼	▼	▼	▼	
	$\lambda = 10^{-1}$			△		△	△		△	△					▼								▼						▼	▼	▼	▼	▼	▼	▼	▼	
	$\lambda = 10^{-2}$		△	△	△	△									▼	▼					▼	▼		△						▼	▼	▼	▼	▼	▼	▼	▼
	$\lambda = 10^{-3}$	△	△	△						▼	▼					▼		△			▼		△						△	▼	▼	▼	▼	▼	▼	▼	▼
	$\lambda = 10^{-4}$	△	△	△						▼	▼															▼				▼	▼	▼	▼	▼	▼	▼	▼
volume	$\lambda = 10^{0}$	▼	▼	▼	▼	▼		▼			△	▼			△	△	▼			△			▼											▼			
	$\lambda = 10^{-1}$	▼	▼				△									△					△	△	▼						▼	▼	▼	▼		▼	▼		
	$\lambda = 10^{-2}$									△										△	△					△				▼	▼	▼	▼	▼	▼	▼	△
	$\lambda = 10^{-3}$	▼													△		▼						▼			△				▼	▼	▼	▼	▼	▼	▼	△
	$\lambda = 10^{-4}$																													▼	▼	▼		▼	▼	▼	△
volume uniformity	$\lambda = 10^{0}$	▼	▼	▼	▼	▼		▼	▼			▼			△					△	△	△												▼			
	$\lambda = 10^{-1}$	▼	▼		△						▼									△					△		△			▼	▼	▼	▼	▼	▼	▼	▼
	$\lambda = 10^{-2}$	△																					△							▼	▼	▼	▼	▼	▼	▼	▼
	$\lambda = 10^{-3}$								▼							▼				▼						▼				▼	▼	▼		▼	▼	▼	▼
	$\lambda = 10^{-4}$																													▼	▼	▼		▼	▼	▼	
position error	$\lambda = 10^{0}$	△					△									▼	△							△	△	△					△			▼			▼
	$\lambda = 10^{-1}$												△	△										△							▼	▼	▼	▼	▼	▼	▼
	$\lambda = 10^{-2}$																	△	△				△						△	▼	▼	▼	▼	▼	▼	▼	▼
	$\lambda = 10^{-3}$	△		△			△				▼																		△	▼	▼	▼	▼	▼	▼	▼	▼
	$\lambda = 10^{-4}$			△							▼											△		△					△	▼	▼	▼	▼	▼	▼	▼	▼
noise susceptibility N_{th}	$\lambda = 10^{0}$	▼	▼	▼	▼	▼	△			△		▼			△	△	▼						▼					▼		▼				▼	▼	▼	△
	$\lambda = 10^{-1}$	▼																						▼							▼		▼	▼	▼	▼	△
	$\lambda = 10^{-2}$																													▼	▼	▼		▼			
	$\lambda = 10^{-3}$																															▼	△		▼		△
	$\lambda = 10^{-4}$								▼		△	▼							△	△			▼	▼		▼	▼			▼	▼	▼	△	▼		▼	△
summary counts	# good	10	11	16	3	8	13	0	5	7	5	0	1	2	6	4	2	4	3	6	3	3	3	7	5	3	1	0	6	0	1	0	2	0	0	0	8
	# bad	12	7	4	6	3	0	5	3	3	11	7	0	0	8	9	9	0	0	3	7	3	13	3	1	4	2	4	6	34	32	32	27	39	35	33	22
	net	-2	4	12	-3	5	13	-5	2	4	-6	-7	1	2	-2	-5	-7	4	3	3	-4	0	-10	4	4	-1	-1	-4	0	-34	-31	-32	-25	-39	-35	-33	-14
summary *without* $\lambda = 10^{0}$	# good	7	10	15	3	8	9	0	3	4	1	0	1	1	1	1	1	4	2	3	2	2	3	6	4	2	1	0	6	0	0	0	2	0	0	0	6
	# bad	7	2	0	0	0	0	0	2	3	11	1	0	0	8	8	3	0	0	3	7	3	7	2	0	4	1	0	5	29	31	31	25	31	30	29	20
	net	0	8	15	3	8	9	0	1	1	-10	-1	1	1	-7	-7	-2	4	2	0	-5	-1	-4	4	4	-2	0	0	1	-29	-31	-31	-23	-31	-30	-29	-14

$\lambda = 1$. (This is a lower-rank pattern among the I–M$_{80+}$, so it is unsuitable for the smallest hyperparameters, e.g. $\lambda = 10^{-6}$, which are not considered in this table.) While its net score of 12 almost tied it with 3–3, those bad ratings removed it from the list of recommended patterns. However, $\lambda = 1$ in this study corresponds to a level of regularization that has limited to no utility since it defocuses the target to such an extent that it covers much of the sensor area. Removing $\lambda = 1$ scores from consideration, the picture changes, as shown in the final three rows of table 7.4. Several additional patterns become good performers, including 2–2, 3–1, 3–2, 4–1, 5–1, 7–5, and 7–6. In fact, 2–2 becomes a better choice than 3–3. If a hyperparameter as small as $\lambda = 10^{-3}$ can be used, the number of acceptable patterns becomes larger, and the optimal I–M patterns change. For example, I–M = 3–3 drops to only one good rating, whereas 2–1, 2–2, and 7–7 have three to four good ratings, the rest being neutral.

7.2.6 Number of electrodes: 13 versus 16

At small λ, symmetries resulted in the deficient performance of a number of the I–M patterns in the 16-electrode system. Lowering the number of electrodes to 15 would remove the highest symmetry patterns, and lowering the number to 13 would eliminate all the symmetries. Prior chapters showed that going from 16 to 12 electrodes may be acceptable, resulting in a relatively small loss in performance compared to the gain in operating speed; the higher speed may even improve performance if noise can be reduced by averaging a larger number of points, allowing the use of a smaller λ. Thus, in this section we examine the I–M patterns in a system with 13 electrodes.

Results for 15 electrodes are shown in appendix G.24. In summary, the 5–5 pattern was highly symmetric and thus had low rank, yielding poor amplitude and resolution performance. However, it was not as bad as 8–4 or 8–8 in the 16-electrode system. Reconstructions using other 5–# and #–5 patterns suffered from position errors. The patterns with the best performance in the 15-electrode configuration were 2–2, 3–2, 4–2, 4–3, 4–4, 6–2, and 6–4. (Note that these patterns are at different angles than were given for the 16-electrode system in table 7.2.)

Peak amplitude and resolution for the 13-electrode system are shown in figure 7.22 for a target near the center of the sensor, using the same *y*-axis scales as figure 7.15. There are several things to note about these data. First, as a group the peak amplitudes and resolutions were comparable to those obtained using the I–M_{80+} with 16 electrodes, although the best among the 16-electrode system outperformed the best among the 13-electrode system. Second, none of the patterns in the 13-electrode system were of low-rank: all of the I–M had a rank of 64. Thus at $\lambda = 10^{-6}$, all performed identically, excepting 2–2, which had a justly slightly smaller peak amplitude.

There were several patterns to avoid using 13 electrodes. As is understood from the physics, the 1–# patterns were outperformed by the others at high λ; the usual series of dips in amplitude can be seen in figure 7.22(b) as well as the corresponding peaks in resolution in figure 7.22(d). The amplitude curve for 1–1 with 13 electrodes was similar to the one for 16 electrodes, starting with a better performance at low regularization and deteriorating rapidly above $\lambda = 10^{-2}$. The high-angle 6–# patterns had notably poor resolution at $\lambda = 1$, especially 6–5. The 4–4 pattern had anomalously poor performance at $\lambda = 10^{-3}$.

Plots for other metrics are shown in appendix G.23. The worst performers on volume conservation at high λ were 1–1, 2–1, 2–2, 3–1, 4–1, 5–1, and 6–5. Position errors were comparable in the 13-electrode system to those in the 16-electrode system. A few patterns fared more poorly than others on this metric, notably 6–5 followed by 4–4 and then 6–#. For the other patterns, errors were less than 4% at $\lambda = 1$. Shape errors for all the patterns were at most 4%.

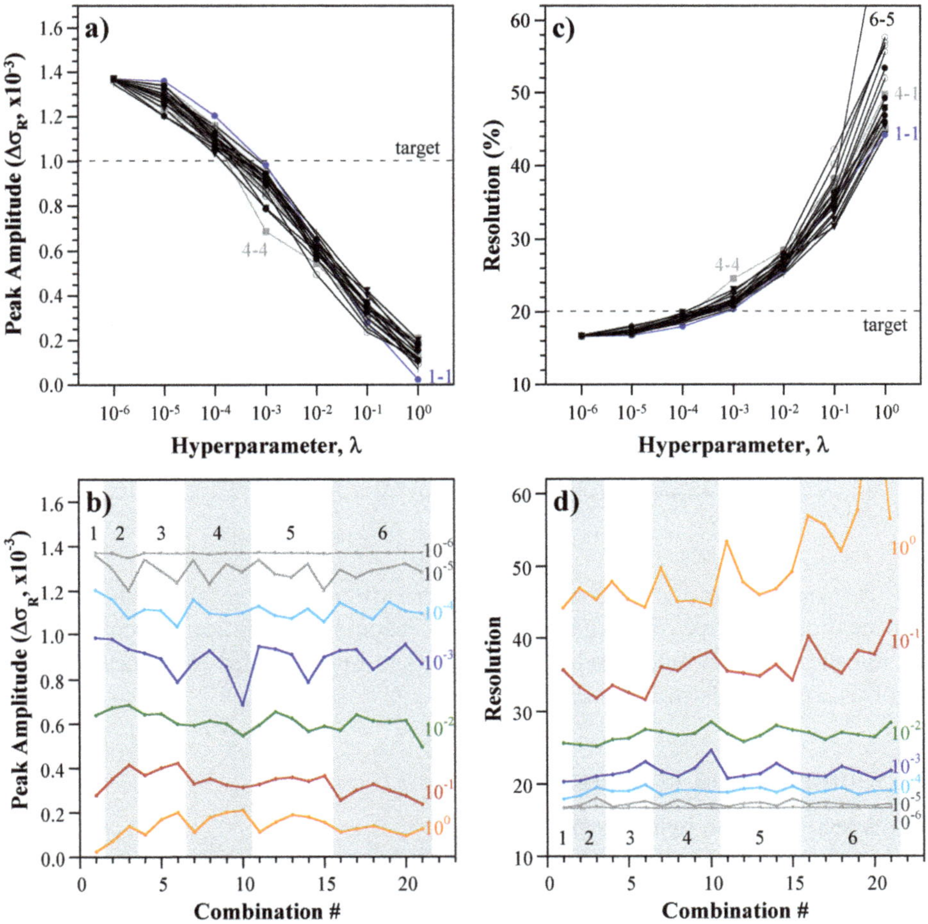

Figure 7.22. For a 13-electrode system with a circular target at $x = 0.1$, the (a), (b) peak amplitude and (c), (d) resolution as function of (a), (c) hyperparameter and (b), (d) I–M pattern. Reproduced from [59].

The best patterns overall for the 13-electrode system were 3–2, 4–2, 4–3, 5–2, and 5–5. However, differences among the I–M patterns, excepting the #–1, were relatively minor.

It was previously shown, in section 6.22, how noise susceptibility depends on the number of electrodes, so that was not examined again here. However, the $\mathbf{U}^T\boldsymbol{\Delta}$ curves are shown in appendix G.23 to allow comparison with the 16-electrode system.

The performance metrics of the best I–M patterns for the two systems are summarized in table 7.5 at one large hyperparameter, $\lambda = 0.1$, and one position, $x = 0.1$. This provides a snapshot near the worst-performing conditions.

The difference between the two best performing patterns, 3–3 for 16 electrodes and 3–2 for 13 electrodes, was a 16% lower amplitude and 7% larger resolution, resulting in a 4% smaller volume; position errors were small for both. Differences in

Table 7.5. Comparison of four metrics for the best performing I–M patterns for the 16- and 13-electrode systems at $x = 0.1$ and $\lambda = 10^{-1}$. The best performing I–M patterns for each are shown in blue. Averages of the rows are shown on the right. The difference between the best and average values is also shown.

16 Electrodes	3–3	5–2	5–3	6–2	6–3	6–6	7–3	7–5	Average
Peak amplitude	0.477	0.399	0.410	0.410	0.426	0.411	0.409	0.374	0.414
Resolution	30.4	33.0	32.7	32.5	32.2	32.8	32.0	33.8	32.4
Volume	0.419	0.409	0.414	0.407	0.416	0.423	0.396	0.407	0.411
Position error	1.6	−0.1	0.1	1.2	1.9	3.1	1.1	−0.9	1.0

13 Electrodes	3–2	4–2	4–3	5–2	5–5	Average		Best Diff.	Av. Diff.
Peak amplitude	0.402	0.353	0.325	0.351	0.365	0.359		−16%	−13%
Resolution	32.6	35.6	37.2	35.2	34.3	35.0		+7%	+8%
Volume	0.401	0.418	0.422	0.408	0.404	0.410		−4%	0%
Position error	0.3	−2.1	−2.7	−0.7	1.5	−0.7		–	–

these metrics for the averages of the top performers were similar. These findings reinforce those shown earlier, that while there is some degradation in performance in reducing the number of electrodes, the benefits in higher speed to reduce noise may make this worthwhile in some cases.

7.3 Summary and conclusions

7.3.1 Selection of the hyperparameter

Section 7.1 examined the issues around choosing a hyperparameter considering the presence of artefacts as a performance criterion for tactile sensing applications. Given the importance of identifying the correct number, locations, and strengths of highly variable sensor contacts, the onset of artifacts in the image was introduced as a metric. Metrics such as resolution, position error, amplitude error, and shape error have been standard in EIT, but there has been relatively little discussion of artefacts. Because artefacts can be large, and because a light touch simultaneous with a heavier one can look like an artefact, artefacts should be considered in evaluating image quality.

As with all EIT images, the challenge is to best balance the problems that arise from overfitting noise with those from hyperparameter-induced blurring, so that the images best represent the input. The particular challenge of tactile sensing is not knowing in advance what an image is supposed to show. This study was based on the premise that the elimination of non-target features is more important for tactile sensing than minor resolution improvements.

A noise threshold $N_{\text{th}}(\lambda)$ was defined as the maximum noise at a given hyperparameter for which there were no artefacts in five trials. Equivalently, the hyperparameter $\lambda_{\text{th}}(N)$ was the smallest λ at a given level of noise before the onset of artefacts. The onset of artefacts was an efficient metric for evaluating the usability of tactile images, requiring only a handful of replicate images for repeatable determination of the onset of instability. If small artefacts can safely be ignored, the threshold could be lowered to 1–2 artefacts in five trials, the determination depending on the nature of the expected stimuli. This metric can be used to compare systems and parameters.

Because a wide range of contacts can be experienced by a tactile sensor, understanding how λ needs to be adjusted is advantageous. First the relationship between λ and N_{th} was found. N_{th} increased as λ^b, where b is a constant that depends on the target and other factors. For example, for I–M = 7–1 and a single target under the specific simulation conditions that were employed, $N_{\text{th}} \sim \lambda^{0.87}$, or an increase by a factor of 7.4 for each factor of 10 increase in λ. The relationship held up to $\lambda = 10^{-2}$; above that N_{th} leveled off. This value of b was for a target of radius 0.2. For a smaller target of radius 0.05, b was also smaller at 0.75, while for a larger target of radius 0.4, b rose to 0.92. larger targets are thus increasingly more immune to noise.

Results from the artefact-based metric were compared to those from the L-curve, GCV, and BestRes. The artefact method was more efficient than BestRes, requiring fewer replicates due to lower variability. Both GCV and BestRes resulted in smaller hyperparameters at higher noise levels, producing images with erroneous tactile information, and both struggled at low SNR. The artefact-based metric and the L-curve resulted in similar hyperparameters. However, the L-curve also failed at low SNR.

Applications that require robots or other systems to make decisions autonomously based on tactile inputs having high dynamic range will require an automated method of hyperparameter selection. Setting λ in advance can be highly sub-optimal unless the dynamic range of SNRs is narrow. Changing λ until the images appear by eye to be reasonable (heuristic selection) is infeasible for an automated system, as is using methods that require prior information about the contacts or averaging data frames. (If time is available, the focus should instead be on improving SNR by averaging more points during data collection to reduce the required hyperparameter.) The L-curve and GCV select the hyperparameter based on the stimulus in a single frame of data. If the computational overhead can be tolerated, using upper and lower limits if the method fails, this would allow considerably more accurate images than setting a fixed λ that is optimal for a worst-case SNR.

Recommendations for future work include understanding how non-idealities in experimental conditions affect EIT performance. In addition, there is a need to determine a low-computational-overhead method of automatic hyperparameter selection for particular application conditions.

7.3.2 Selection of the injection–measurement pattern

A key conclusion of section 7.2 is that the relative performance among the I–M patterns is strongly dependent on the hyperparameter (table 7.4). At small λ, performance is dominated by rank, while at large λ, by sensitivity at the center of the sensor. It is through the understanding of the role of hyperparameter in shifting the relative merits of the I–M patterns that one can understand the conflicting advice in the literature on the topic of I–M patterns.

Secondly, it must be emphasized that even more important than choosing the best I–M pattern (excluding the low-rank patterns) is keeping the hyperparameter small by keeping noise low. Differences in metrics such as peak amplitude and resolution among the patterns were smaller than differences resulting from changing λ by a factor of 10.

If the noise level and signal strength, and thus the hyperparameter, for a given experiment are consistent, and if the metrics critical to the given application have been identified, then the plots presented here can guide the choice of an I–M pattern. On the other hand, if the required hyperparameter is highly variable, then a pattern that gives good overall performance across the entire studied range of regularization and metrics can be chosen. For the 16-electrode system 3–3 was the best overall compromise with other good choices being 6–2, 6–3, and 7–3. If hyperparameters greater than 10^{-1} are not required (this value being appropriately scaled to the system of interest), then 2–2 becomes a good overall choice, followed by 3–2 and 3–3, and then 6–2 and 7–3.

There are several reasons that the pseudo-polar (PP, nearly-opposite, 7) injection position, I, has been recommended in the literature. First, due to the greater injection electrode separation, the measured voltage drops are larger than for more closely spaced electrodes. This is advantageous for hardware requirements and power consumption. Second, for PP the distribution of the electric field lines results in higher sensitivity to changes in conductivity at the center of the sensor than ADJ. This was manifested here at large hyperparameters in better conservation of volume, or peak energy, and uniformity of volume across the sensor, as well as better noise immunity. Third, due to the position's asymmetry, the number of independent measurements is greater than for more symmetric high-angle positions, especially the polar, which has the highest symmetry. However, the associated measurement position M must also be considered. At large hyperparameter 7–1 had poor peak amplitude and resolution, as well as low uniformity, and its noise susceptibility was also one of the worst. A better choice is 7–3, which had no serious drawbacks and several areas of superior performance.

There are also reasons that the adjacent (ADJ, 1–1) pattern has been recommended. The hardware was easier to implement in former times, and it has superior performance on several of the metrics, including amplitude and resolution, at small hyperparameter: defocusing becomes severe only at larger λ, needed at high noise levels. (It has been previously noted [1] that 1–1 performs poorly in the presence of noise, which is another way of saying that it performs poorly at large λ.) It is on the basis of poor performance at the largest $\lambda \geqslant 0.1$, which represents a high level of regularization, that the #−1 patterns are discouraged here.

It has been suggested that different I–M patterns be used depending on the target position. The present study shows how the spatial dependences of the metrics vary with the I–M pattern. However, these results do not provide support for switching among I–M patterns. Examining the position dependence of peak amplitude (figure 7.13(a)), resolution (figure 7.13(b)), and volume (figure 7.18(a)) shows that differences among the I–M_{80+} patterns at the periphery were relatively small and that all the I–M_{80+} patterns experienced a monotonic drop in performance from the perimeter to the center, albeit with different steepness and plateau radii. This finding is consistent with the results in [2]. Thus the question here became, which patterns dropped the least? This question is important both for detecting contacts at the center of the sensor and for detecting multiple simultaneous touches at different locations (minimizing masking, figure 7.12(b)).

The overall best compromise performance of 3–3 (or 2–2) contradicts earlier advice to employ high-angle patterns. Some of those studies were based on the distinguishability metric using a point target, and others examined changes in I, keeping M = 1. In fact, the low-angle patterns perform well in terms of amplitude and resolution at small λ, whereas the mid- to high-angle patterns perform well on the volume metrics. Thus, depending on the particular use case, the optimal pattern may vary.

The use of 13 electrodes eliminates high-symmetry patterns. More importantly, the reduction in the number of required measurements (allowing either more time at each position to reduce noise or a faster frame rate) and the smaller size of the matrices that need to be manipulated may be advantageous. The best overall pattern with 13 electrodes was 3–2.

A review of the 53 publications in the tactile sensing literature using bipolar injection patterns with 16 electrodes at the periphery of the sensor showed that just over half of the papers used 1–1, one used 8–1, one 8–8, and three compared several patterns; in approximately 40% of the publications the I–M pattern was unclear or unspecified. Based on the ranks in figure 7.10, the sensitivity maps in figure 7.11, and the relative amplitudes of the potential drops, all of which have been known, this is surprising, particularly given that the experimental systems are frequently described as suffering from high noise. The predominant use of 1–1 may go a little way toward explaining the recurring criticism of EIT as being low resolution, as well as the increasing number of publications using machine learning for reconstruction.

The simulations performed here were limited to a particular target, a circular sensor of uniform and isotropic baseline conductivity, a step conductivity change, and a certain inverse algorithm and prior, and they assumed ideal point electrodes and normally-distributed noise. It is anticipated that the results will be valid for similar targets and for multiple targets, since superposition holds for EIT images, although for larger targets the metrics are less strongly degraded by regularization. In future work, the generality of these findings to other scenarios (e.g. square or irregular sensor geometries, other algorithms and priors, etc) should be explored.

This study showed what would be expected in the ideal, generic case. Sensitivity studies that seek to understand how various perturbations to the forward problem affect the solution would be helpful to understanding various non-idealities. For example, an early study showed that difference imaging is relatively insensitive to contact impedance [3]. Another study found that bipolar patterns were less sensitive to errors in contact impedance and electrode size when voltages were measured only on non-current-carrying electrodes, and that image deterioration due to these effects could be reduced by greater regularization [4].

In future work the findings presented here should also be compared with experiments. For example, tactile materials can be non-uniform and anisotropic, and the consequences of that on the choice of I–M pattern are unknown. These issues can be tackled by combining physics-based modeling with EIT to handle such effects as irregular geometries of sensors and anisotropic conductivity, as shown in [5]. Noise that depends on electrode position or electrode pair separation may strongly affect the noise performance of some patterns. Stress on the electrodes due to contacts may shift the advantage to higher angle I–M combinations that rely less on peripheral information. However, it is clear that the tactile sensing community should move away from the adjacent configuration that has been the norm.

References

[1] Booth M J 2000 Design and development of a distributed planar pressure sensor utilising electrical impedance tomography *PhD Thesis* Sheffield Hallam University

[2] Nagakubo A, Alirezaei H and Kuniyoshi Y 2007 A deformable and deformation sensitive tactile distribution sensor *IEEE Int. Conf. Robot. Biomimetics (ROBIO) (Sanya, China, Dec. 15–18)* pp 1301–8

[3] Kato Y, Mukai T, Hayakawa T and Shibata T 2007 Tactile sensor without wire and sensing element in the tactile region based on EIT method *IEEE Sensors (Atlanta, GA, Oct. 28–31)* pp 792–5

[4] Elsanadedy A 2012 Application of electrical impedance tomography to robotic tactile sensing *MS Thesis* Mechanical Engineering, Carleton University

[5] Tawil D S, Rye D and Velonaki M 2012 Interpretation of the modality of touch on an artificial arm covered with an EIT-based sensitive skin *Int. J. Robot. Res.* **31** 1627–41

[6] Yao A, Yang C L, Seo J K and Soleimani M 2013 EIT-based fabric pressure sensing *Comput. Math. Method. Medicine* **2013** 405325

[7] Pugach G, Pitti A and Gaussier P 2015 Neural learning of the topographic tactile sensory information of an artificial skin through a self-organizing map *Adv. Robotics* **29** 1393–409

[8] Tallman T N, Gungor S, Wang K W and Bakis C E 2015 Tactile imaging and distributed strain sensing in highly flexible carbon nanofiber/polyurethane nanocomposites *Carbon* **95** 485–93

[9] Visentin F, Fiorini P and Suzuki K 2016 A deformable smart skin for continuous sensing based on electrical impedance tomography *Sensors* **16** ARTN 1928

[10] Lee H, Kwon D, Cho H, Park I and Kim J 2017 Soft nanocomposite based multi-point, multi-directional strain mapping sensor using anisotropic electrical impedance tomography *Sci. Rep.* **7** 39837

[11] Russo S, Nefti-Meziani S, Carbonaro N and Tognetti A 2017 Development of a high-speed current injection and voltage measurement system for electrical impedance tomography-based stretchable sensors *Technologies* **5** 48

[12] Chen Y, Yu M, Bruck H A and Smela E 2018 Compliant multi-layer tactile sensing for enhanced identification of human touch *Smart Mater. Struct.* **27** 125009

[13] Tawil D S, Rye D and Velonaki M 2011 Improved image reconstruction for an EIT-based sensitive skin with multiple internal electrodes *IEEE Trans. Robot.* **27** 425–35

[14] Liu K, Wu Y, Wang S, Wang H, Chen H, Chen B and Yao J 2020 Artificial sensitive skin for robotics based on electrical impedance tomography *Adv. Intell. Syst.* **2** 1900161

[15] Gaggero P O 2011 Miniaturization and distinguishability limits of electrical impedance tomography for biomedical application *PhD Thesis* Landquart, Switzerland: Nanomedecine Division, Centre Suisse d'Electronique et de Microtechnique (CSEM), University of Neuchâtel

[16] Hansen P C 2010 *Discrete Inverse Problems: Insight and Algorithms, Fundamentals of Algorithms* (Philadelphia, PA: Society for Industrial and Applied Mathematics (SIAM))

[17] Graham B M and Adler A 2006 Objective selection of hyperparameter for EIT *Physiol. Meas.* **27** S65–79

[18] Correia T, Gibson A, Schweiger M and Hebden J 2009 Selection of regularization parameter for optical topography *J. Biomed. Opt.* **14** 034044

[19] Chen Y 2018 Tactile Sensing with Compliant Structures for Human-Robot Interaction *PhD Thesis* Department of Mechanical Engineering, University of Maryland

[20] Islam M R and Kiber M A 2014 Electrical impedance tomography imaging using Gauss-Newton algorithm *Int. Conf. Informatics, Electronics & Vision (ICIEV) (Dhaka, 23–24 May)* pp 1–4

[21] Zhou Z, Malone E, dos Santos G S, Li N, Xu H and Holder D 2014 Comparison of different quadratic regularization for electrical impedance tomography *6th Eur. Conf. Intl. Fed. Medical and Biological Engineering (MBEC 2014)* vol 45 *(Dubrovnik, Sept. 7–11)* I Lacković and D Vasic pp 200–3

[22] Smela E 2022 EIT for tactile sensing: considering artefacts in hyperparameter selection *Eng. Res. Expr* **4** 035057

[23] Adler A, Dai T and Lionheart W R B 2007 Temporal image reconstruction in electrical impedance tomography *Physiol. Meas.* **28** S1–S11

[24] Braun F, Proença M, Solà J, Thiran J-P and Adler A 2017 A versatile noise performance metric for electrical impedance tomography algorithms *IEEE Trans. Biomed. Eng.* **64** 2321–30

[25] Brinckerhoff M 2018 Comparison of electrical impedance tomography reconstruction algorithms with EIDORS reconstruction software *MS Thesis* Mathematics, Clemson University

[26] Chaves L M, Carvalho L D D, Reis C J D and Souza D J D 2019 Explaining the generalized cross-validation on linear models *J. Math. Stat* **15** 298–307

[27] Buccini A and Reichel L 2021 Generalized cross validation for ℓ^p-ℓ^q minimization *Numer. Algor.* **88** 1595–616

[28] Hansen P C 2001 The L-curve and its use in the numerical treatment of inverse problems *Computational Inverse Problems in Electrocardiology* ed P R Johnston (Ashurst, Southampton: WIT Press) vol 4 pp 119–42

[29] Hansen P C 1994 Regularization tools: a Matlab package for analysis and solution of discrete ill-posed problems *Numer. Algor* **6** 1–35

[30] Hansen P C 2007 Regularization Tools version 4.0 for Matlab 7.3 *Numer. Algor.* **46** 189–94

[31] Hansen P C 2008 *Regularization Tools: A Matlab Package for Analysis and Solution of Discrete Ill-Posed Problems*, Version 4.1 for Matlab 7.3, MATLAB Central File Exchange

[32] Hamilton S J, Lionheart R B and Adler A 2019 Comparing D-bar and common regularization-based methods for electrical impedance tomography *Physiol. Meas.* **40** ARTN 044004

[33] Tawil D S, Rye D and Velonaki M 2011 Improved EIT drive patterns for a robotics sensitive skin *Australasian Conf. Robotics and Automation (ACRA) (Sydney, Dec. 2–4)* pap 112s111

[34] Tawil D S 2012 Artificial skin and the interpretation of touch in human-robot interaction *PhD Thesis* School of Aerospace, Mechanical and Mechatronic Engineering, University of Sydney
[35] Silvera-Tawil D, Rye D, Soleimani M and Velonaki M 2015 Electrical impedance tomography for artificial sensitive robotic skin: a review *IEEE Sens. J.* **15** 2001–16
[36] Chen Y, Yu M, Bruck H A and Smela E 2018 Characterization of a compliant multi-layer system for tactile sensing with enhanced sensitivity and range *Smart Mater. Struct.* **27** 065005
[37] Dai H B and Thostenson E T 2019 Large-area carbon nanotube-based flexible composites for ultra-wide range pressure sensing and spatial pressure mapping *ACS Appl. Mater. Interfaces* **11** 48370–80
[38] Adler A and Boyle A 2017 Electrical impedance tomography: tissue properties to image measures *IEEE Trans. Biomed. Eng.* **64** 2494–504
[39] Dickin F and Wang M 1996 Electrical resistance tomography for process applications *Meas. Sci. Technol.* **7** 247–60
[40] Avis N J and Barber D C 1994 Image reconstruction using non-adjacent drive configurations *Physiol. Meas.* **15** A153–60
[41] Schuessler T F and Bates J H T 1998 Current patterns and electrode types for single-source electrical impedance tomography of the thorax *Ann. Biomed. Eng.* **26** 253–9
[42] Kauppinen P, Hyttinen J and Malmivuo J 2006 Sensitivity distribution visualizations of impedance tomography measurement strategies *Int. J. Bioelectromag.* **8** 63–71
[43] Shi X T, Dong X Z, Shuai W J, You F S, Fu F and Liu R G 2006 Pseudo-polar drive patterns for brain electrical impedance tomography *Physiol. Meas.* **27** 1071–80
[44] Xu C, Dong X, Shi X, Fu F, Shuai W, Liu R and You F 2008 Comparison of drive patterns for single current source EIT in computational phantom *2nd Int. Conf. Bioinformatics and Biomedical Engineering (Shanghai, 16–18 May)* pp 1500–3
[45] He Y-B, Wang H-X and Sankowski D 2008 Analysis of electrial impedance tomography sensitive field based on multi-terminal network *Automatyka* **12** 903–9
[46] Zhang L, Wang H and Zhang L 2010 Single source current drive patterns for electrical impedance tomography IEEE Instrumentation & Measurement Technology Conf. Proc *(Austin, TX, 3–6 May)* pp 1477–80
[47] Adler A, Gaggero P O and Maimaitijiang Y 2011 Adjacent stimulation and measurement patterns considered harmful *Physiol. Meas.* **32** 731–44
[48] Bera T K and Nagaraju J 2012 Studying the resistivity imaging of chicken tissue phantoms with different current patterns in Electrical Impedance Tomography (EIT) *Measurement* **45** 663–82
[49] Liu J, Lin L, Zhang W and Li G 2013 A novel combined regularization algorithm of total variation and Tikhonov regularization for open electrical impedance tomography *Physiol. Meas.* **34** 823–38
[50] Wang M, Wang Q and Karki B 2016 Arts of electrical impedance tomographic sensing *Philosoph. Trans.* A **374** 20150329
[51] Luppi Silva O, Gonzalez Lima R, Castro Martins T, Silva de Moura F, Seiji Tavares R and Sales Guerra Tsuzuki M 2017 Influence of current injection pattern and electric potential measurement strategies in electrical impedance tomography *Control Eng. Pract.* **58** 276–86
[52] Russo S, Nefti-Meziani S, Carbonaro N and Tognetti A 2017 A quantitative evaluation of drive pattern selection for optimizing EIT-based stretchable sensors *Sensors* **17** ARTN 1999

[53] Barber D C 2005 EIT: the view from Sheffield *Electrical Impedance Tomography: Methods, History and Applications of the series Series in Medical Physics and Biomedical Engineering* ed C G Orton, J H Nagel and J G Webster (Bristol: IOP Publishing) ch 11

[54] Vauhkonen M, Lionheart W R, Heikkinen L M, Vauhkonen P J and Kaipio J P 2001 A MATLAB package for the EIDORS project to reconstruct two-dimensional EIT images *Physiol. Meas.* **22** 107–11

[55] Adler A and Lionheart W R B 2006 Uses and abuses of EIDORS: an extensible software base for EIT *Physiol. Meas.* **27** S25–42

[56] Adler A 2019 EIDORS: Electrical Impedance Tomography and Diffuse Optical Tomography Reconstruction Software, http://eidors3d.sourceforge.net/

[57] Wu H, Zheng B, Wang H and Ye J 2022 New flexible tactile sensor based on electrical impedance tomography *Micromachines* **13** 185

[58] Lionheart W, Polydorides N and Borsic A 2005 The reconstruction problem *Electrical Impedance Tomography: Methods, History and Applications, Series in Medical Physics and Biomedical Engineering* ed C G Orton, J H Nagel and J G Webster (Bristol: IOP Publishing) ch 1

[59] Smela E 2022 EIT for tactile sensing:considerations regarding the injection-measurement pattern *Eng. Res. Express* **4** 045041

Appendix A

EIT for structural health monitoring

Table A.1. Selected studies that have used EIT for structural health monitoring (SHM), focusing on applications.

References	Year	Application	Sensing
[1–3]	2008	Spatial tensile-compressive strain during cycling loading, impact damage location and severity, corrosion monitoring by byproduct formation of metallic structures	Carbon nanotube (CNT)-polyelectrolyte composite deposited on glass, aluminum 6061-T6, and carbon steel
[4]	2012	Impact damage and holes detected in carbon fiber-reinforced polymer (CFRP) composites	Electrodes mounted directly onto the CFRP sample
[5]	2013	Strain detection in carbon fiber-reinforced polymer (CFRP) composites	CNT-polyvinylidene fluoride (PVDF) latex-composite spray-coated onto CFRP
[6]	2013	Damage in the form of holes detected in glass fiber-reinforced polymer (GFRP) composites	CNT-PVDF latex spray-coated onto glass fiber mat, stacked with other mats and infused with epoxy to form panels
[7]	2013	Impact and holes detected GFRP panel	CNT-PVDF latex spray-coated onto GFRP panel
[5]	2013	Strain detection in GFRP	CNT-PVDF latex spray-coated onto GFRP panel
[8]	2014	Holes in glass fiber/epoxy laminate plate	Carbon black (CB) added to epoxy used in forming glass fiber/epoxy laminate
[9]	2015	Impact damage of glass fiber/epoxy laminate plate	Same as [8]

(*Continued*)

doi:10.1088/978-0-7503-5402-8ch8

Table A.1. (*Continued*)

References	Year	Application	Sensing
[10]	2015	Holes and impact damage of glass fiber/epoxy laminate plate	Same as [8]
[11]	2016	Holes, cut in sensor; impact damage of GFRP panel	Nonwoven aramid fabric filled with CNTs and infused with epoxy, attached with epoxy to GFRP
[12, 13]	2016	Impact damage, delamination of GFRP	Unidirectional glass nonwoven fabric filled with CNTs and infused with epoxy, used singly or in stacks; electrodes attached directly
[14]	2016	Monitor deformation, holes in fabric for inflatable structures	CNT-latex mounted on fabric
[15]	2016	Strain in lap joint	Inkjet-printed CNT film embedded between glossy photo paper and adhesive in the bonding area
[16]	2017	Detect corrosion, cracking of polymeric and concrete substrates	Multi-layer sensor of Cu and Ag paint (Cu reacts with chlorides, Ag does not)
[17]	2017	Detect strain, holes, impact using different minimization than usual EIT	Carbon nanofiber (CNF) in PU; CNF in epoxy; glass fiber/epoxy laminate with CB filler
[18]	2019	Monitor effects of UV irradiation on film by decrease in conductivity	DNA and graphene mixed with conducting polymer (PEDOT: PSS), deposited on CFRP plate
[19]	2019	Identify stress concentrations in piezoresistive composites by induced conductivity changes	CNF/epoxy samples, electrodes attached directly
[20]	2020	Damage and hole detection in CFRP composite	Electrodes attached directly to the laminate
[21]	2020	Review	
[22]	2022	Delamination and holes in CNF-modified GFRP laminates; use genetic algorithm integrated with realistic physics-based damage models	Same as [8]

References

[1] Loh K J, Hou T C, Lynch J P and Kotov N A 2008 Spatial structural sensing by carbon nanotube-based skins *Conf. on Sensors and Smart Structures Technologies for Civil, Mechanical, and Aerospace Systems* SPIE vol 6932 *(San Diego, CA, Mar 10–13)*

[2] Loh K J, Hou T C, Lynch J P and Kotov N A 2009 Carbon nanotube sensing skins for spatial strain and impact damage identification *J. Nondestruct. Eval.* **28** 9–25

[3] Pyo S, Loh K J, Hou T C, Jarva E and Lynch J P 2011 A wireless impedance analyzer for automated tomographic mapping of a nanoengineered sensing skin *Smart. Struct. Syst.* **8** 139–55

[4] Loyola B R, Arronche L, La Saponara V and Loh K J 2012 Conductivity-based damage detection in carbon fiber composites *ASME Conf. on Smart Materials, Adaptive Structures and Intelligent Systems (Stone Mountain, GA, Sep 19–21)* pp 671–8

[5] Loyola B R, La Saponara V, Loh K J, Briggs T M, O'Bryan G and Skinner J L 2013 Spatial sensing using electrical impedance tomography *IEEE Sens. J.* **13** 2357–67

[6] Loyola B R, Briggs T M, Arronche L, Loh K J, La Saponara V, O'Bryan G and Skinner J L 2013 Detection of spatially distributed damage in fiber-reinforced polymer composites *Struct. Health Monit.* **12** 225–39

[7] Loyola B R, Arronche L, LaFord M, La Saponara V and Loh K J 2013 Evaluation of the damage detection characteristics of electrical impedance tomography *ASME Conf. on Smart Materials, Adaptive Structures and Intelligent Systems (SMASIS2013) (Snowbird, UT, Sept. 16–18)* p 3317

[8] Tallman T N and Wang K W 2014 Damage sensitivity and multiple damage detection in glass fiber/epoxy laminates with carbon black filler via electrical impedance tomography *7th Ann. ASME Conf. Smart Materials, Adaptive Structures and Intelligent Systems (SMASIS)/ Symp. on Modeling, Simulation and Control (MSC) (Newport, RI, Sep 8–10)*

[9] Tallman T N and Wang K W 2015 Impact damage identification in glass fiber/epoxy laminates with carbon black filler via electrical impedance tomography *10th Int. Workshop on Structural Health Monitoring (IWSHM) (Stanford, CA, Sept. 1–3)* (DEStech Publications, Inc.) pp 1689–96

[10] Tallman T N, Gungor S, Wang K W and Bakis C E 2015 Damage detection via electrical impedance tomography in glass fiber/epoxy laminates with carbon black filler *Struct. Health Monit.* **14** 100–9

[11] Dai H B, Gallo G J, Schumacher T and Thostenson E T 2016 A novel methodology for spatial damage detection and imaging using a distributed carbon nanotube-based composite sensor combined with electrical impedance tomography *J. Nondestruct. Eval.* **35** 15

[12] Gallo G J and Thostenson E T 2016 Spatial damage detection in electrically anisotropic fiber-reinforced composites using carbon nanotube networks *Compos. Struct.* **141** 14–23

[13] Tallman T N 2016 Electrical resistance tomography with constrained sine wave solutions for impact damage identification in glass fiber/epoxy/carbon black laminate composites *Conf. on Sensors and Smart Structures Technologies for Civil, Mechanical, and Aerospace Systems* SPIE vol 9803 *(Las Vegas, NV, Mar 21–24)*

[14] Wang L, Gupta S, Loh K J and Koo H S 2016 Nanocomposite fabric sensors for monitoring inflatable and deployable space structures *ASME Conf. on Smart Materials, Adaptive Structures and Intelligent Systems (Stowe, VT, Sep 28–30)*

[15] Zhao Y J, Schagerl M, Gschossmann S and Kralovec C 2019 In situ spatial strain monitoring of a single-lap joint using inkjet-printed carbon nanotube embedded thin films *Struct. Health Monit.* **18** 1479–90

[16] Seppänen A, Hallaji M and Pour-Ghaz M 2017 A functionally layered sensing skin for the detection of corrosive elements and cracking *Struct. Health Monit.* **16** 215–24

[17] Tallman T N and Hernandez J A 2017 The effect of error and regularization norms on strain and damage identification via electrical impedance tomography in piezoresistive nano-composites *NDT E Int.* **91** 156–63

[18] Clausi M, Toto E, Botti S, Laurenzi S, La Saponara V and Santonicola M G 2019 Direct effects of UV irradiation on graphene-based nanocomposite films revealed by electrical resistance tomography *Compos. Sci. Technol.* **183** 8

[19] Hassan H and Tallman T N 2019 Experimental identification of stress concentrations in piezoresistive nanocomposites via electrical impedance tomography *Conf. on Sensors and Smart Structures Technologies for Civil, Mechanical, and Aerospace Systems* SPIE vol 10970 *(Denver, CO, Mar 4–7)*

[20] Cagáň J and Michalcová L 2020 Impact damage detection in CFRP composite via electrical resistance tomography by means of statistical processing *J. Nondestruct. Eval.* **39** 12

[21] Tallman T N and Smyl D J 2020 Structural health and condition monitoring via electrical impedance tomography in self-sensing materials: a review *Smart Mater. Struct.* **29** 25

[22] Hassan H and Tallman T N 2022 Precise damage shaping in self-sensing composites using electrical impedance tomography and genetic algorithms *Struct. Health Monit.* **16** 372–87

IOP Publishing

Electrical Impedance Tomography for Tactile Imaging
A primer for experimentalists
Elisabeth Smela

Appendix B

Eigen-images

Eigen-images for I–M pattern 1–1

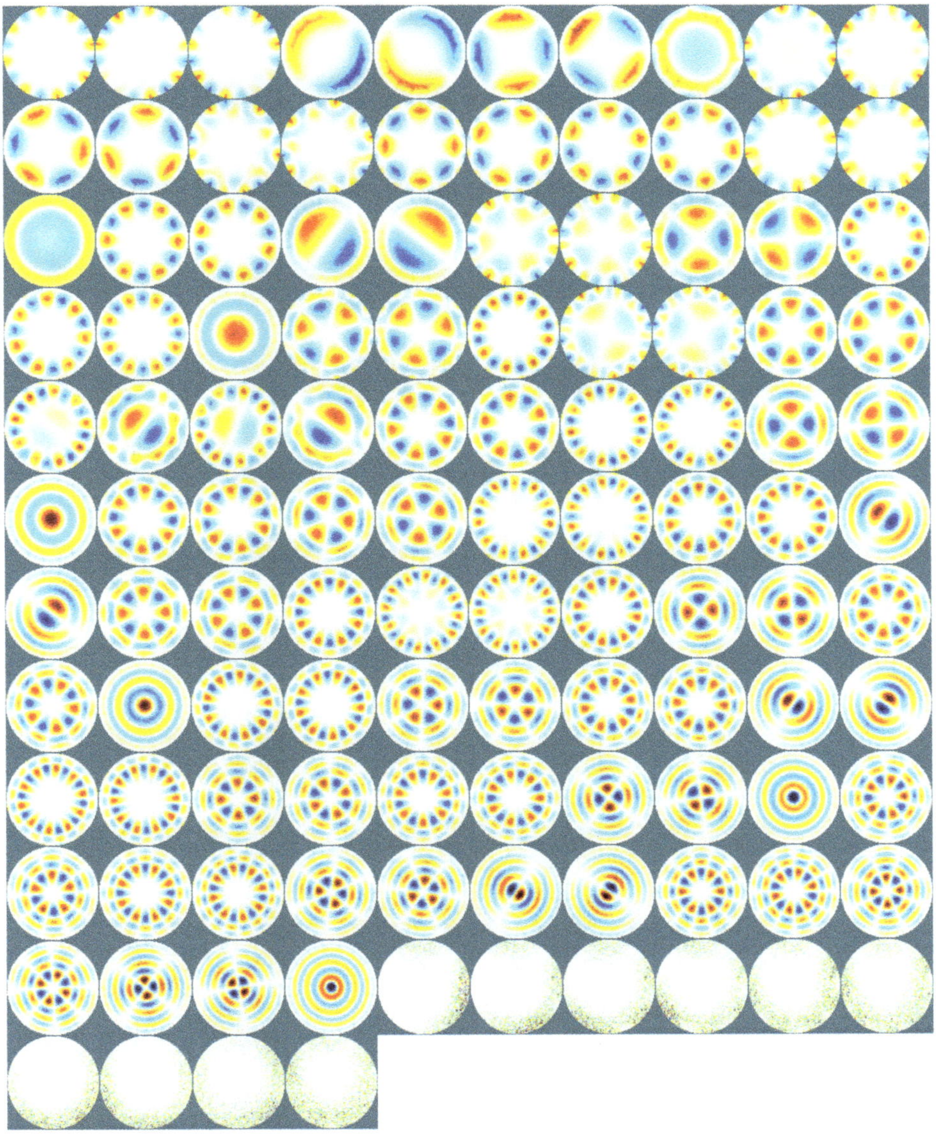

Figure B.1. All the $\mathbf{v}_i$ for I–M = 1–1.

Eigen-images for I–M pattern 7–1

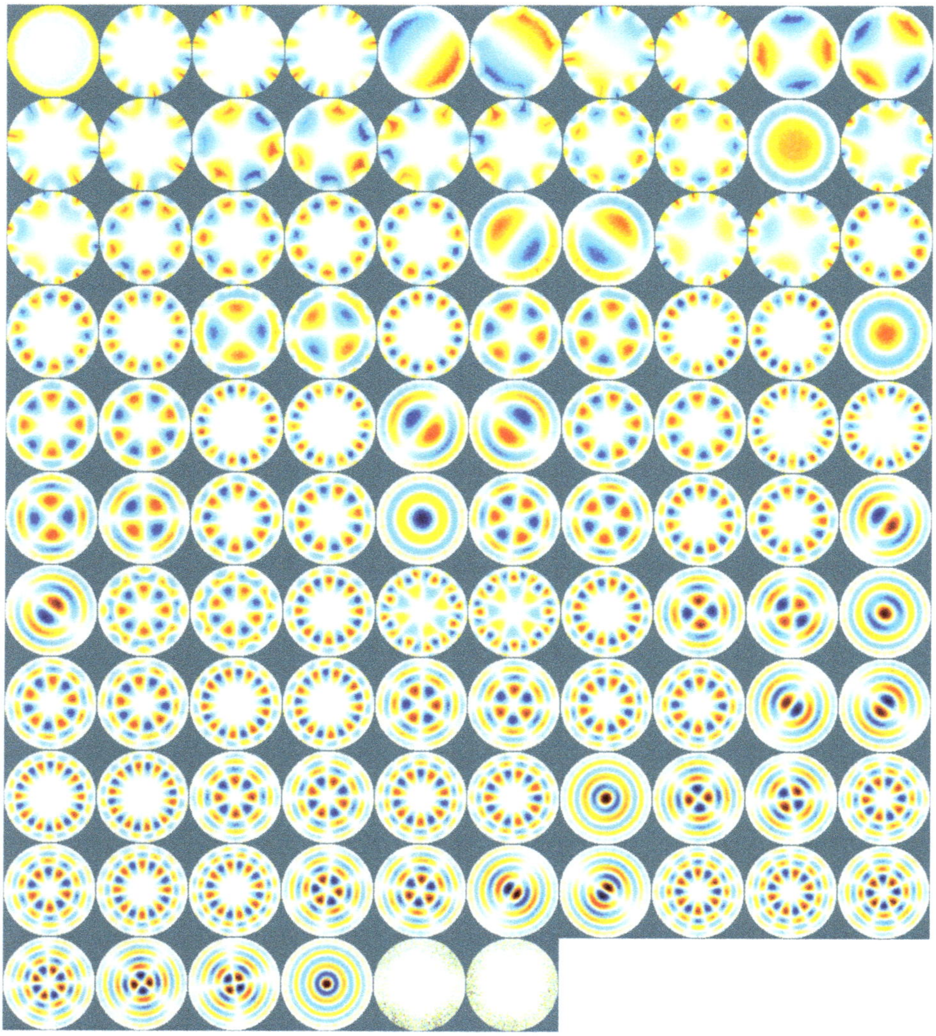

Figure B.2. All the $\mathbf{v}_i$ for I–M = 7–1.

Appendix C

Sensitivity maps of J for all I–M, first seven measurement positions

The same color scale was used for all images below (figure C.1). Code for displaying **J** is given here: http://eidors3d.sourceforge.net/tutorial/EIDORS_basics/sensitivity_-map.shtml

doi:10.1088/978-0-7503-5402-8ch10

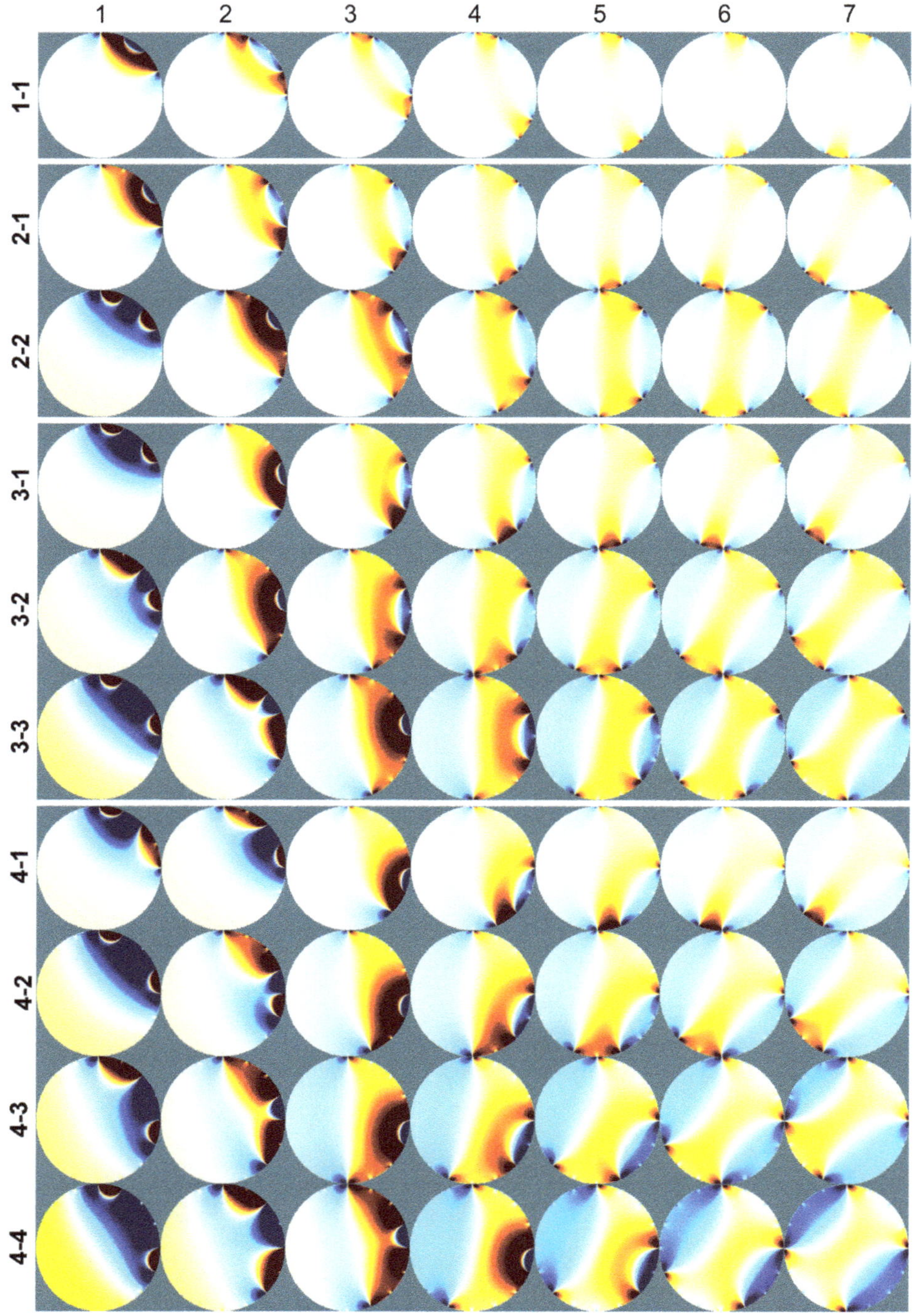

Figure C.1. Visualization of the first seven rows of the Jacobian **J** for all the I–M patterns for a sensor with uniform conductivity.

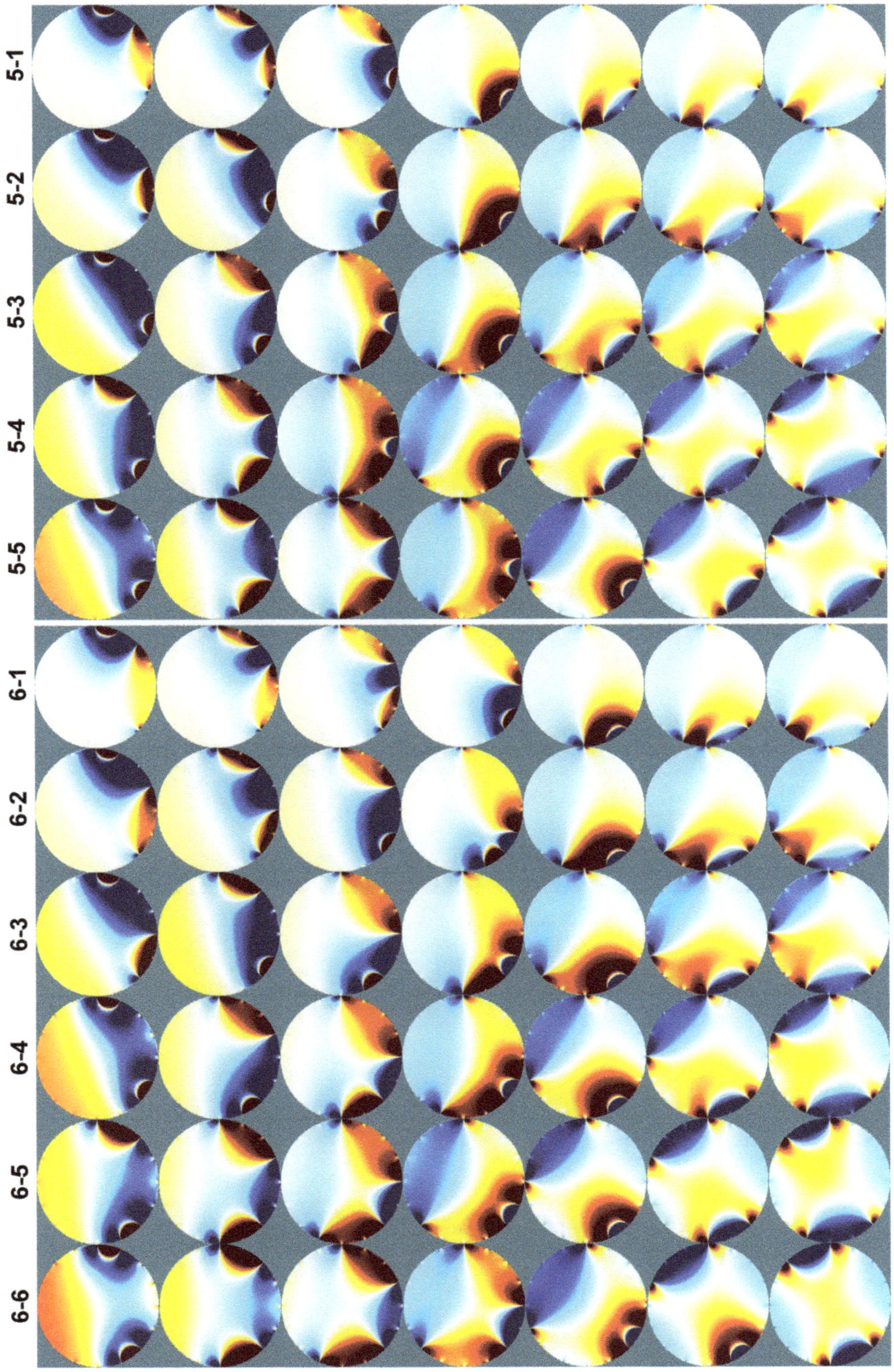

Figure C.1. (Continued.)

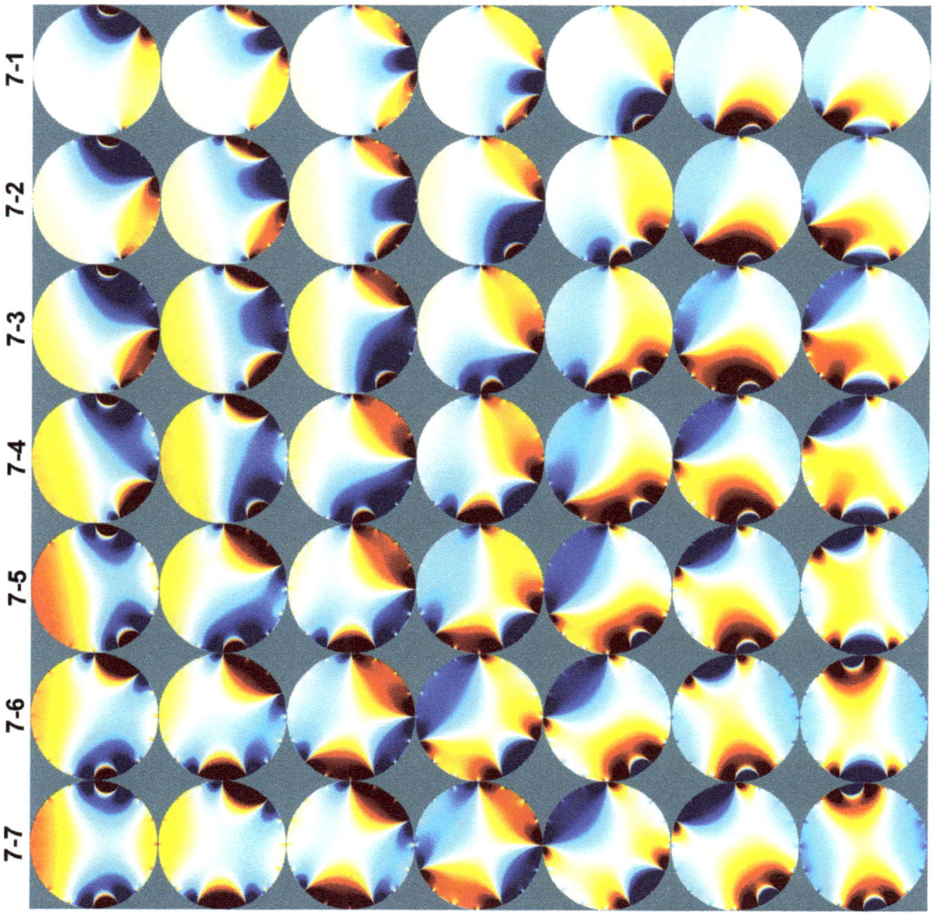

Figure C.1. (Continued.)

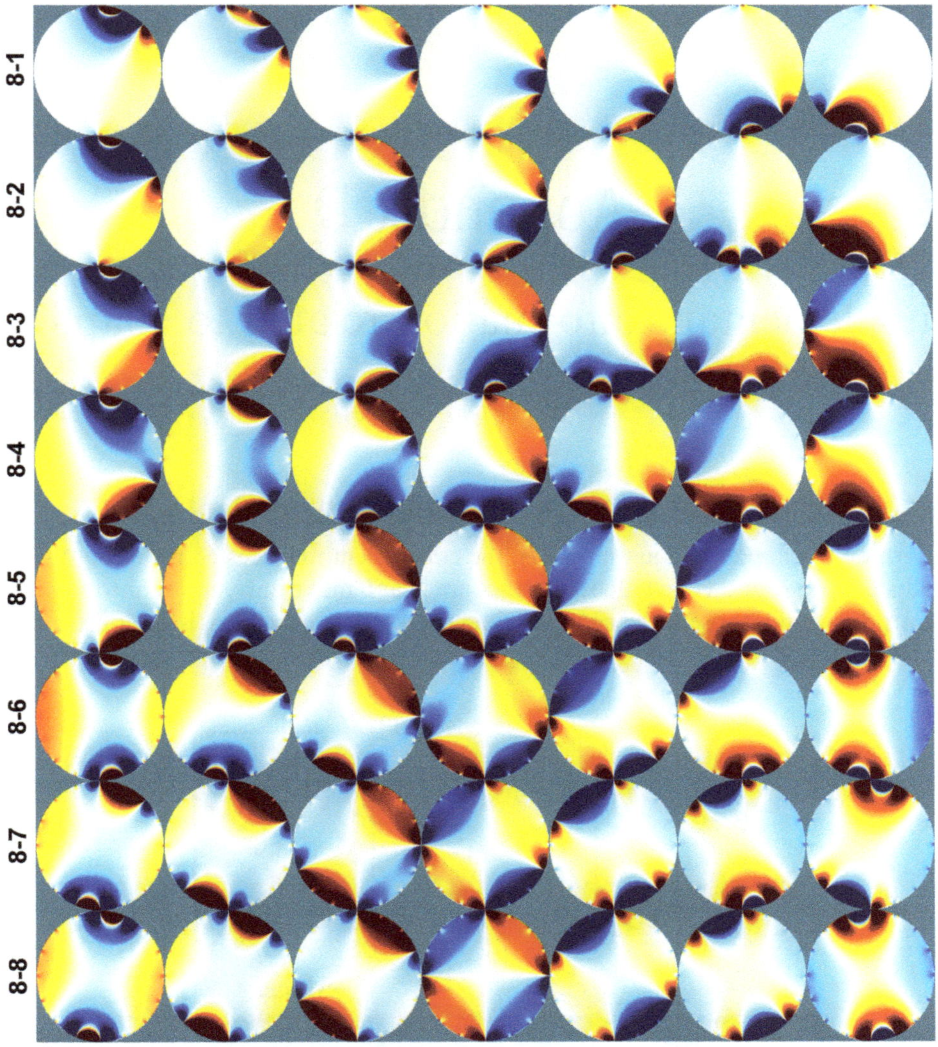

Figure C.1. (Continued.)

IOP Publishing

Electrical Impedance Tomography for Tactile Imaging
A primer for experimentalists
Elisabeth Smela

Appendix D

Supplementary information related to chapter 4

D.1 The component matrices of J (related to section 4.3)

Returning to chapter 4, equation (4.7), the component matrices contributing to **J** are products of $\mathbf{u}_i$, s_i, and $\mathbf{v}_i$, so values in $\mathbf{u}_i$ that are near 0 make only small contributions to this product, while those with negative values reverse the image. This is demonstrated for

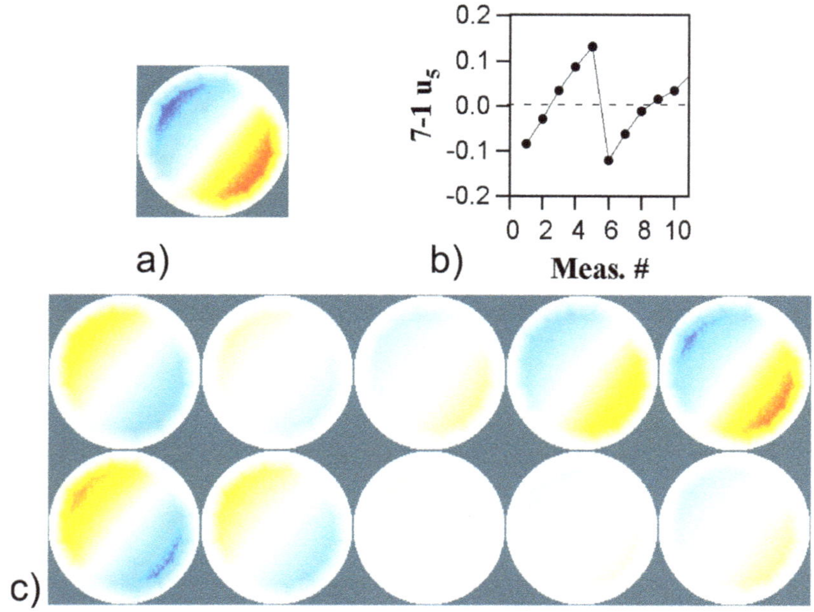

Figure D.1. Images of the first 10 terms in $s_5\mathbf{u}_5\mathbf{v}_5^{\mathrm{T}}$ for I–M = 7–1. (a) The fifth image from figure 4.7(e), $\mathbf{v}_5$. (b) A close-up of the first 10 points of the fifth plot of figure 4.10, $\mathbf{u}_5$. (c) The first 10 terms of $s_5\mathbf{u}_5\mathbf{v}_5^{\mathrm{T}}$; color scale differs from (a). ($I = 3 \times 10^{-5}$, $\sigma_0 = 0.01$).

doi:10.1088/978-0-7503-5402-8ch11

illustration in figure D.1 by the first 10 entries of $s_5\mathbf{u}_5\mathbf{v}_5$ for I–M = 7–1, for which $s_5 = 6.5 \times 10^{-3}$; $\mathbf{u}_5$ was shown in figure 4.10 and its first 10 terms are repeated in figure D.1(b), while $\mathbf{v}_5$ was shown in figure 4.7(e) and is repeated in figure D.1(a) Note how the amplitude of first image in figure D.1(c) is reversed from that of figure D.1(a) because of the negative sign of the first point in figure D.1(b). The third image has a small but positive amplitude, which increases in going to the fifth image, and between the fifth and sixth images there is another reversal. (These are not to be confused with the component matrices of the image.)

D.2 Components in the GN one-step calculation of equation (4.12) (related to section 4.3)

Examples of matrix values are given in table D.1 for a relatively large hyper-parameter, i.e. $\lambda^2 > \mathbf{J}^T\mathbf{W}\mathbf{J}(1,1)$, showing how it affects the sum in the denominator of chapter 4, equation (4.12).

Table D.1. Example matrix values, the first five row and column entries, for six components used in the GN one-step calculation of chapter 4, equation (4.12) with the Laplace prior found using inv_solve_diff_GN_one_step.m. The last matrix, 'sum', is the sum in the denominator of chapter 4, equation (4.12): $\mathbf{J}^T\mathbf{W}\mathbf{J} + \lambda^2\mathbf{R}^T\mathbf{R}$. (I–M = 7–1, $I = 3 \times 10^{-5}$, $\sigma_0 = 0.01$, $\lambda = 10^{-3}$.)

R^TR	1	2	3	4	5	λ^2R^TR	1	2	3	4	5
1	**6**	0	−2	0	0	**1**	**6E-6**	0	−2E-6	0	0
2	0	**6**	−2	0	0	**2**	0	**6E−6**	−2E−6	0	0
3	−2	−2	**6**	−2	0	**3**	−2E−6	−2E−6	**6E−6**	−2E−6	0
4	0	0	−2	**6**	0	**4**	0	0	−2E−6	**6E−6**	0
5	0	0	0	0	**4**	**5**	0	0	0	0	**4E−6**
W	**1**	**2**	**3**	**4**	**5**	**J**	**1**	**2**	**3**	**4**	**5**
1	**1**	0	0	0	0	**1**	**−7E−8**	−6E−8	−1E−7	−1E−7	1E−4
2	0	**1**	0	0	0	**2**	−2E−7	**−2E−7**	−3E−7	−4E−7	−4E−5
3	0	0	**1**	0	0	**3**	−4E−6	7E−7	**−2E−6**	−2E−6	−8E−6
4	0	0	0	**1**	0	**4**	5E−6	−2E−8	4E−6	**3E−6**	−4E−6
5	0	0	0	0	**1**	**5**	−2E−7	−2E−7	−3E−7	−4E−7	**−2E−6**
J^TWJ	**1**	**2**	**3**	**4**	**5**	**sum**	**1**	**2**	**3**	**4**	**5**
1	**1E−9**	5E−11	7E−10	6E−10	1E−10	**1**	**6E−6**	5E−11	−2E−6	6E−10	1E−10
2	5E−11	**1E−10**	8E−11	1E−10	−5E−11	**2**	5E−11	**6E−6**	−2E−6	1E−10	−5E−11
3	7E−10	8E−11	**5E−10**	5E−10	1E−10	**3**	−2E−6	−2E−6	**6E−6**	−2E−6	1E−10
4	6E−10	1E−10	5E−10	**4E−10**	7E−11	**4**	6E−10	1E−10	−2E−6	**6E−6**	7E−11
5	1E−10	−5E−11	1E−10	7E−11	**1E−7**	**5**	1E−10	−5E−11	1E−10	7E−11	**4E−6**

D.3 Tikhonov regularization (related to section 4.4)

In this work, we start from the premise that we can use $\mathbf{J\sigma} = \mathbf{\Delta}$; in other words, that we can use a linear approximation for the relationship between conductivity and voltages, since **J** holds an array of slopes:

$$J_{i,k} = \left.\frac{\partial V_i}{\partial \sigma_k}\right|_{\sigma_0}. \tag{D.1}$$

For large changes in conductivity (more than about 20% [1]), this approximation may cease to be sufficiently valid.

The inverse algorithms (excluding the Sheffield back-propagation method) is basically about how to invert the

$$\mathbf{Ax} = \mathbf{b} \tag{D.2}$$

(for us, $\mathbf{J\sigma} = \mathbf{\Delta}$) to find **x** when **A** (for us **J**) when the number of columns (for us, m is the number of columns, or measurements), is less than the number of rows (for us, n is the number of rows, or mesh elements), and **A** is ill-conditioned (the ratio of the largest to the smallest singular values s_i of **A** is large) so that $\mathbf{Ax} = \mathbf{b}$ has no unique solution. To manage this, constraints can be put on the problem (e.g. no negative values for $x(\boldsymbol{\sigma})$ [2, 3], **x** expressed by sine waves [4], etc), but normally regularization of some kind is used. Regularization can be considered to be a kind of filter to remove various undesired solution components. For sensors, the undesired components are image artefacts or image break-up due to noise, as illustrated in sections 4.6.1 and 6.1.2. Different types of filters have been developed that have different effects on the image.

The following derivation is based on a lecture by Strang [5]. The usual approach to dealing with noisy data, if the columns of **A** are independent (the rank r of **A** is equal to the number of columns), is to solve a linear least-squares problem, minimizing the difference (Euclidian distances) between an approximate solution and the measured, noise-contaminated data **b**.

$$\min \|Ax - b\|_2^2 \tag{D.3}$$

Expanding equation (D.3):

$$\min \|Ax - b\|_2^2 = (Ax - b)^T(Ax - b) = x^T A^T Ax - 2A^T x^T b + b^T b \tag{D.4}$$

The minimum is obtained by taking the derivative and setting it to zero,

$$\frac{d}{dx}(x^T A^T Ax - 2A^T x^T b + b^T b) = 2A^T Ax - 2A^T b = 0$$

giving for the best estimate or 'minimal-norm' $\hat{x}$:

$$\hat{x} = (A^T A)^{-1} A^T b \tag{D.5}$$

This is known at the Moore–Penrose generalized inverse [6].

However, with an ill-conditioned **A**, obtaining $\hat{x}$ (for us, getting a meaningful image $\boldsymbol{\sigma}$) requires making an adjustment to the problem. This has been described as replacing the problem in equation (D.3) with another one that is less sensitive to the noise in **b** (for us, in $\boldsymbol{\Delta}$) [7]. In *Tikhonov regularization* (or ridge regression) the new problem is [5]:

$$\min\{\|Ax - b\|_2^2 - \alpha\|x\|_2^2\} \tag{D.6}$$

where $\alpha > 0$ is the regularization parameter. If there is a known approximation of **x**, $\mathbf{x}_0$, then one can use [7]:

$$\min\{\|Ax - b\|_2^2 - \alpha\|x - x_0\|_2^2\} \tag{D.7}$$

The solution can be improved by using [7]

$$\min\{\|Ax - b_{\text{meas}}\|_2^2 - \alpha\|L(x - x_0)\|_2^2\} \tag{D.8}$$

where L is a regularization matrix, sometimes called a Tikhonov matrix (see also [8]). (The Tikhonov matrix is for us the so-called 'prior'.) This is known as *generalized Tikhonov regularization.* In electrical impedance tomography for tactile imaging, $(\mathbf{x}-\mathbf{x}_0)$ (for us, $(\boldsymbol{\sigma}-\boldsymbol{\sigma}_0)$) can be used if the background conductivity $\boldsymbol{\sigma}_0$ is not substantially spatially uniform.

Setting $\mathbf{x}_0 = 0$ (i.e. assuming a uniform background conductivity), and expanding

$$\begin{aligned}\min\{\|Ax - b\|_2^2 - \alpha\|L(x)\|_2^2\} &= \min\{(Ax - b)^T(Ax - b) - \alpha(Lx)^T(Lx)\} \\ &= \min\{x^TA^TAx - 2A^Tx^Tb + b^Tb - \alpha L^Tx^TLx\}\end{aligned} \tag{D.9}$$

followed by taking the derivative and setting it to zero

$$\frac{d}{dx}(x^TA^TAx - 2A^Tx^Tb + b^Tb - \alpha L^Tx^TLx) = A^TAx - 2A^Tb - \alpha L^TLx = 0 \tag{D.10}$$

gives

$$(A^TA - \alpha L^TL)x - A^Tb = 0 \tag{D.11}$$

which means:

$$\hat{x} = \{(A^TA - \alpha L^TL)^{-1}A^T\}b \tag{D.12}$$

Recalling that

$$\sigma = \mathbf{J}_{\mathbf{reg}}^{-1}\Delta \tag{D.13}$$

and comparing to equation (D.12) in section 4.4.2, repeated here,

$$\mathbf{J}_{\mathbf{reg}}^{-1} = (\mathbf{J}^{\mathbf{T}}\mathbf{W}\mathbf{J} + \lambda^2\mathbf{R}^{\mathbf{T}}\mathbf{R})^{-1}\mathbf{J}^{\mathbf{T}}\mathbf{W} \tag{D.14}$$

one sees that expression in brackets in equation (D.12) and chapter 4's equation (4.12) have the same form, but with an additional covariance matrix **W**, which is the identity **I** by default. In our case $\alpha = \lambda^2$.

D.4 Amplitude, resolution, and volume versus position for various regularization methods (related to section 4.5)

For TSVD, the number of terms retained under the simulation conditions of section 4.5 is as shown in table D.2 (figures D.2–D.4).

Table D.2. For the specified hyperparameter, the number of terms retained in TSVD.

$\lambda = 10^{-3}$	all 192
$\lambda = 10^{-2}$	86
$\lambda = 10^{-1}$	67
$\lambda = 10^{0}$	50
$\lambda = 10^{+1}$	31

Figure 4.17 showed peak amplitude, resolution, and half-amplitude volume as a function of x-position for the four regularization methods at $\lambda = 0.1$. Figures D.2–D.4 show the results over a range of λ using the same simulation conditions.

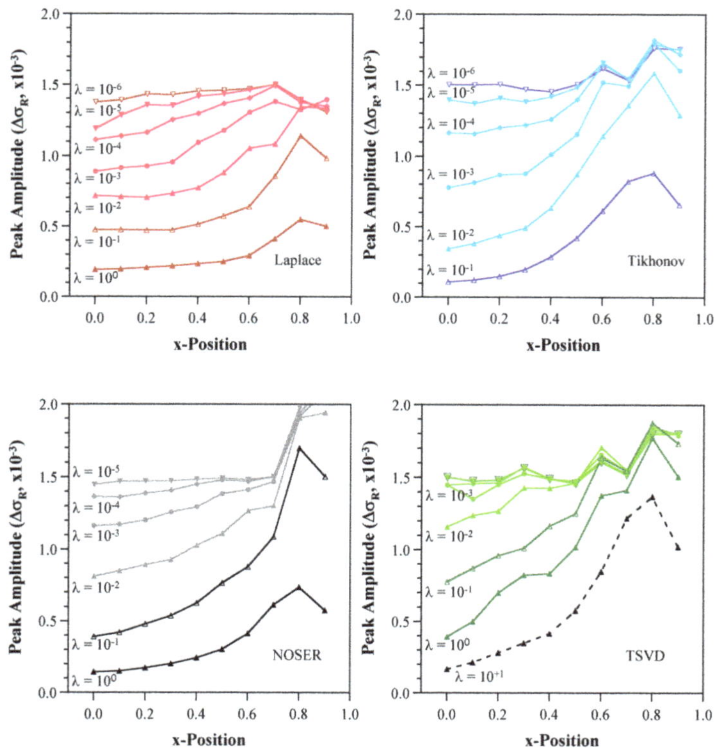

Figure D.2. Peak amplitude as a function of position for different values of λ using four regularization methods.

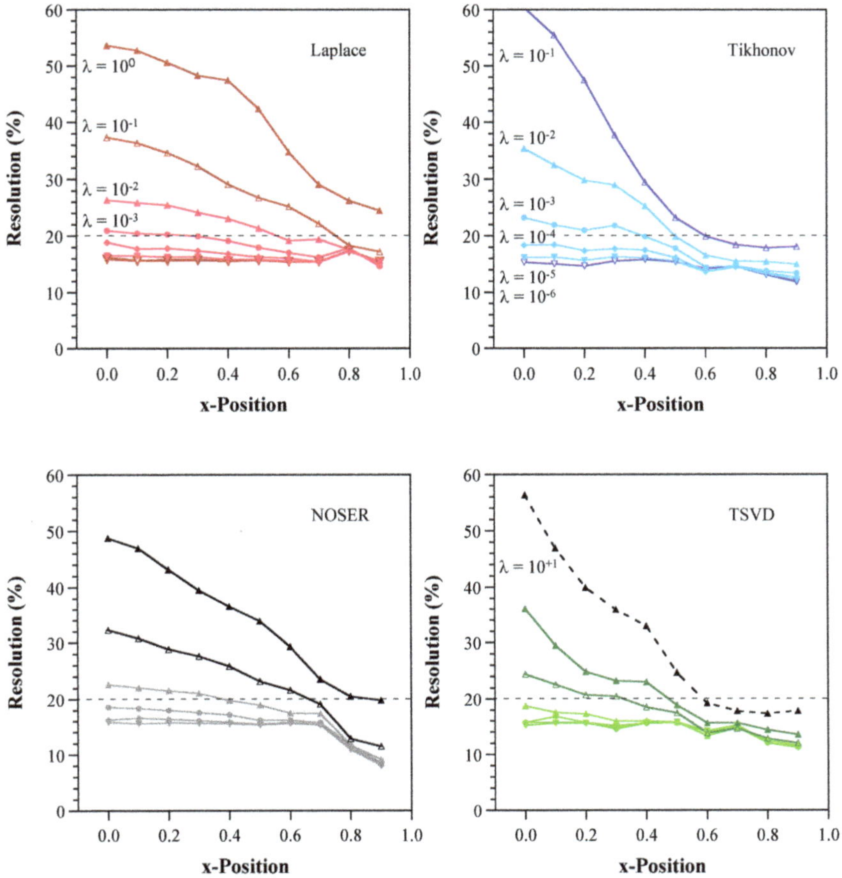

Figure D.3. Resolution as a function of position for different values of λ using four regularization methods.

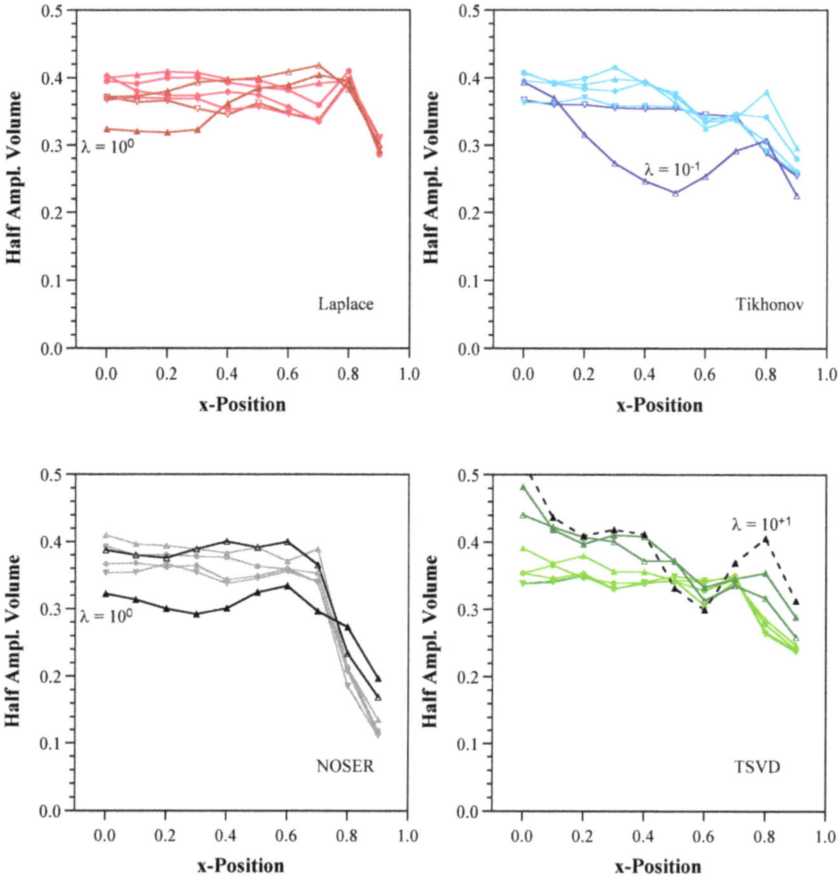

Figure D.4. Feature volume as a function of position for different values of λ using four regularization methods.

D.5 $\mathbf{U}^{\mathrm{T}}\boldsymbol{\Delta}$ versus singular values for three I–M patterns (related to section 4.6)

Figure D.5 compares the coefficients P_i ($\mathbf{U}^{\mathrm{T}}\boldsymbol{\Delta}$ terms) and the singular values s_i for three I–M configurations with 16 electrodes, a current $I = 0.003$, and $\sigma_0 = 0.01$. The target was circular, $r = 0.2$ at $x = 0.5$, contrast = 40%. Note that the singular values do not incorporate target information.

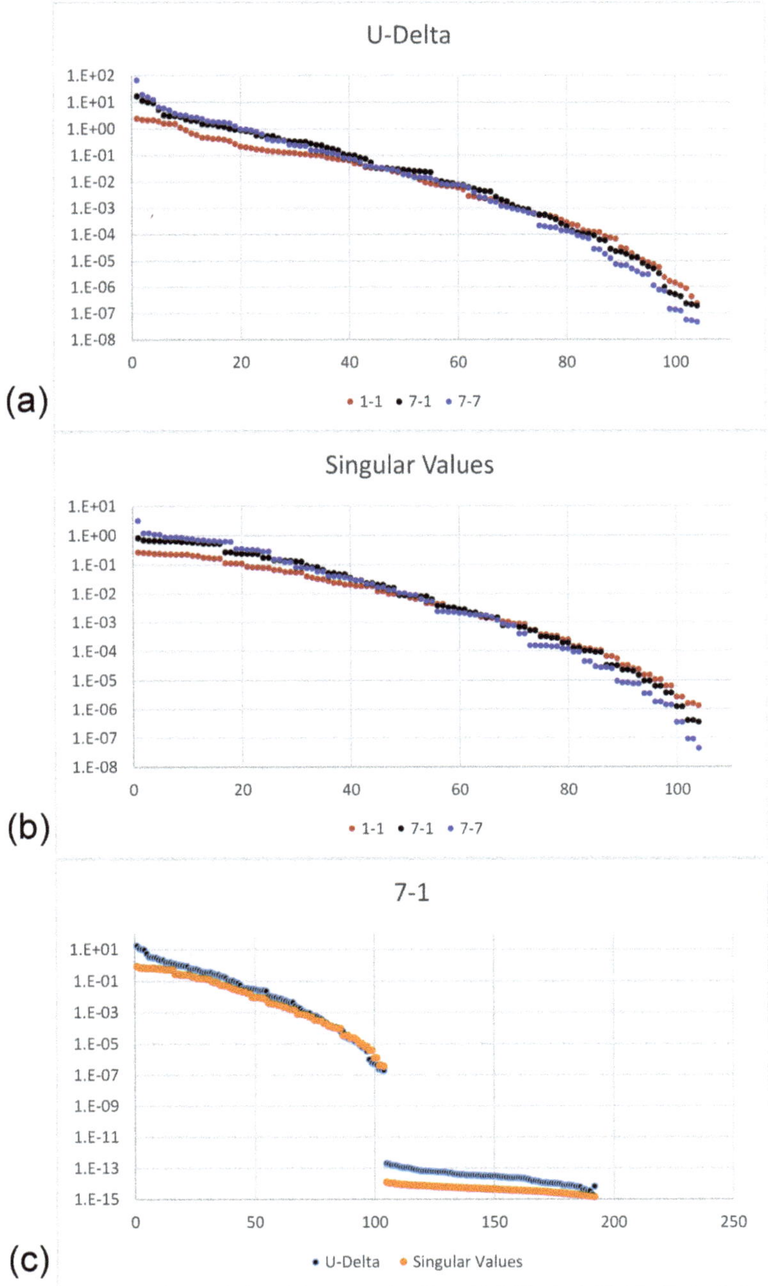

Figure D.5. (a) Comparison of values of $|\mathbf{U}^T\mathbf{\Delta}|$ for I–M = 1–1, 7–1, and 7–7. (b) Comparison of values of **S** for I–M = 1–1, 7–1, and 7–7. (c) Comparison of values of $|\mathbf{U}^T\mathbf{\Delta}|$ and **S** for I–M = 7–1.

D.6 Comparison of $P_i = \mathbf{U}^\mathrm{T}\boldsymbol{\Delta}$, $C_i = \mathbf{V}^\mathrm{T}\boldsymbol{\sigma}$, $\mathbf{U}^\mathrm{T}\boldsymbol{\Delta}/s_i$, and s_i (related to section 4.6)

At small λ, $C_i = P_i/s_i$ is shown in figure D.6.

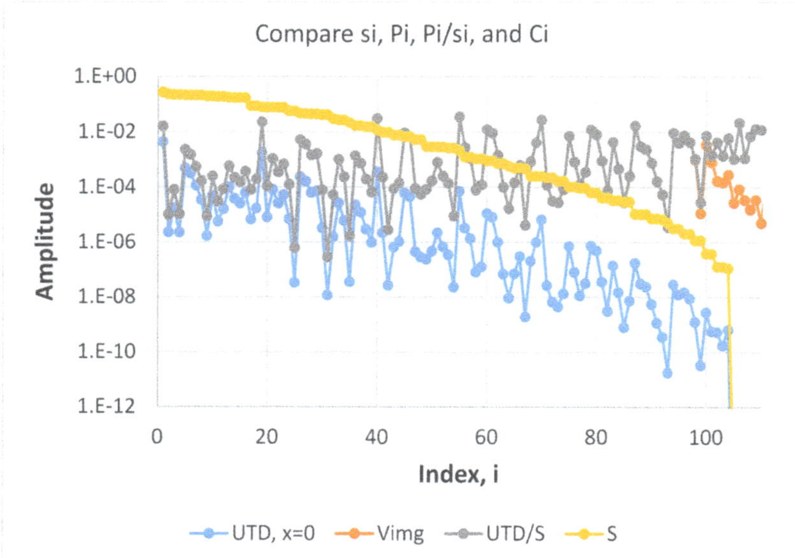

Figure D.6. Comparison of noise-free spectra for $\mathbf{U}^\mathrm{T}\boldsymbol{\Delta} = P_i$ (blue), $\mathbf{V}^\mathrm{T}\boldsymbol{\sigma} = C_i$ (orange), $\mathbf{U}^\mathrm{T}\boldsymbol{\Delta}/s_i = P_i/s_i$ (gray), and s_i (yellow) for I–M = 7–1 for a triangular target at $x = 0$ and $\lambda = 10^{-6}$.

D.7 $|V^T\sigma|$ spectra for different regularization approaches (related to section 4.6)

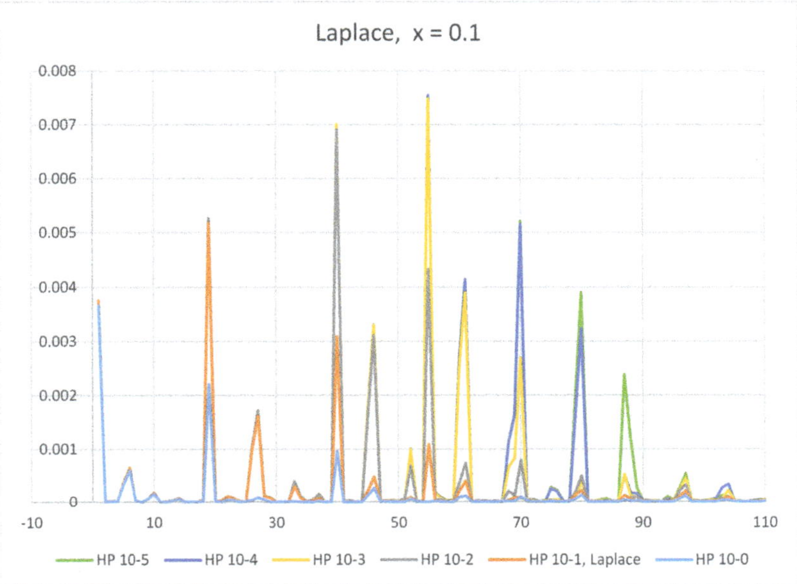

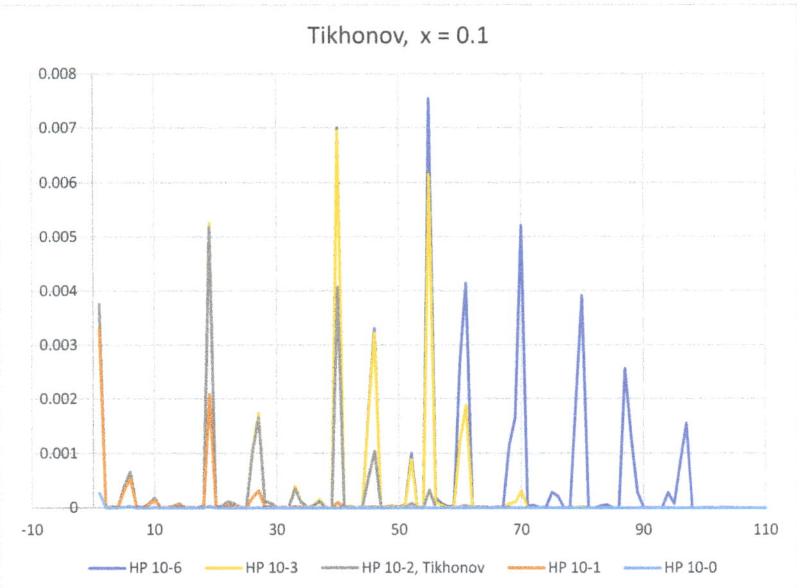

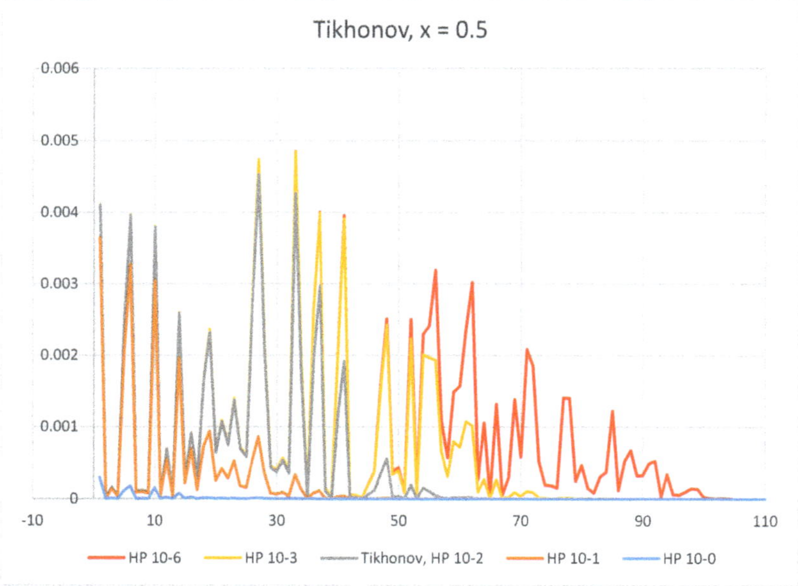
Tikhonov, x = 0.5
0.006
0.005
0.004
0.003
0.002
0.001
0
-10
10
30
50
70
90
110
HP 10-6
HP 10-3
Tikhonov, HP 10-2
HP 10-1
HP 10-0

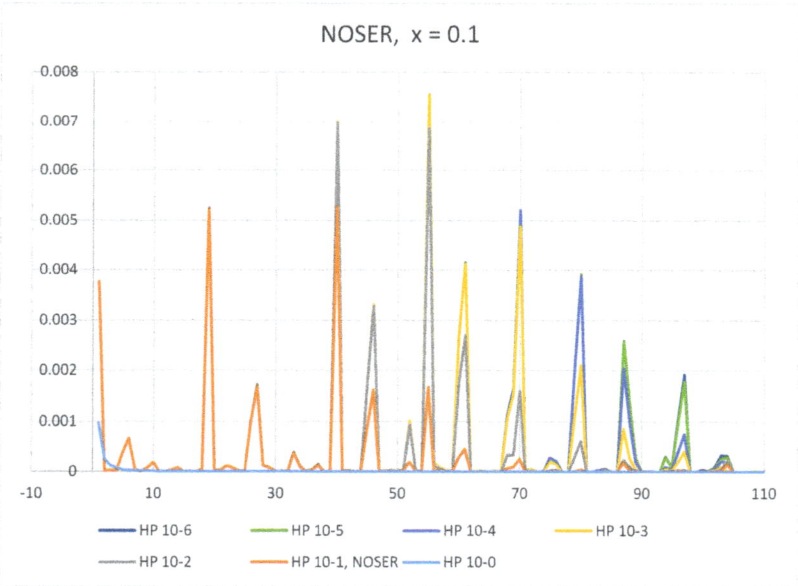
NOSER, x = 0.1
0.008
0.007
0.006
0.005
0.004
0.003
0.002
0.001
0
-10
10
30
50
70
90
110
HP 10-6
HP 10-5
HP 10-4
HP 10-3
HP 10-2
HP 10-1, NOSER
HP 10-0

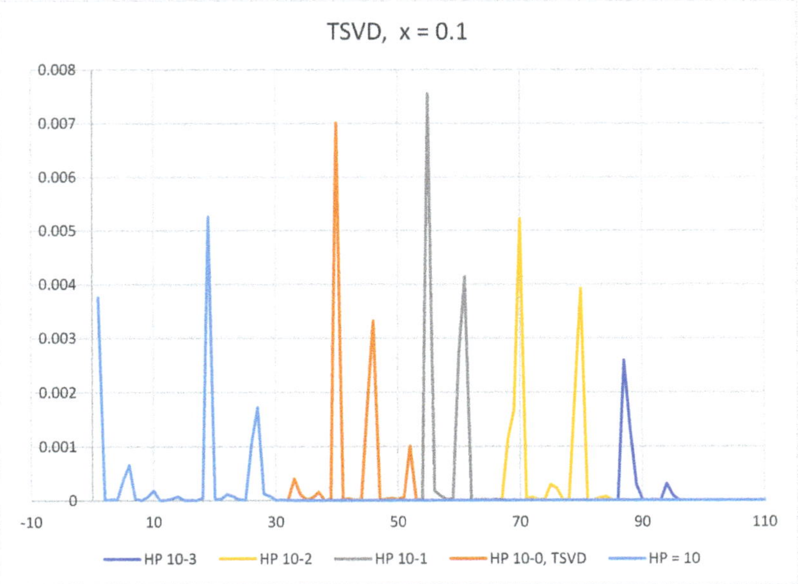
TSVD, x = 0.1
0.008
0.007
0.006
0.005
0.004
0.003
0.002
0.001
0
-10
10
30
50
70
90
110
HP 10-3
HP 10-2
HP 10-1
HP 10-0, TSVD
HP = 10

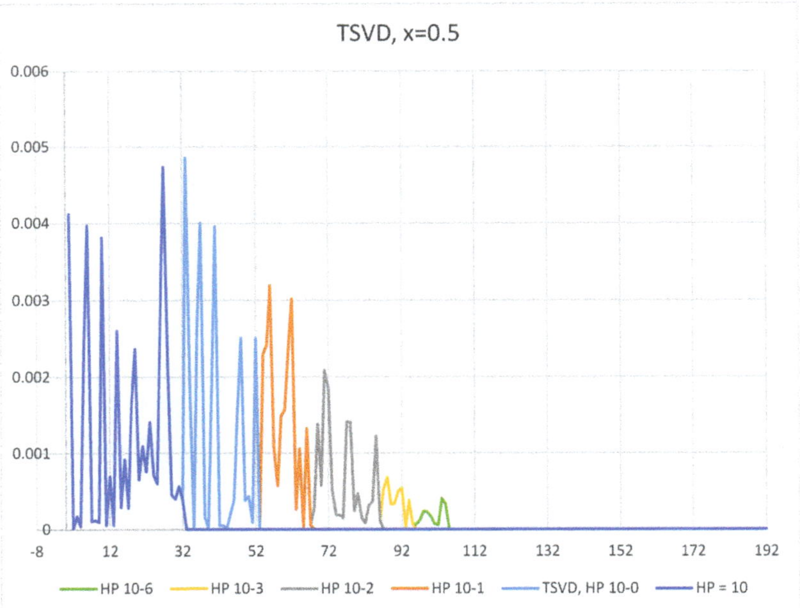
TSVD, x=0.5
0.006
0.005
0.004
0.003
0.002
0.001
0
-8
12
32
52
72
92
112
132
152
172
192
HP 10-6
HP 10-3
HP 10-2
HP 10-1
TSVD, HP 10-0
HP = 10

References

[1] Holder D S 2005 Introduction to biomedical electrical impedance tomography *Electrical Impedance Tomography: Methods, History and Applications, Series in Medical Physics and Biomedical Engineering* ed C G Orton, J H Nagel and J G Webster (Bristol: IOP Publishing) appendix B

[2] Kato Y, Mukai T, Hayakawa T and Shibata T 2007 Tactile sensor without wire and sensing element in the tactile region based on EIT method *IEEE Sensors (Atlanta, GA, Oct. 28–31)* pp 792–5

[3] Tallman T N, Gungor S, Koo G M and Bakis C E 2017 On the inverse determination of displacements, strains, and stresses in a carbon nanofiber/polyurethane nanocomposite from conductivity data obtained via electrical impedance tomography *J. Intell. Material Syst. Struct.* **28** 2617–29

[4] Tallman T N and Wang K W 2016 Damage and strain identification in multifunctional materials via electrical impedance tomography with constrained sine wave solutions *Struct. Health Monit.* **15** 235–44

[5] Strang G 2018 9. Four Ways to Solve Least Squares Problems, MIT 18.065 Matrix Methods in Data Analysis, Signal Processing, and Machine Learning, https://youtube.com/watch?v=ZUU57Q3CFOU&t=183s

[6] Lionheart W, Polydorides N and Borsic A 2005 The reconstruction problem *Electrical Impedance Tomography: Methods, History and Applications, Series in Medical Physics and Biomedical Engineering* ed C G Orton, J H Nagel and J G Webster (Bristol: IOP Publishing) ch 1

[7] Buccini A, Donatelli M and Reichel L 2017 Iterated Tikhonov regularization with a general penalty term *Numer. Linear Algebra Appl.* **24** e2089

[8] Silvera-Tawil D, Rye D, Soleimani M and Velonaki M 2015 Electrical impedance tomography for artificial sensitive robotic skin: a review *IEEE Sens. J.* **15** 2001–16

IOP Publishing

Electrical Impedance Tomography for Tactile Imaging
A primer for experimentalists
Elisabeth Smela

Appendix E

Supplementary information related to chapter 5

E.1 Scaling, comparison of peak cross-sections for varying currents (related to section 5.1)

Comparison of three different currents under otherwise identical simulation conditions. The effective λ are different. To have the same regularization, for a smaller current λ needs to be reduced, since λ has a larger effect on smaller currents. Even though the N_{th} for the different currents at the same λ are the same, the lower-current images have lower resolution at the same hyperparameter (figure E.1).

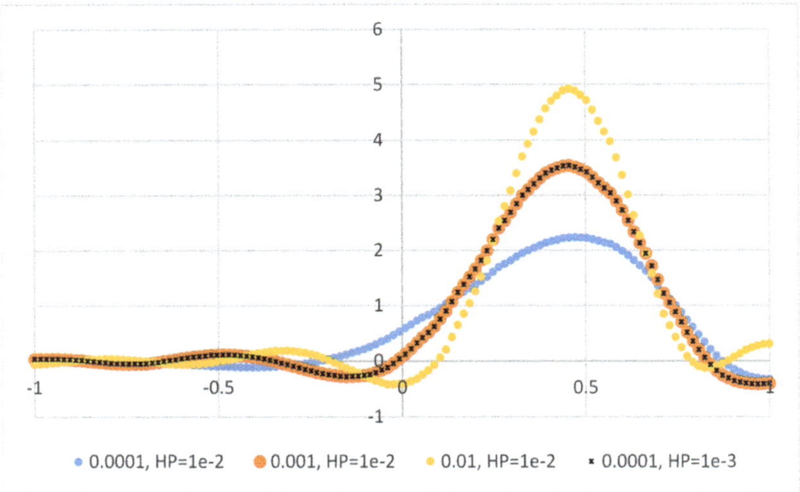

Figure E.1. Cross-sections showing the amplitude of the reconstructed feature as a function of position for different injected currents and hyperparameters, indicated in the legend. (16 electrodes, I–M = 7–1, $\sigma_0 = 0.01$, $\lambda = 10^{-2}$, triangular target, $\sigma_T = 0.006$, $x = 0.5$, $r_T = 0.2$, $N = 1 \times 10^{-12}$)

doi:10.1088/978-0-7503-5402-8ch12

E.2 Scaling, comparison of peak cross-sections for varying sensor conductivity (related to section 5.1)

Figures E.2 and E.3 show cross sections along the x-axis ($y = 0$) for a circular target at three sensor baseline conductivities σ_0, all using $\lambda = 10^{-2}$ and minimal noise ($N = 1 \times 10^{-12}$). The amplitudes are adjusted to account for the difference in $\Delta\sigma$, which is based on σ_0. The amplitude of $\sigma_0 = 0.001$ is multiplied by 10, and the amplitude of $\sigma_0 = 0.0001$ is multiplied by 100. The smaller the baseline conductivity (the higher the resistivity), the larger the effective hyperparameter is (figure E.2). To have the same effective hyperparameter, then for each reduction in σ_0 by a factor of 10 the hyperparameter needs to be reduced by a factor of 100. This is shown in figure E.3.

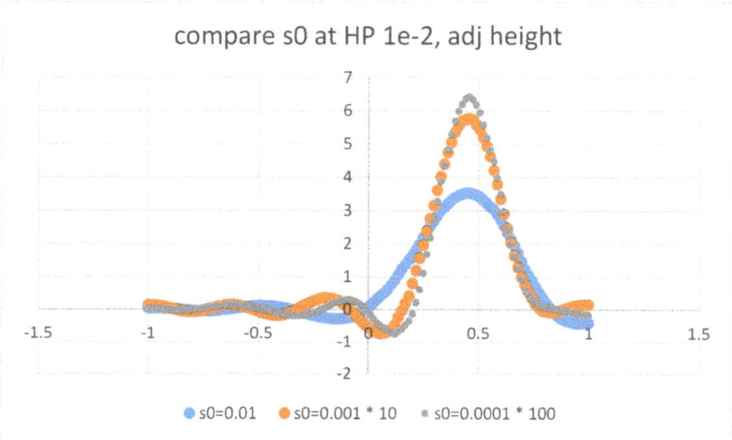

Figure E.2. Cross-sections showing the amplitude of the reconstructed feature as a function of position for different sensor baseline conductivities using $\lambda = 10^{-2}$. Heights in the figure have been adjusted to allow comparison of the curves: the legend indicates the conductivity as well as the amplitude multiplier. (16 electrodes, I–M = 7–1, $I = 10^{-3}$, triangular target, $\sigma_T = 0.6\sigma_0$, $x = 0.5$, $r_T = 0.2$, $N = 1 \times 10^{-12}$)

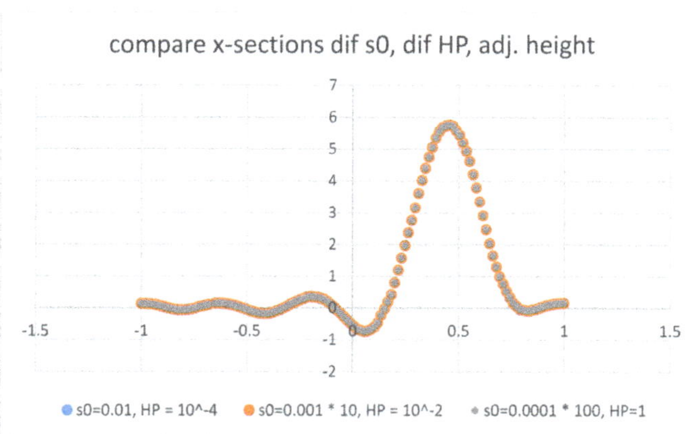

Figure E.3. Cross-sections for different sensor conductivities with λ adjusted as indicated in the legend. The legend also indicates the amplitude multiplier in the figure, required because of the proportional change in $\Delta\sigma_T$. (16 electrodes, I–M = 7–1, $I = 10^{-3}$, triangular target, $\sigma_T = 0.6\sigma_0$, $x = 0.5$, $r_T = 0.2$, N = 1×10^{-12})

E.3 Curve-fitting amplitude and resolution (related to section 5.2)

Feature amplitudes as a function of x for different λ, r_T = 0.2, I–M = 7–1

The amplitude error data of figure 5.5(b) in the main text are shown with curve fits in figure E.4, beginning at $\lambda = 10^{-4}$ when the hyperparameter began to have an effect

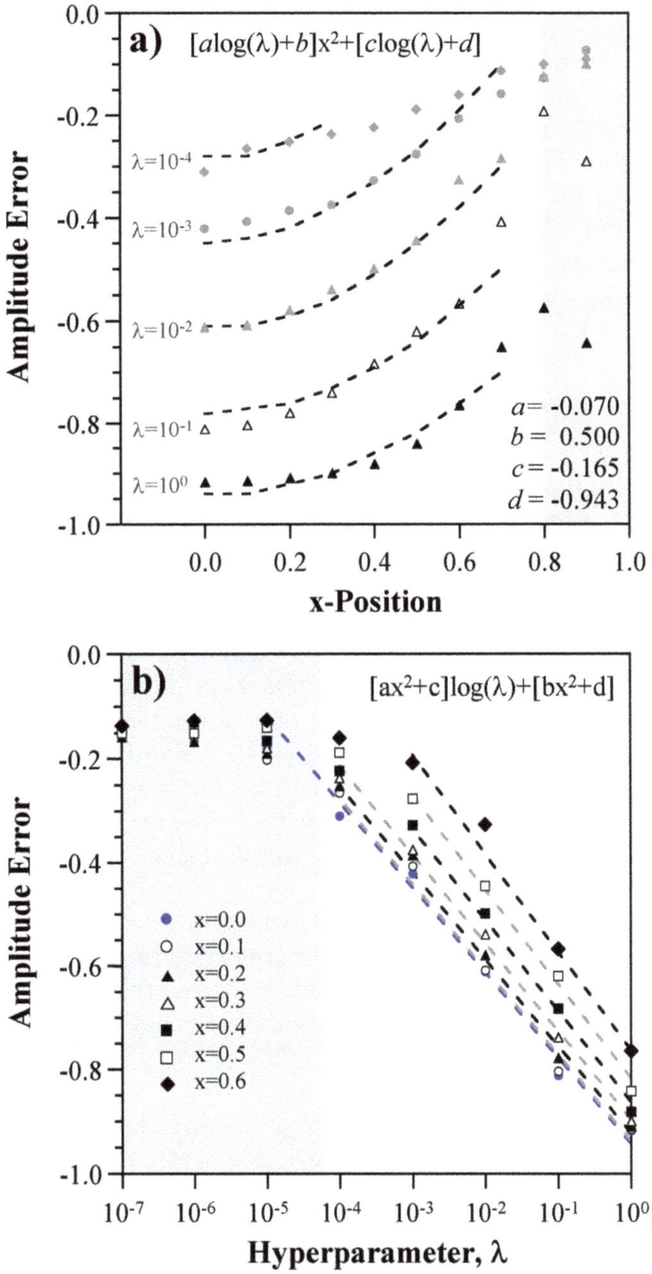

Figure E.4. Curve fits for amplitude error (a) as a function of position for different hyperparameters and (b) as a function of hyperparameter for different positions. Curve fits and coefficients are shown.

and excluding x-positions at the periphery. The hyperparameter exerted an effect on the amplitude that went as the square of the radial position, *Amplitude Error* = $a'x^2 + b'$. Both the curvature a' and the intercept b' could be expressed as linear functions of logλ:

$$\text{Amplitude Error} = [a \log \lambda + b]x^2 + [c \log \lambda + d].$$

As mentioned in the main text, for these simulation parameters, the coefficients for curvature were $a = -0.070$, $b = 0.500$ and those for the intercept were $c = -0.165$, $d = -0.943$). The logλ dependence is evident from looking at figure E.4(b), where the same data are plotted as a function of λ instead of x.

In figure E.4(b) the slopes for $\lambda > 10^{-4}$, below which λ had little effect, were almost the same for all x. Since the data in figures E.4(a) and (b) are the same, the expression for fitting in figure E.4(b) is just a rearrangement of the one in chapter 5, equation (5.1), with the constants being the same.

$$\text{Amplitude Error} = [ax^2 + c]\log \lambda + [bx^2 + d]$$

Given the wiggles in the data and the small number of constants used for fitting, these expressions gave reasonable estimates. The fitting process is illustrated step by step in the next section.

Different ways of representing the effect of the hyperparameter on the amplitude are shown in figure E.5; parts (a) and (b) are repeated from the main text.

The average amplitude (figure E.5(c)) was smaller than that of the target, while the peak amplitude was larger (figure E.5(a)). Otherwise they were similar except when $x > 0.7$. These two metrics are largely redundant. As shown in figure 5.5, the peak amplitude curves had the almost the same shape as the amplitude error curves, and they could be fit by an equation of the same form, the coefficients changing to $a = -0.12 \times 10^{-3}$, $b = 0.82 \times 10^{-3}$, $c = -0.29 \times 10^{-3}$, $d = 0.07 \times 10^{-3}$. Likewise, the average amplitude curves could be described the same way, with $a = -0.04 \times 10^{-3}$, $b = 0.53 \times 10^{-3}$, $c = -0.16 \times 10^{-3}$, $d = 0.06 \times 10^{-3}$. (The average amplitude is related to the amplitude error by *Av. Ampl.* = *Ampl. Error**0.001 + 0.001 for these simulation conditions.)

When the amplitude error was normalized to the peak value at $x = 0.8$ (figure E.5(d)), the order of the curves changed: the error at the center compared to that at the perimeter was largest for $\lambda = 10^{-2}$ and 10^{-1}. This is therefore *not* a useful method of displaying the information. (The normalized amplitude error differs from the uniformity.)

Curve-fitting peak amplitude, I–M = 7–1

The raw peak amplitude data are shown in figure E.6. The parts that are to be fit are those between $\lambda = 10^{-4}$ and 10°, when λ begins to have an effect on the amplitude. Each curve plotted as a function of log(λ) is separately fit with a linear approximation, as shown in figure E.7. The coefficients are pulled from the linear fits, as shown in table E.1. The coefficients are then fit with equations of the form $ax^2 + b$,

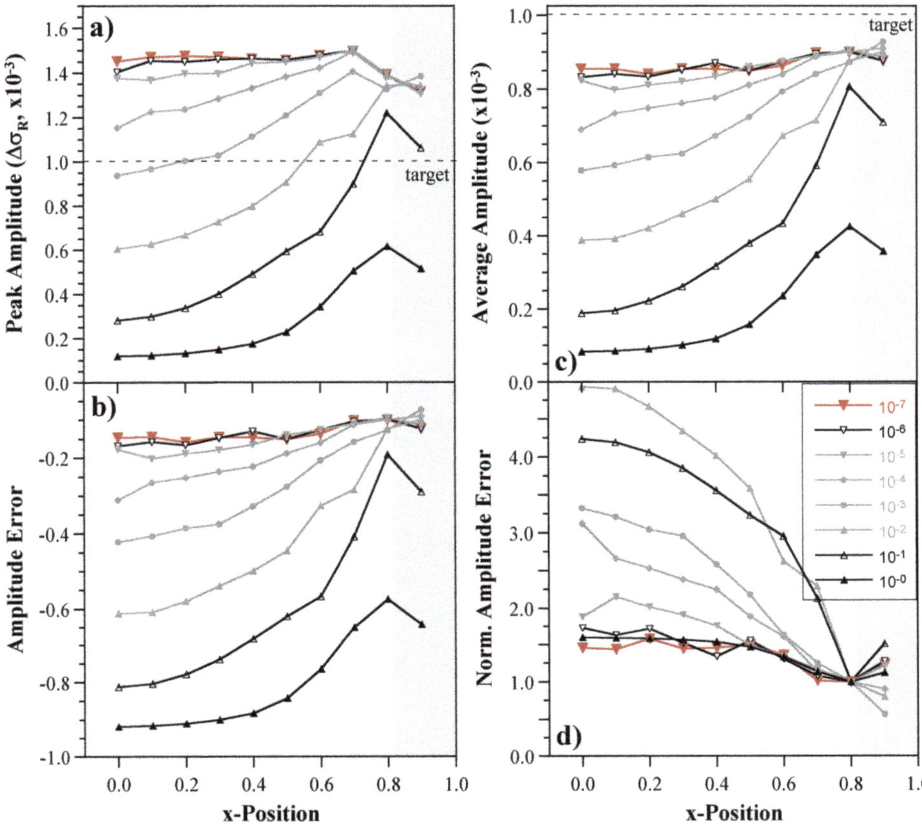

Figure E.5. Different ways of representing the effect of the hyperparameter on the amplitude: (a) peak amplitude, (b) amplitude error, (c) average amplitude, and (d) normalized amplitude error.

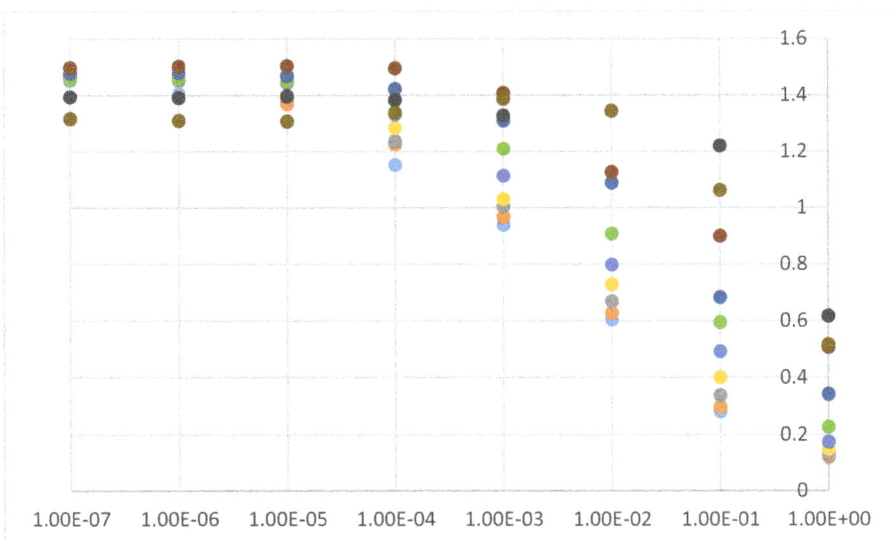

Figure E.6. Peak amplitude as a function of hyperparameter λ for different values of position, x.

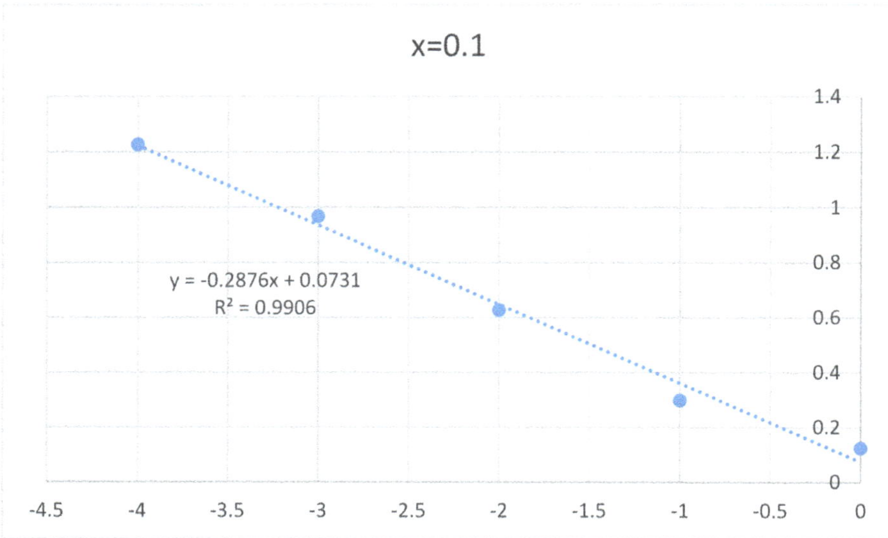

Figure E.7. Example of a linear approximation for the $x = 0.1$ data.

Table E.1. The coefficients in the linear approximations.

x	0	0.1	0.2	0.3	0.4	0.5	0.6	0.7
a	−0.26	−0.29	−0.29	−0.29	−0.31	−0.33	−0.33	−0.29
b	0.087	0.07	0.1	0.14	0.17	0.25	0.36	0.55

as shown in figure E.8. Fitting of the data as a function of position is performed similarly, and the results are compared.

Curve-fitting of resolution, I–M = 7–1

Figure E.9(a) shows linear curve fits, $Resolution = ax + b$. The dependence on λ is shown in figure E.9(b), again fitting hyperparameters from 10^{-4} to 10^{-1} and x between 0.1 and 0.7.

$$(a'x + c')\sqrt{\left|\frac{1}{\log \lambda}\right|} + (b'x + d') \tag{E.1}$$

For these simulation conditions, for 7–1 $a' = -40$, $b' = 41$, $a' = 15$, $b' = -2$, the same as for figure E.9(a), as must be the case, since equation (E.1) is a rearrangement of chapter 5 equation (5.2).

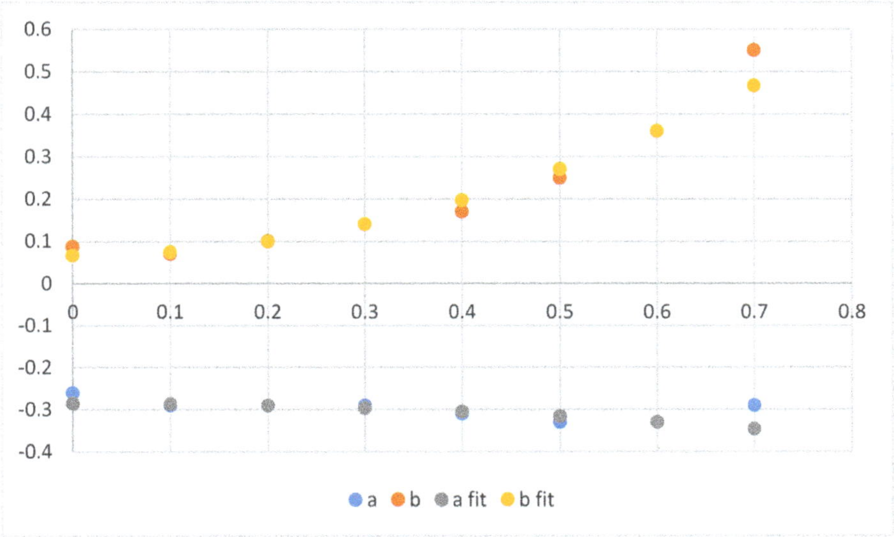

Figure E.8. Fitting the coefficients in the linear approximations as $ax^2 + b$.

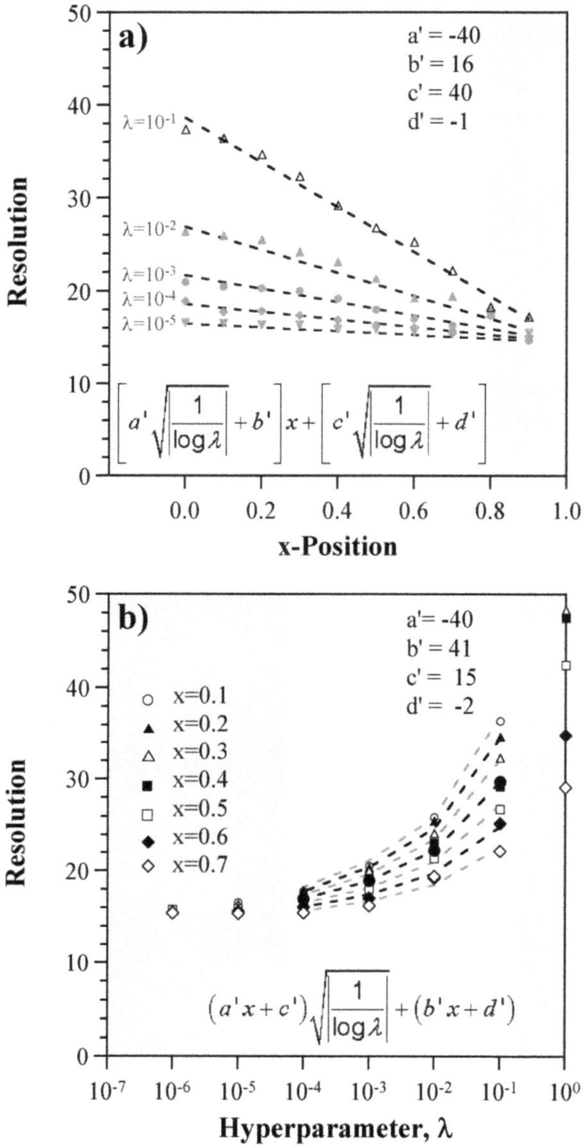

Figure E.9. Curve fits for resolution (a) as a function of position for different hyperparameters and (b) as a function of hyperparameter for different positions. Curve fits and coefficients are shown.

Curve-fitting process for peak amplitude, I–M = 3–3

The resolution could be reasonably well fit by $1/\ |\log(\lambda)|^{0.5}$ for 3–3 for any given value of x, but there was no simple pattern regarding the position dependence, the coefficient between $x = 0$ and 0.3 increasing with a slope of $7x$ and the coefficient between $x = 0.5$ and 0.7 decreasing with a larger slope of $-31x$ (figure E.10).

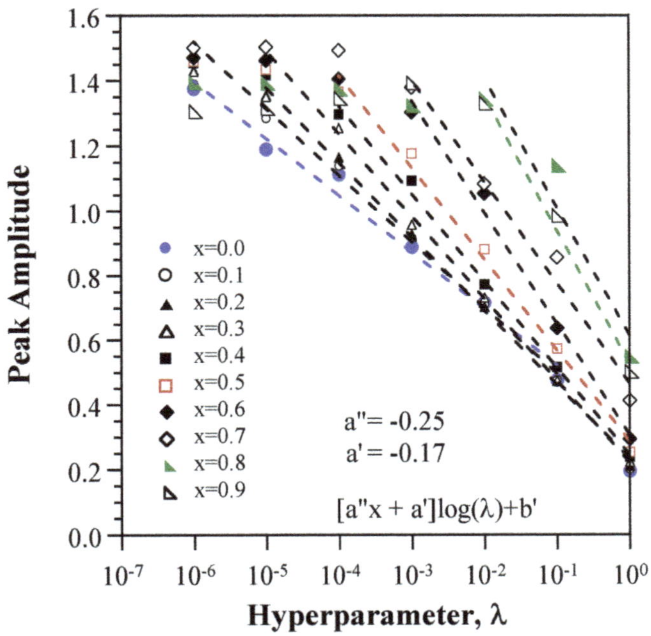

Figure E.10. Curve fits for peak amplitude as a function of hyperparameter for different target positions. Curve fits and coefficients are shown.

E.4 Other size errors as a function of target position (related to section 5.2)

Figure E.11 shows other size errors: radius error, area error, and x- and y-resolution errors.

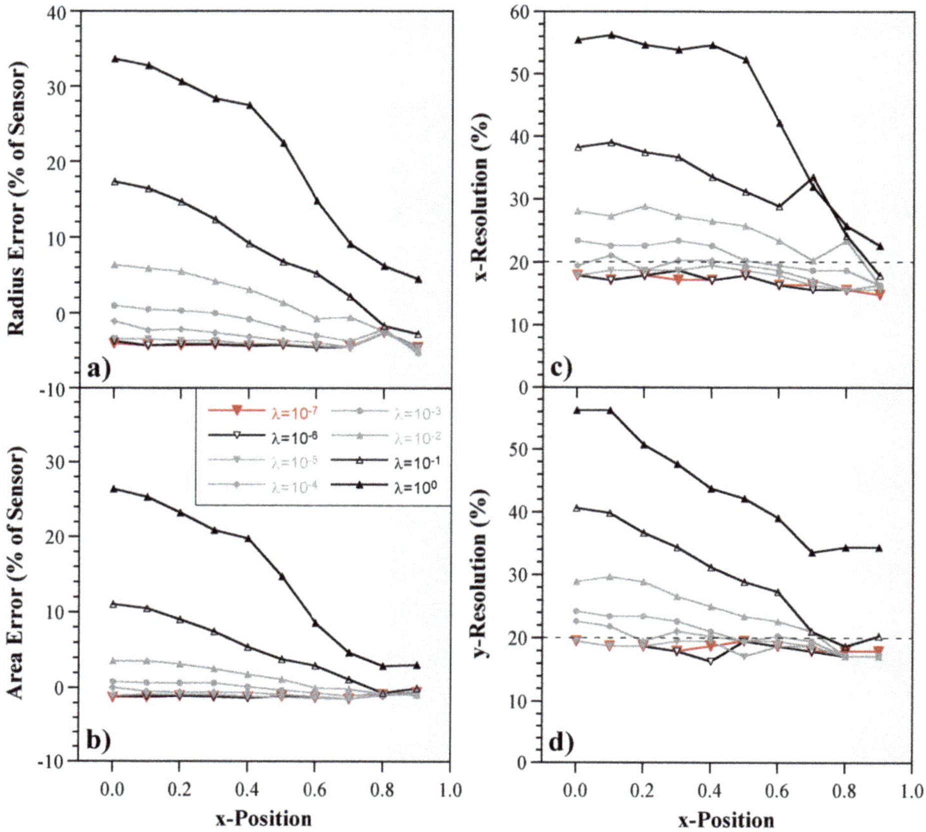

Figure E.11. Various additional size error metrics for single circle target as a function of position for different hyperparameters λ. (a) Radius error, normalized by the sensor radius. (b) The same information shown as a normalized area error. (c) x-Resolution and d) y-resolution shown separately. (Compare to figure 5.5 in the main text) (16 electrodes, I–M = 7–1, $r_T = 0.2$, $x = 0.5$, $\sigma_0 = 10^{-2}$, $\sigma_T = 0.9\sigma_0$ (−10% target contrast), $I = 10^{-3}$, $N = 10^{-12}$).

IOP Publishing

Electrical Impedance Tomography for Tactile Imaging
A primer for experimentalists
Elisabeth Smela

Appendix F

Supplementary information related to chapter 6

F.1 The voltage signal Δ for three I–M patterns (related to section 6.1.3)

The **Δ**s for four injection patterns at two target positions are shown in figure F.1 for a target of $r_T = 0.2$ having a conductivity change of −40% ($\sigma_0 = 10$ mS m^{-1}, $\Delta\sigma = -4$ mS m^{-1}, corresponding to an increase in resistance). The voltage changes for a target at the center of the sensor are smaller than for a target at the edge. The smallest signals are from ADJ. The signals from using PP for both injection and measurement, PP–PP, which are by far the largest.

Figure F.1 shows **Δ**s for three I–M patterns for circular targets at two positions. Since 7–1 uses data from fewer electrodes each cycle (13 versus 14 for the other two, as shown in section 4.2.1), it oscillates with a different period. For all three I–M, when the target is at $x = 0$ the pattern of **Δ** is periodic and symmetric. When $x = 0.7$, the signal is larger at some electrodes than others. The largest Δ_i for 1–1 are concentrated near the third–sixth cycles, while for 7–1 the Δ_i switch sign between the fourth and sixth cycles and again between the 14th and 16th, and for 7–7 the Δ_i show large positive and negative changes in every cycle.

F.2 Noise figure, NF (related to section 6.1.1)

The noise figure NF is a frequently employed metric to measures noise amplification in reconstructions [1]. It is determined for a specific measurement (**Δ**) and a given value of the hyperparameter. It is defined as the ratio of the voltage SNR to the image SNR, specifically the ratio of $E(|\mathbf{\Delta}|)$/std(voltage noise) to E(image amplitude)/std(image noise) [1, 2]. The NF can be calculated in EIDORS (calc_noise_figure.m). It compares the volume (for a 2D sensor) in the target image to the volume that would result if a voltage vector $\mathbf{\Delta}_N$ comprising only zero mean Gaussian noise with a standard deviation of **Δ**, were added to the reference voltages. Since $\mathbf{\Delta}_N$ has an amplitude std(**Δ**), the noise image scales with $E(|\mathbf{\Delta}|)$.

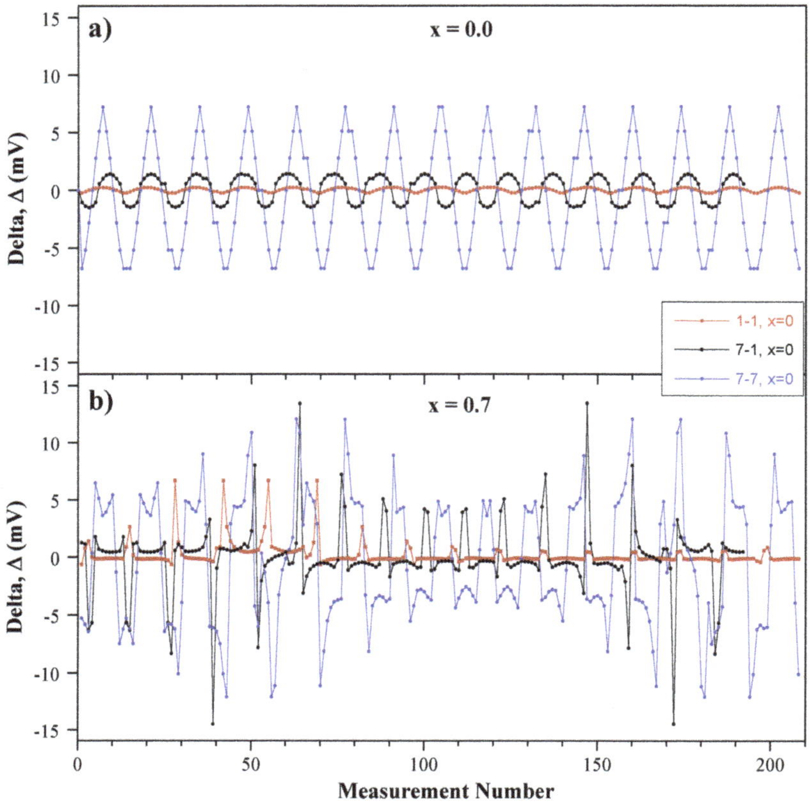

Figure F.1. For three I–M patterns, the values in $\mathbf{\Delta}$ for a circular target at (a) $x = 0$ and (b) $x = 0.7$. ($r_T = 0.2$, $\sigma_0 = 0.01$, $\sigma_T = 0.6\sigma_0$, $I = 1 \times 10^{-3}$, noise $= 10^{-9}$ V)

The usual EIT image is created from $\mathbf{\Delta}$, and the volume v_{img} of each image element is then found as the product of the amplitude of the element and its area. The signal amplitude S.A. is defined as the absolute value of the mean of the image volumes divided by the mean of $|\mathbf{\Delta}|$. A series of images of noise are then created from different $\mathbf{\Delta}_N$, and the volumes v_N of the image elements are again found. The noise amplitude N.A. is defined differently from S.A., however, as std($|v_N|$)/std($|\mathbf{\Delta}_N|$) Finally the average of the trials is found:

$$\mathrm{NF} = E(\mathrm{N.\,A.}/\mathrm{S.\,A.}) = \frac{\mathrm{std}(|\,v_N\,|)}{\mathrm{std}(|\,\Delta_N\,|)} / \frac{E\left(\left|\,v_{img}\,\right|\right)}{E(|\,\Delta\,|)} = \frac{\mathrm{std}(|\,v_N\,|)}{E\left(\left|\,v_{img}\,\right|\right)} \frac{E(|\,\Delta\,|)}{\mathrm{std}(|\,\Delta_N\,|)} \quad \text{(F.1)}$$

The noise figure includes both voltage and image information since it is based on the extent to which voltage noise is amplified in the image.

It has previously been noted that NF does not work well for comparing I–M patterns [3]. (A different noise performance (NP) metric was suggested, but it requires a model of likely noise [3].) The NF for I–M = 1–1, 7–1, and 7–7 at two hyperparameters are shown in figure F.2(a). The NFs were obtained by running 100

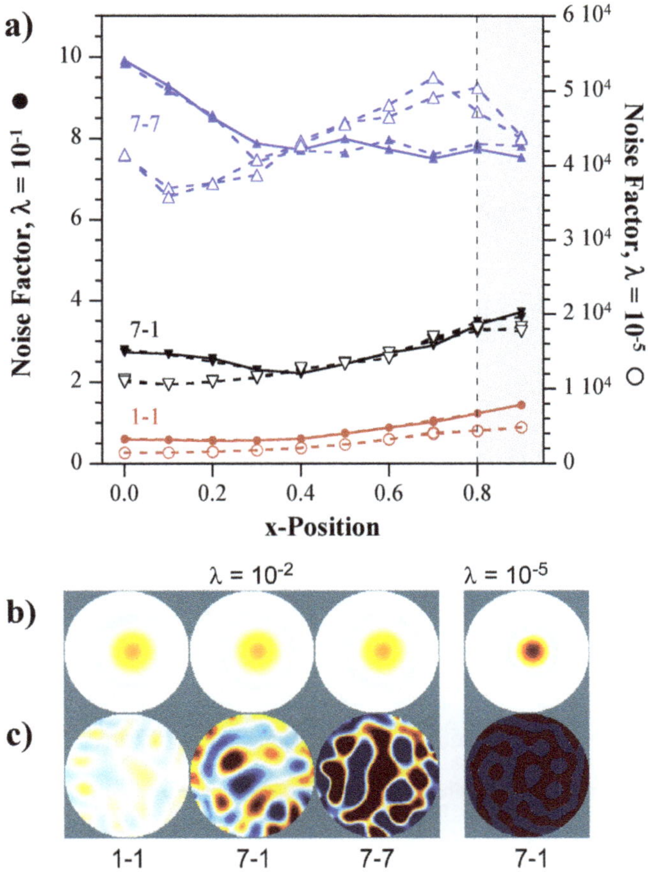

Figure F.2. (a) NF, as a function of x-position for a circular target for I–M = 1–1, 7–1, and 7–7 at $\lambda = 10^{-1}$ (filled symbols, left axis) and $\lambda = 10^{-5}$ (open symbols, right axis); two replicates are shown. (b) EIT images at two hyperparameters for $x = 0.1$ and (c) the corresponding noise images. (16 electrodes, $\sigma_0 = 10^{-2}$, $\sigma_T = 0.9\sigma_0$, $I = 1 \times 10^{-3}$, circular target, $r_T = 0.2$)

trials at each point to reduce the standard deviation; two replicates are shown to indicate the variation still present. The NF for the smaller hyperparameter was orders of magnitude higher (right axis); the NF scaled as log(NF) ~ 0.9log(λ) for all three I–M patterns. The NF and λ scale together because λ controls the trade-off between image fidelity and noise suppression. Since all the terms in equation (16) scale with $\mathbf{\Delta}$, the NF did not depend on the target contrast. EIT images at two hyperparameters and the corresponding noise images are shown in figure F.2(b),(c), illustrating the noise scaling.

As expected, the overall amplitude of the NF followed $E(|\mathbf{\Delta}|)$ (compare figure 6.7), although the spatial dependence of the NF differed and the spatial dependence varied with λ. The NF was dominated by $E(|\mathbf{\Delta}|)$ because the ratio of input noise to output noise is almost constant, while the image amplitude is nearly the same for

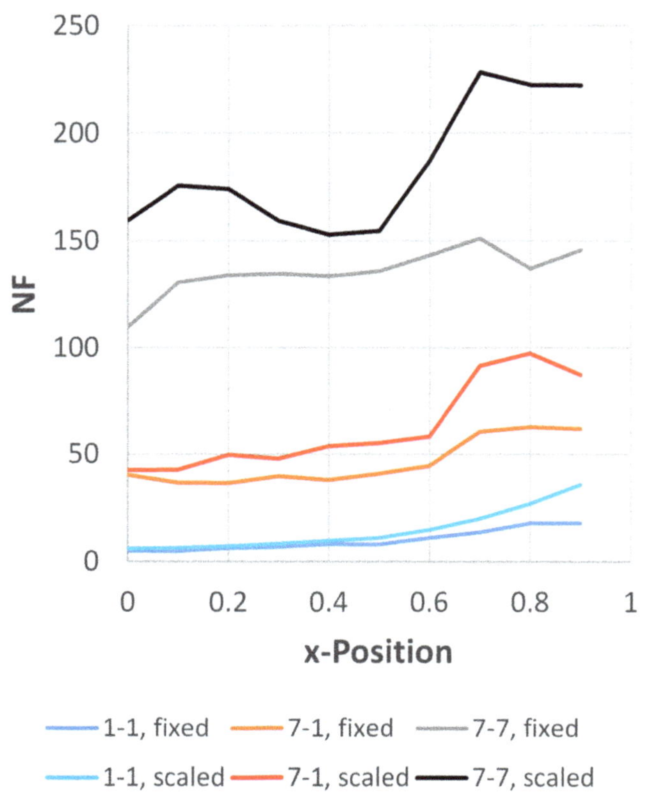

Figure F.3. (a) NF, as a function of x-position for a circular target for I–M = 1–1, 7–1, and 7–7 at $\lambda = 10^{-5}$ using noise that scaled with $\mathbf{\Delta}$, following equation (16), and a fixed value of noise of 2×10^{-5}. (16 electrodes, $\sigma_0 = 10^{-2}$, $\sigma_T = 0.6\sigma_0$, $I = 3 \times 10^{-3}$, circular target, $r_T = 0.2$)

every I–M. Thus, since 7–7 had the highest mean $\mathbf{\Delta}$ of the three patterns, it had the highest NF (figure F.2(a)).

When the NF was calculated using fixed noise instead of noise that scaled with $\mathbf{\Delta}$, it was smaller, as shown in figure F.3, and the position dependence was also reduced, both as expected.

F.3 Some $\mathbf{u}_i$ associated with triangular and circular targets (related to section 6.1.3)

Examples of the component vectors $\mathbf{u}_i$ are shown in figure F.4 for I–M = 7–1. $\mathbf{U}$ varies with the I–M pattern, but it does not vary with the target or with current or σ_0. However, the P_i depend on the target and measurement conditions through the multiplication by $\mathbf{\Delta}$.

For triangular and circular targets of the same size and at the same position (figure 4.19(a)), the $\mathbf{u}_i$ corresponding to the largest two P_i are the same for circular

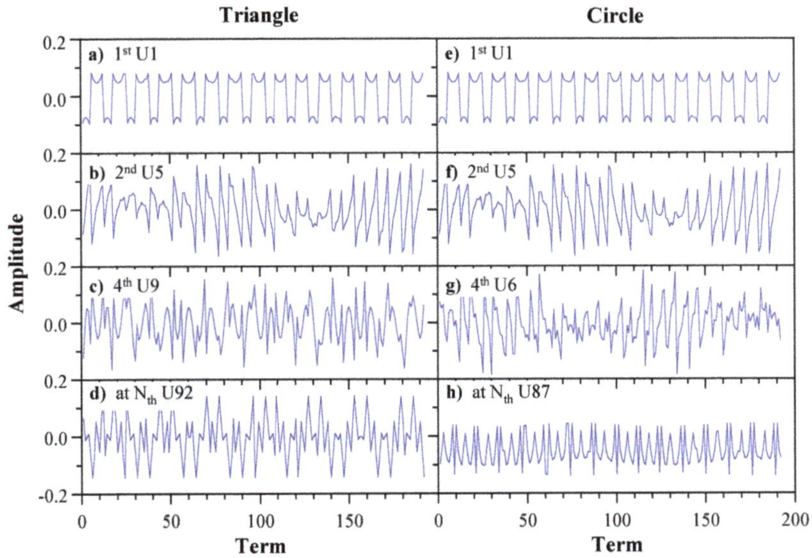

Figure F.4. Some of the $\mathbf{u}_i$ for I–M = 7–1. (a) For a triangular target at $x = 0.5$, the largest coefficient is P_1 corresponding to $\mathbf{u}_1$ and (b) the second largest is P_5, corresponding to $\mathbf{u}_5$. (c) The fourth largest coefficient is P_9 corresponding to $\mathbf{u}_9$. (d) Just below the noise threshold N_{th}, the 85th largest term is P_{92} corresponding to $\mathbf{u}_{92}$. (e),(f) The two largest coefficients for a circular target are also P_1 and $\mathbf{P}_5$. (g) However, the fourth largest term for a circular target is P_6, corresponding to $\mathbf{u}_6$, while (h) the 85th largest term is $\mathbf{P}_{87}$. (16 electrodes, I–M = 7–1, $\sigma_0 = 10^{-2}$, $\sigma_T = 0.6\sigma_0$, $I = 1 \times 10^{-3}$, $r_T = 0.2$, $x = 0.5$)

and triangular targets (compare figures F.4(a),(e), and F.4(b),(f)), but thereafter they differ (compare figure F.4(c),(g)). Recall that $\mathbf{u}_1$ corresponds to the largest singular value, and that the relative importance of the $\mathbf{u}_i$ to the sensitivity **J** decreases with i. The $\mathbf{u}_i$ corresponding to the 85th largest P_i are also shown, which are $\mathbf{u}_{92}$ for the triangle and $\mathbf{u}_{87}$ for the circle. Their amplitudes are corrupted at $N = 10^{-7}$ V, along with those corresponding to even smaller P_i. Noise results in incorrect amplitudes for some of the patterns $\mathbf{u}_i$ that are used to express the voltage signal, leading to a misrepresentation of the target.

F.4 Effect of contrast, conductivity, and current on $\mathbf{U}^{\mathrm{T}}\boldsymbol{\Delta}$ (related to section 6.1.3)

The effect of changing injection current, sensor conductivity, and contrast on the $\mathbf{U}^{\mathrm{T}}\boldsymbol{\Delta}$ spectra are illustrated in figure F.5. Figure F.5(a) shows the P_i as the contrast was varied. As would be expected, changes in contrast resulted in a proportional up or down shifting of these curves, since contrast is linearly related to $\boldsymbol{\Delta}$: lowering the contrast from 10% to 1% to 0.1% moved the curve downward by an order of magnitude each time. Therefore, the noise that can be tolerated by the system increases linearly with the contrast, all other parameters being equal. Likewise (figure F.5(b)), increasing the baseline conductivity σ_0 by an order of magnitude

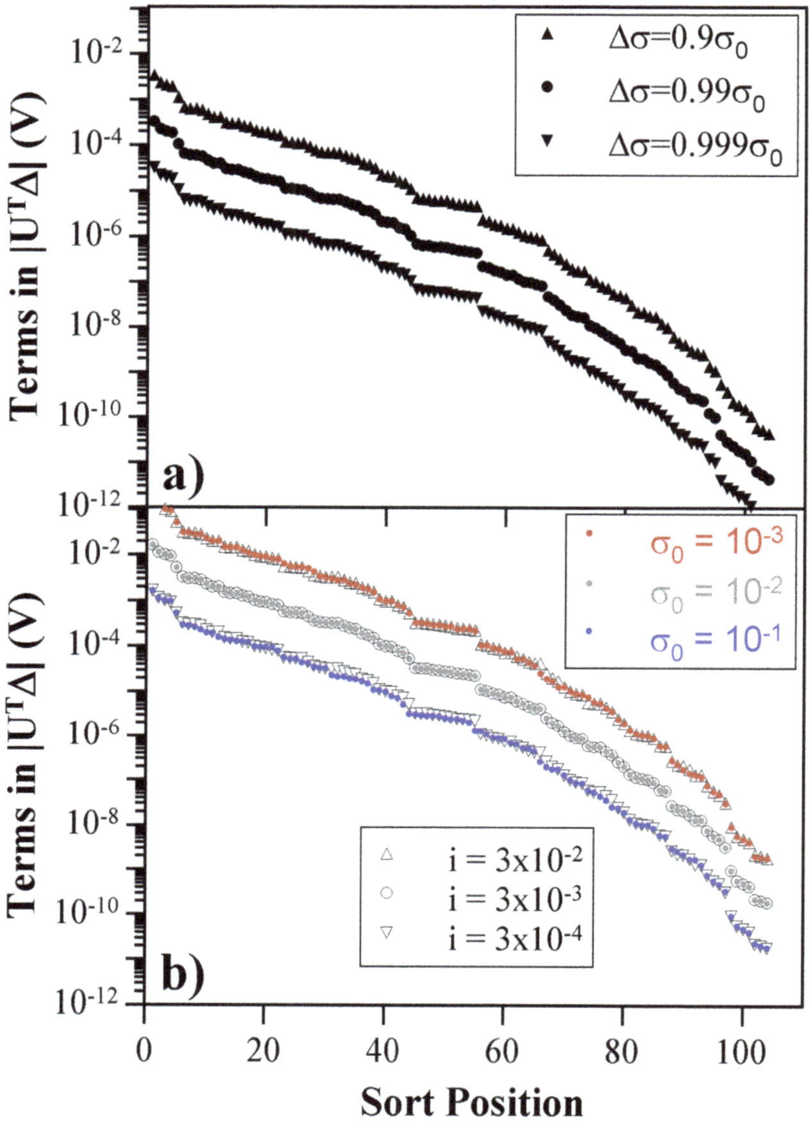

Figure F.5. Terms in $|\mathbf{U}^T\mathbf{\Delta}|$ with a circular target at $x = 0.5$. (a) Varying contrast between 10% and 0.1% (fixing $\sigma_0 = 10^{-2}$, $I = 3 \times 10^{-3}$). (b) Varying sensor conductivity (fixing $\sigma_T = 0.6\sigma_0$, $I = 3 \times 10^{-3}$) and varying current (fixing $\sigma_T = 0.6\sigma_0$, $\sigma_0 = 10^{-2}$). (16 electrodes, I–M = 7–1, $r_T = 0.2$)

shifted the $|\mathbf{U}^T\mathbf{\Delta}|$ curve downward by an order of magnitude, making the system more susceptible to noise; this also simply reflected the inverse relationship between conductivity and $\mathbf{\Delta}$. Increasing the current had an effect identical in magnitude but in the opposite direction, shifting the curves upward, also reflecting the linear dependence of $\mathbf{\Delta}$ on current.

F.5 Comparison of $U^T\Delta$, $V^T\sigma$, $U^T\Delta/s_i$, and s_i (related to section 6.1.3)

At small λ, $C_i = P_i/s_i$, as shown in figure D.6 (repeated here as figure F.6).

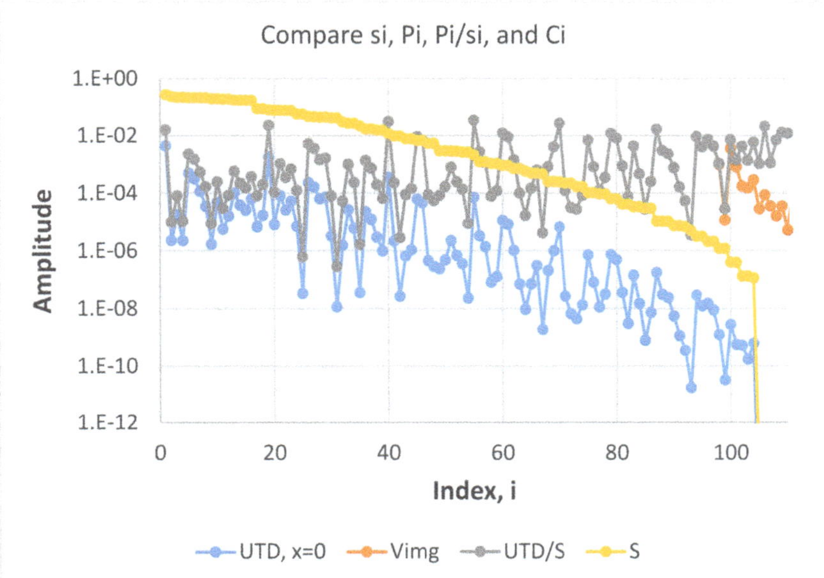

Figure F.6. Comparison of noise-free spectra for $U^T\Delta = P_i$ (blue), $V^T\sigma = C_i$ (orange), $U^T\Delta/s_i = P_i/s_i$ (gray), and s_i (yellow) for I–M = 7–1 for a triangular target at $x = 0$ and $\lambda = 10^{-6}$.

F.6 Peak amplitude with noise at different λ for three I–M patterns (related to section 6.1.3)

As another confirmation of the qualitative data in the EIT images, a reconstructed feature was examined to determine whether there was a clear difference among the three patterns in the effect of noise at N_{th}. The peak amplitude of the reconstructed feature was found at different hyperparameters and target positions with noise at N_{th} added. Thirty trials were run for each point and the average and standard deviations obtained. Figure F.7 shows the results. The peak amplitude for the noise-free case is also indicated. The noise performance of all three patterns was again similar: differences among them were smaller than the standard deviations. (Differences in the peak amplitudes for the three patterns at $\lambda = 10°$ were due to the hyperparameter, not the noise.) The effect of noise on the target feature for the three patterns was not notably different, consistent with figure 6.8 and inconsistent with $E(|\mathbf{\Delta}|)$.

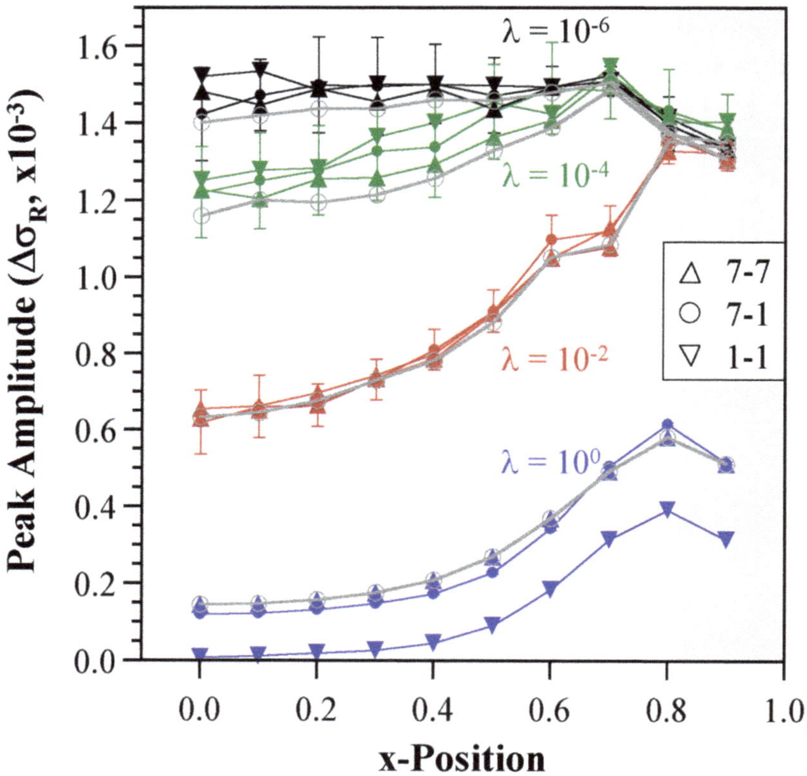

Figure F.7. Peak amplitude of the reconstructed feature for three I–M patterns in the presence of noise (filled symbols) and without noise ($N = 1 \times 10^{-12}$) for 7–1 (open gray symbols) at four values of λ. The same amount of noise, at or below the N_{th} found for 1–1, was added to the three patterns. Each point is the average of 30 trials and error bars show the standard deviation for 7–1. The standard deviation of the noise at $\lambda = 10°$ was smaller than the symbol size. ($N = 2 \times 10^{-9}$ for $\lambda = 10^{-6}$, $N = 1.5 \times 10^{-7}$ for $\lambda = 10^{-4}$, $N = 5 \times 10^{-6}$ for $\lambda = 10^{-2}$, $N = 1.5 \times 10^{-5}$ for $\lambda = 10°$) (16 electrodes, $\sigma_0 = 10^{-2}$, $\sigma_T = 0.9\sigma_0$, $I = 1 \times 10^{-3}$, circular target, $r_T = 0.2$)

F.7 $U^T\Delta$ versus singular values for three I–M patterns (related to section 6.1.3)

Figure F.8 (also figure D.5, repeated here) compares the coefficients P_i ($\mathbf{U}^T\mathbf{\Delta}$ terms) and the singular values s_i for three I–M configurations with 16 electrodes, a current $I = 0.003$, and $\sigma_0 = 0.01$. The target was circular, $r_T = 0.2$ at $x = 0.5$, contrast = 40%. Note that the singular values do not incorporate target information.

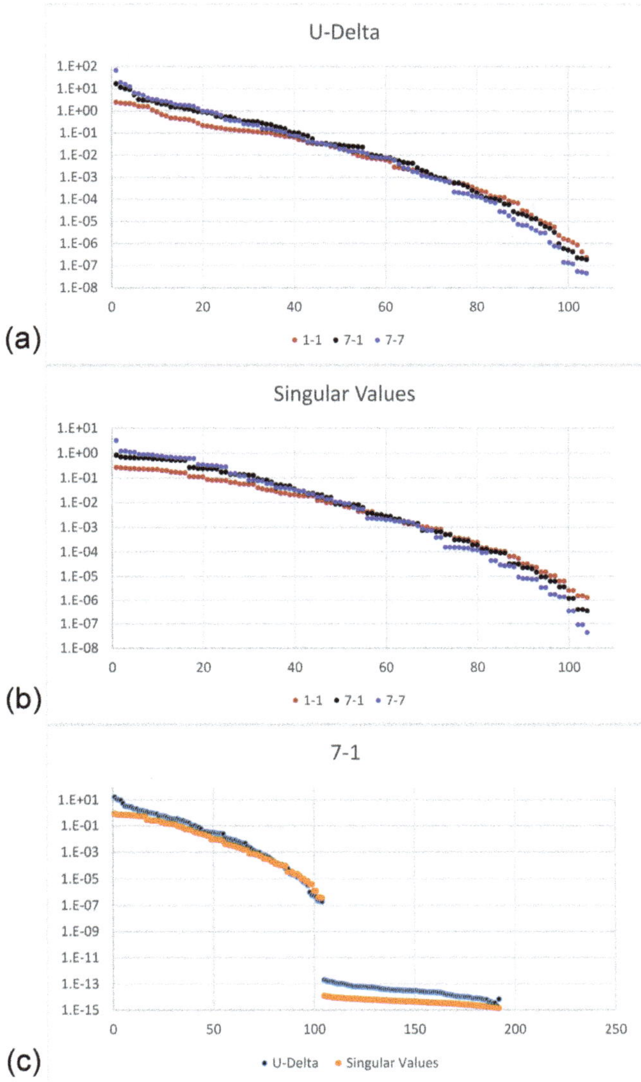

Figure F.8. (a) Size-sorted values of $|\mathbf{U}^T\mathbf{\Delta}|$ for I–M = 1–1, 7–1, and 7–7. Same as figure 6.11(a) in the main text. (b) Comparison of values of **S** for I–M = 1–1, 7–1, and 7–7. (c) Comparison of values of $|\mathbf{U}^T\mathbf{\Delta}|$ and **S** for I–M = 7–1.

F.8 $\mathbf{SV}^T\sigma$ at four hyperparameters (related to section 6.1.3)

The $\mathbf{SV}^T\boldsymbol{\sigma}$ spectra were generated using the same mesh for the forward and inverse problems: j2d4c. As λ increased, the higher sort order terms decreased, with the location of the divergence moving to lower sort number for higher λ (figure F.9). These spectra show how the contribution of higher-order eigen-images to the reconstruction drops, resulting in loss of detail in the EIT images.

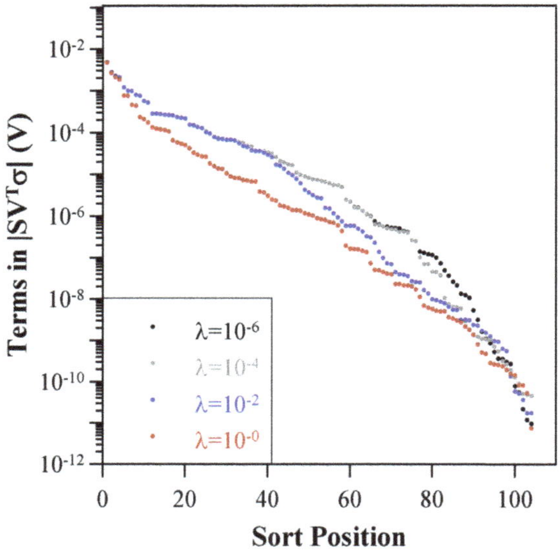

Figure F.9. The size-sorted absolute values of the terms in $\mathbf{SV}^{\mathrm{T}}\boldsymbol{\sigma}$ with negligible noise for I–M = 7–1 with a triangular target at $x = 0.5$ for as λ increases. (16 electrodes, $\sigma_0 = 10^{-2}$, $\sigma_{\mathrm{T}} = 0.6\sigma_0$, $I = 1 \times 10^{-3}$, $r_{\mathrm{T}} = 0.2$)

F.9 Comparison of N_{th} with $E(|\Delta|)$ for different target sizes (related to section 6.2.4)

The values of N_{th} and $E(|\Delta|)$, normalized to their values at $r_{\mathrm{T}} = 0.05$, are shown in figure F.10 as a function of target radius. It is clear that $E(|\Delta|)$ does not have the same dependence on position as the N_{th} does. The measured N_{th} (blue) at $\lambda = 10^{-2}$ and the expected N_{th} (orange) based on the target area ($\sim r_{\mathrm{T}}^2$), shown on linear and log scales in figure F.11. The latter is reasonable model up to $r_{\mathrm{T}} = 0.3$.

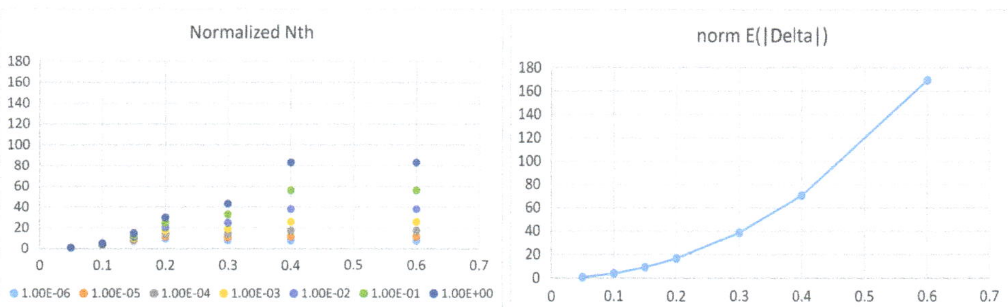

Figure F.10. N_{th} and $E(|\Delta|)$ for a circular target, normalized to their values at $r_{\mathrm{T}} = 0.05$, as a function of target radius. (16 electrodes, I–M = 7–1, $\sigma_0 = 10^{-2}$, $\sigma_{\mathrm{T}} = 0.6\sigma_0$ (40% contrast), $I = 10^{-3}$, noise = 10^{-12}, $r_{\mathrm{T}} = 0.2$, $x = 0.3$)

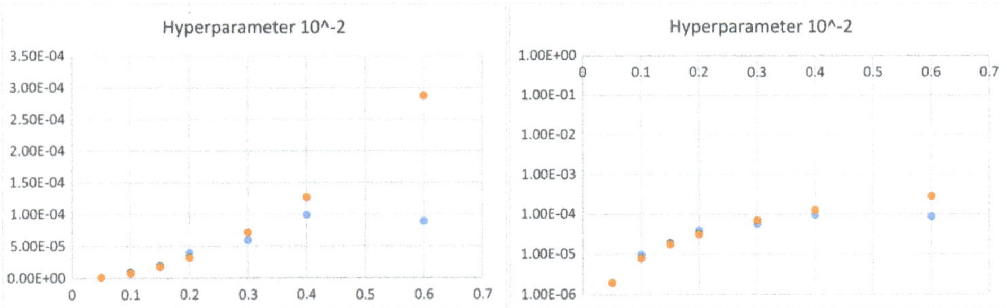

Figure F.11. Measured N_{th} (blue) at $\lambda = 10^{-2}$ and expected N_{th} (orange) based on the target area ($\sim r_{\mathrm{T}}^2$), shown on linear and log scales. (16 electrodes, I–M = 7–1, $\sigma_0 = 10^{-2}$, $\sigma_{\mathrm{T}} = 0.6\sigma_0$ (40% contrast), $I = 10^{-3}$, noise = 10^{-12}, $r_{\mathrm{T}} = 0.2$, $x = 0.3$)

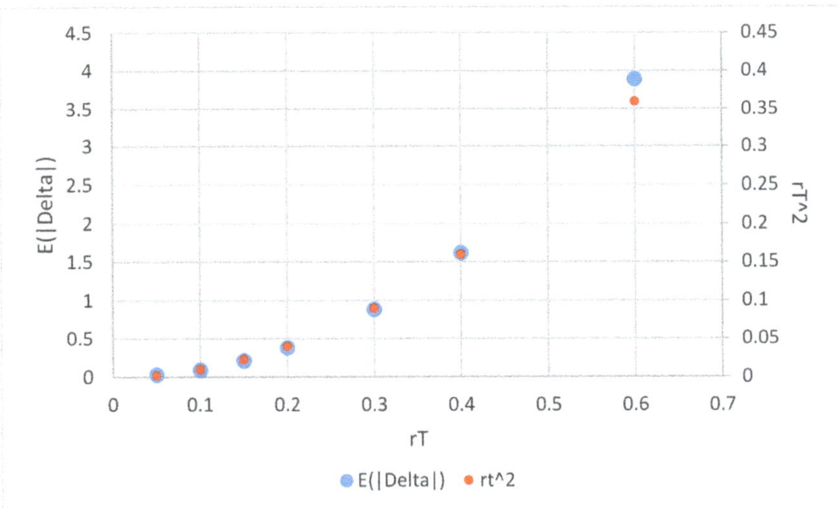

Figure F.12. $E(|\Delta|)$ (blue) and r_{T}^2 (orange) versus r_{T}. (16 electrodes, I–M = 7–1, $\sigma_0 = 10^{-2}$, $\sigma_T = 0.6\sigma_0$ (40% contrast), $I = 10^{-3}$, noise = 10^{-12}, $r_{\mathrm{T}} = 0.2$, $x = 0.3$)

Figure F.12 compares $E(|\Delta|)$ with r_{T}^2. They track perfectly up to $r_{\mathrm{T}} = 0.4$, and then $E(|\Delta|)$ increases even faster.

F.10 Additional EIT images for targets at different positions (related to section 6.1.2)

Figure F.13 shows EIT images of circular and triangular targets for the conditions of figure 6.2 at additional *x*-positions, noise levels, and hyperparameters.

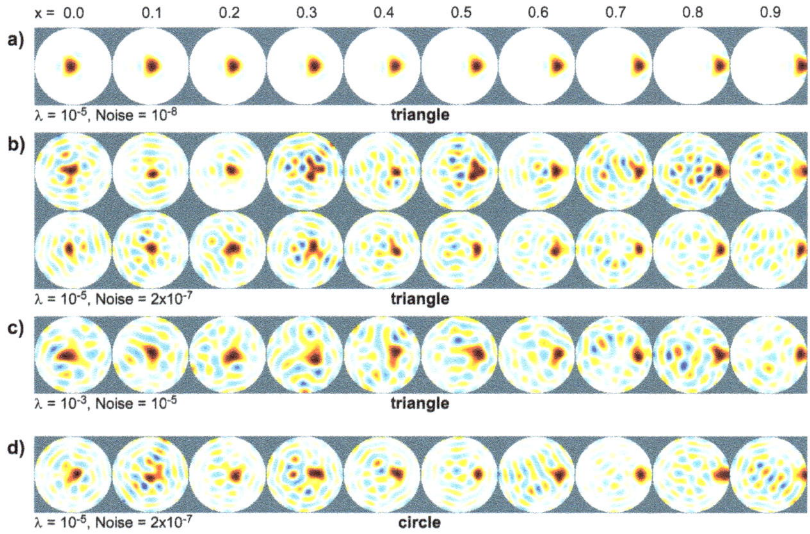

Figure F.13. Reconstructions of the (a)–(c) triangular and (d) circular targets of figure 6.2 at different x positions at increasing x. For a hyperparameter of $\lambda = 10^{-5}$, noise levels of (a) 10^{-8} and (b) 2 runs at 2×10^{-7}. (c) For a larger $\lambda = 10^{-3}$ and noise = 10^{-5}. (d) For a circular target and the noise conditions of (b), $\lambda = 10^{-5}$, noise 2×10^{-7}.

References

[1] Adler A *et al* 2009 GREIT: a unified approach to 2D linear EIT reconstruction of lung images *Physiol. Meas.* **30** S35–55

[2] Adler A and Boyle A 2017 Electrical impedance tomography: tissue properties to image measures *IEEE Trans. Biomed. Eng.* **64** 2494–504

[3] Braun F, Proença M, Solà J, Thiran J-P and Adler A 2017 A versatile noise performance metric for electrical impedance tomography algorithms *IEEE Trans. Biomed. Eng.* **64** 2321–30

Appendix G

Supplementary information related to chapter 7

The sections in this appendix appeared in the Supporting Information associated with the two papers reproduced in chapter 7.

G.1 Number of artefacts as a function of noise, fixed λ (related to section 7.1)

Figure G.1(a) shows histograms of the number of artefacts at six levels of noise. Figure G.1(b) shows the means and standard deviations of the number of artefacts,

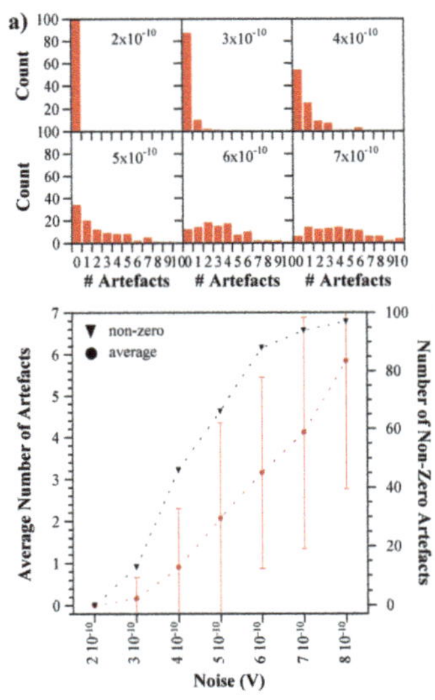

Figure G.1. Number of artefacts in 100 trials at different noise levels for a circular target at $x = 0$. (a) Histograms showing counts of the number of artefacts for six noise levels. (b) The average number of artefacts as a function of noise, with standard deviations indicated (circular symbols, left axis) and the number of images with one or more artefacts (triangular symbols). (16 electrodes, I–M = 7–1, $\sigma_0 = 10^{-2}$, $\sigma_T = 0.999\sigma_0$, circular target, $r_T = 0.2$, $I = 3 \times 10^{-3}$, $x = 0$, $\chi = 10^{-5}$).

as well as the number of non-zero artefacts as a function of noise. Note that the y-axis for latter is reversed from the one figure 7.3(a). Even with 100 trials, the standard deviations are large.

G.2 EIT Images corresponding to figure 7.3 (related to section 7.1)

EIT images corresponding to figure 7.3 are shown in figure G.2.

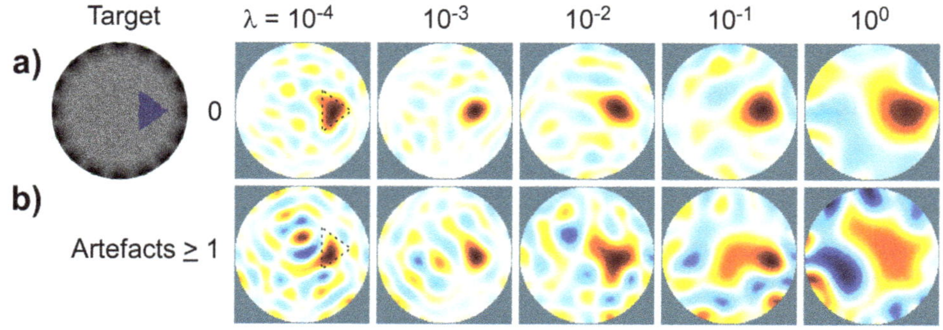

Figure G.2. Using I–M = 7–1, EIT images at N_{th} and just above N_{th} for different values of λ, corresponding to figure 7.3 in the main text. (16 electrodes, $\sigma_0 = 10^{-2}$, $\sigma_T = 0.6\sigma_0$, $I = 3 \times 10^{-3}$, $r_{\text{T}} = 0.2$, triangular target, $x = 0.5$.)

G.3 Effect on N_{th} of varying the forward and inverse mesh sizes (related to section 7.1)

In the code, mesh sizes were specified as:

a–j => mesh density (see table below)
2d => use 2d Distmesh model
0–4 => element refinement
c => use a circular mesh

letter	# mesh elements
j	20 230
i	17 420
h	15 790
g	14 084
f	12 996
e	10 065
d	6894
c	1754
b	603
a	282

The results of varying the size of the inverse mesh are shown in figure G.3(a) for one value of the hyperparameter, $\lambda = 10^{-4}$, and the corresponding values of N_{th} obtained from these data are shown as a function of the number of mesh elements in figure G.3(b). The reconstructions at a noise level $N = 7 \times 10^{-7}$ are shown in figure G.4 for meshes a, c,

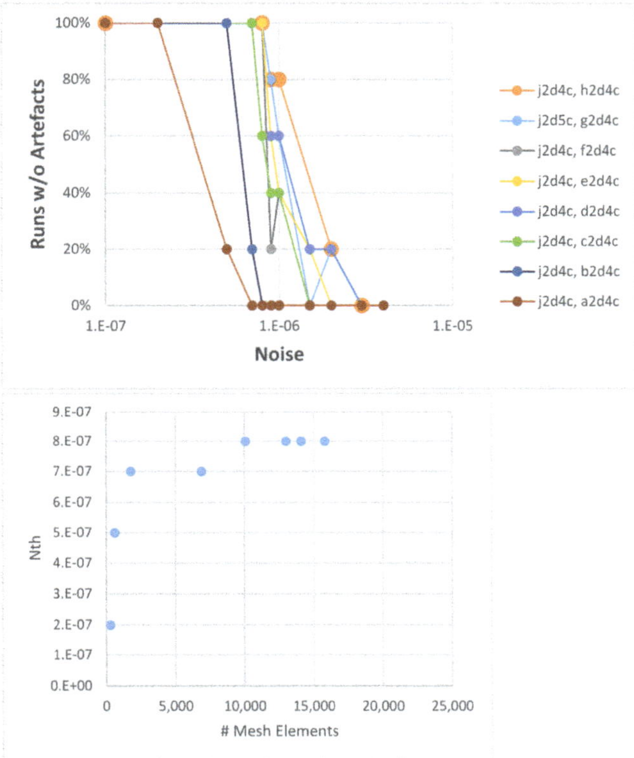

Figure G.3. (a) At a fixed $\lambda = 10^{-4}$, the number of runs without artefacts using the finest mesh for the forward problem (j2d4c) and varying the mesh for the inverse problem (from a2d4c to h2d4c). (b) The value of N_{th} obtained from the data in (a) as a function of the number of mesh elements. (16 electrodes, triangular target, $I = 1 \times 10^{-3}$, I–M = 7–1, $\sigma_0 = 10^{-2}$, $\sigma_T = 0.6\sigma_0$, $r_T = 0.2$, $x = 0.5$)

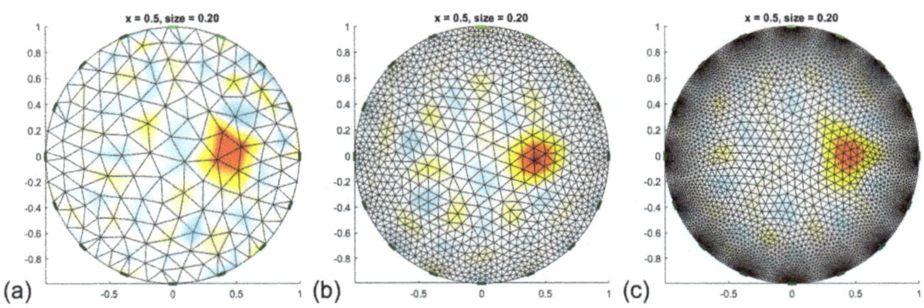

Figure G.4. Reconstructions at noise $N = 7 \times 10^{-7}$ using the conditions in figure G.3 for mesh sizes (a) a, (b) c, and (c) e.

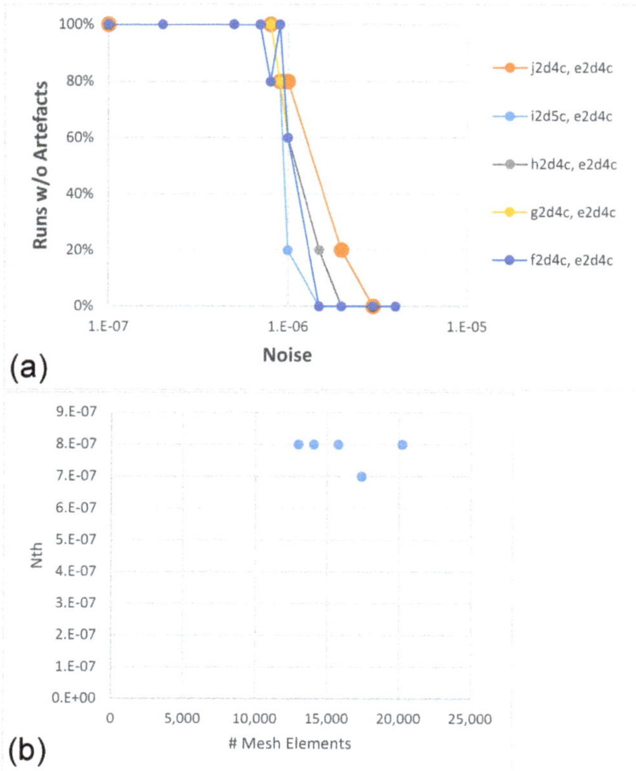

Figure G.5. (a) At a fixed $\lambda = 10^{-4}$, the number of runs without artefacts using mesh size 'e' for the inverse problem (e2d4c) and varying the mesh for the forward problem (from j2d4c to f2d4c), keeping the inverse mesh coarser than the forward mesh. (b) The value of N_{th} obtained from the data in (a) as a function of the number of mesh elements. (16 electrodes, triangular target, $I = 1 \times 10^{-3}$, I–M = 7–1, $\sigma_0 = 10^{-2}$, $\sigma_T = 0.6\sigma_0$, $r_T = 0.2$, $x = 0.5$.)

and e. In these images, there are no artefacts and only the target is seen. (The target is larger than the smallest possible artefact.) For fine meshes, the value of N_{th} was invariant with the size of the inverse mesh. The value of N_{th} was affected when the size of the mesh was not small compared to the smallest EIT feature sizes.

The results of varying the size of the forward mesh are shown in figure G.5(a) for one value of the hyperparameter, $\lambda = 10^{-4}$, and the corresponding values of N_{th} obtained from those data are shown as a function of the number of mesh elements in figure G.5(b). For these meshes, which had mesh elements that were small compared to the smallest EIT feature size, the value of N_{th} was invariant with the size of the forward mesh.

G.4 EIT images and cross-sections for different hyperparameters (related to section 7.1)

Figure G.6 shows examples of overfitting (which gives a large image norm), optimally fitting, and over-regularizing (which gives a large residual norm). The 'size' of the image in figure G.6(a) is larger than the ones in figures G.6(b) and (c).

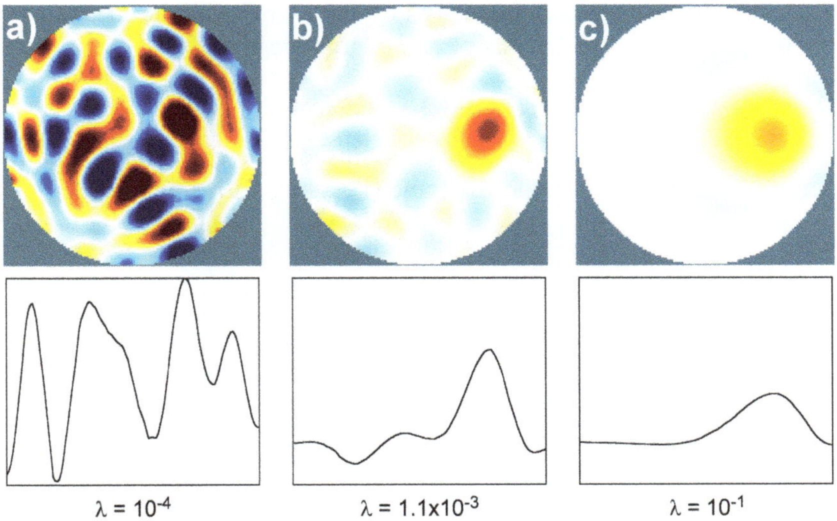

Figure G.6. EIT images (top, same color scales) and corresponding cross-sections (bottom, amplitude versus position, same scales) for hyperparameters that are (a) too small, (b) close to optimal, and (c) too large.

G.5 Residual for different hyperparameters (related to section 7.1)

The Picard coefficients for the conditions of figure G.6 are shown in figure G.7. The residual is the difference between the noisy data (gray, note the noise floor at $N = 10^{-6}$ V) and the damped Picard coefficients (black, red, blue). The residual increases with λ.

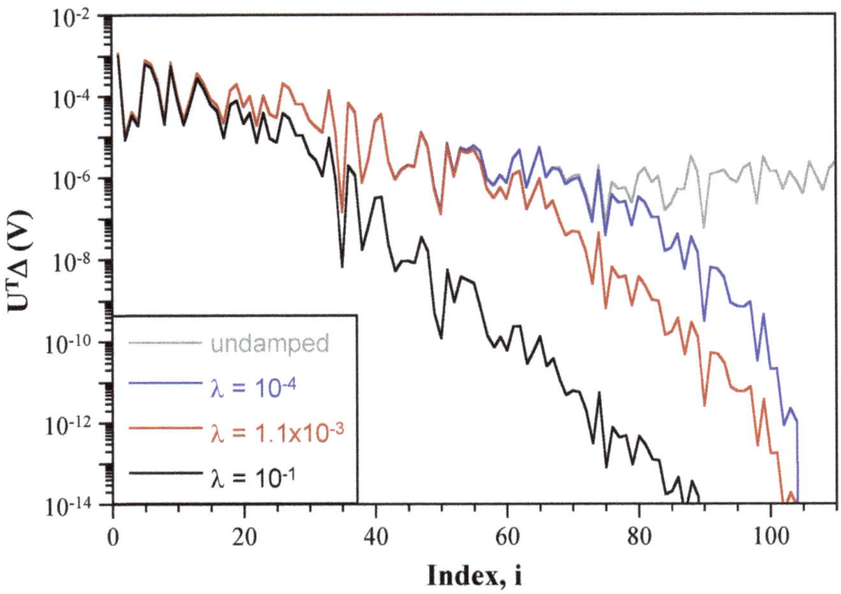

Figure G.7. Picard coefficients P_i (gray) with increasing levels of damping $\frac{s_i^2}{s_i^2 + \lambda_j^2} P_i$ (blue, red, black). (Note the log scale).

At $\lambda = 10^{-4}$, most of the noise is damped. By $\lambda = 1 \times 10^{-1}$, many of the target components are also damped, resulting in defocusing and a larger residual.

G.6 L-curve calculation (related to section 7.1)

The table below translates the notation used in the code *l_curve.m* to the notation used in an introductory primer on the topic [1], along with some notes.

Code	Translation	Notes, sizes
beta = U'*b	**beta** = $\mathbf{U}^T\boldsymbol{\Delta} = \mathbf{P}$	$b = \boldsymbol{\Delta}$, both $\boldsymbol{\Delta}$ and **beta** are 192 × 1 **P** is the vector holding the signed Picard coefficients—*without taking the absolute values.*
beta2 = norm(b)^2—norm(beta)^2	$\sum_{i=1}^{r}(\Delta_i)^2 - \sum_{i=1}^{r}(P_i)^2$	norm(v) returns the Euclidean norm of vector v: $\sqrt{\sum_{j=1}^{n}(v_j)^2}$ a single value, e.g. −4.235e−22
p	*r*	the rank, 192 for injection measurement pattern I–M = 7–1
s2 = s.^2	s2 = $\mathbf{S}^2$	every element of S (to rank r) is squared, 192 × 1
xi = beta(1:p)./s	$\mathbf{P/S} = \mathbf{C}_u$ xi(i) = $C_{u,i}$	Divide the Picard coefficients by the singular values, 192 × 1 In the absence of regularization, $C_i = P_i/s_i$. C_u indicates undamped C_i. Again, note that these are signed, not abs. This division flattens the Picard coefficients so they don't fall with increasing index *i*. They are equal to the amplitudes C_i for the image components $\mathbf{v}_i$.
regparam	λ_j *j* goes to numpoints	A vector of numpoints = 200 λ_j covering a huge range based on the larger of s_r or s_1*(16*the precision of floating numbers), 200 × 1
ratio	$s_1/\lambda_{200}{}^{1/199}$	This will be the ratio of each regparam to the last, based on the largest s_1. e.g. ratio = 1.182
f = s2./(s2 + reg_param (i)^2)	$f_j = \mathbf{S}^2/(\mathbf{S}^2 + \lambda_j^2)$	Divide each element of $\mathbf{S}^2$ by $\mathbf{S}^2 + \lambda^2$. This dampens the singular values, the number dampened depending on λ. Note that there is no f_j as such—only 1 continuously overwritten value of f.

eta(i) = norm(f.*xi)	eta(j) = norm[C_u*S^2/($S^2 + \lambda_j^2$)] $eta_j = C_u/[1+ (\lambda_j/S)^2]$ = norm[**P**/**S*****S**^{2}/(**S**$^2 + \lambda_j^2$)] = $\sqrt{\sum_{i=1}^{r}(\frac{s_i^2}{s_i^2+\lambda_j^2}\frac{P_i}{s_i})^2}$	C is the vector of image component amplitudes. Down-weight the components of the solution for which $s_i < \lambda$. This is how the size of the image is obtained. Thus eta is the norm of the C_i (which are damped), eta = $\sqrt{\sum_{i=1}^{r} C_i^2}$. Note that this damping is NOT the same as what we actually use (Laplace prior).
rho(i) = norm((1−f).*beta(1:p))	$\text{rho}_j = \sqrt{\sum_{i=1}^{r}((1-\frac{s_i^2}{s_i^2+\lambda_j^2})P_i)_i^2}$	When λ is large, the length of the Picard coefficients. When λ is small, 0. When λ is medium, the length of the P_i for which the corresponding $s_i > \lambda$ (not damped). Large rho corresponds to large λ. Use the P_i since the residual refers to the difference between the $\mathbf{J}\sigma$ and $\mathbf{\Delta}$, and the normalized solution is given by the ratio $S^2/(S^2 + \lambda_j^2)$. The difference between the data and the 'regularized data'.

G.7 Onset of diminution of $|V^T\sigma|$ peaks and dampening calculated for the L-curve (related to section 7.1)

Tikhonov regularization is described as filtering out components for which $s_i^2 < \lambda^2$ [2] or, alternatively, as damping the eigen-images $\mathbf{v}_i$ by $s_i^2/(s_i^2 + \lambda^2)$ [3]. Figure G.8 (red) shows the indices i_f at various λ of a circular target at $x = 0.5$. At i_f the most significant image modes $\mathbf{v}_i$ were first lowered by more than 5% relative to their values at $\lambda = 10^{-6}$, where the most significant contributors to the final image were defined as those having amplitudes $|\mathbf{v}_i\boldsymbol{\sigma}| = C_i > 2 \times 10^{-4}$. For hyperparameters between 10^{-4} and 10^0 the relationship between log(λ) and i_f was linear. This relationship allows one to estimate the number of coefficients C_i affected at a given λ: the i_f are a measure of the 'reach' of λ toward the lower-index image modes. Figure G.8 also shows the indices at which $s_i^2/(s_i^2 + \lambda^2)$ was reduced by more than 5% for different values of λ. This curve showed a stronger damping (leftward shift).

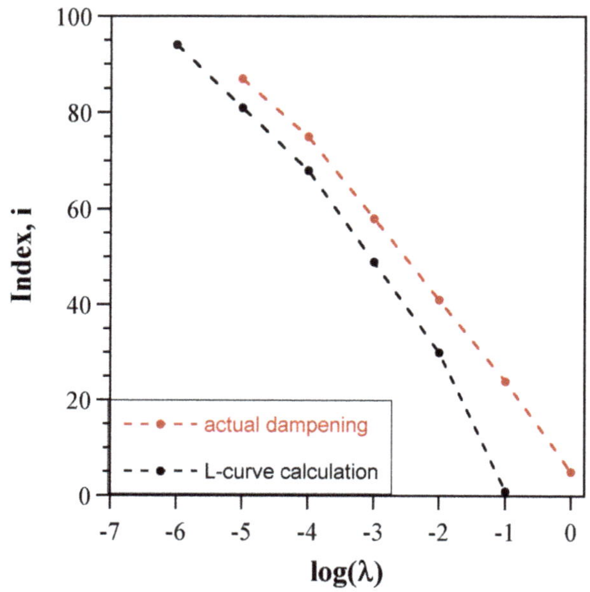

Figure G.8. Index i_f (red) as a function of log(λ) measured from the coefficients C_i for a circular target at $x = 0.5$ at various λ for I–M = 7–1. Also shown is i_f obtained from $s_i^2/(s_i^2+\lambda^2)$ (black). (16 electrodes, $I = 10^{-3}$, $\sigma_0 = 10^{-2}$, $\sigma_T = 0.6\sigma_0$, $N = 10^{-12}$, $r_T = 0.2$)

G.8 GCV, or G(λ), Calculation (related to section 7.1)

Table G.1 translates the notation used in the codes *gcv.m* and *gcvfun.m* to the notation used in our introductory primer on the topic [31], along with some notes.

Table G.1.

code	translation	notes, sizes
beta = U'*b	**beta** = $\mathbf{U}^T\mathbf{\Delta} = \mathbf{P}$	same as for L-curve calculation, b = $\mathbf{\Delta}$
beta2 = norm(b)^2 – norm(beta)^2	$\sum_{i=1}^{r}(\Delta_i)^2 - \sum_{i=1}^{r}(P_i)^2$	same as for L-curve calculation
p	r	the rank, same as for L-curve calculation
ps	1	since the data are 192 x 1 for I–M = 7–1
s2 = s.^2	s2 = $\mathbf{S}^2$	every element of S (to rank r) is squared, 192 x 1 for 7–1
m, n	size(**U**)	for 7–1, both are 192 since U is 192 x 192
delta0	0	since $m = n$
reg_param	λ_j j goes to numpoints	A vector of numpoints = 200 λ_j covering a huge range based on the larger of s_r or s_1* (16*the precision of floating numbers), 200 x 1
f = (lambda^2)./(s2 + lambda^2)	$\lambda_j^2/(\mathbf{S}^2 + \lambda_j^2)$	this is the filter – compare with f for L-curve, which is $f = \mathbf{S}^2/(\mathbf{S}^2 + \lambda_j^2)$
G = norm(f.*beta)^2/sum(f)^2	norm(f*$\mathbf{U}^T\mathbf{\Delta}$)^2 / sum($f$)^2	this is the function to be minimized

G.9 Results of GCV: G(λ) Curves (related to section 7.1)

G(λ) curves for five replicates at the four levels of noise in figure 5 are shown in figures G.9 and G.10. Curves vary depending on the noise in **Δ**, as do the resulting optimal λ.

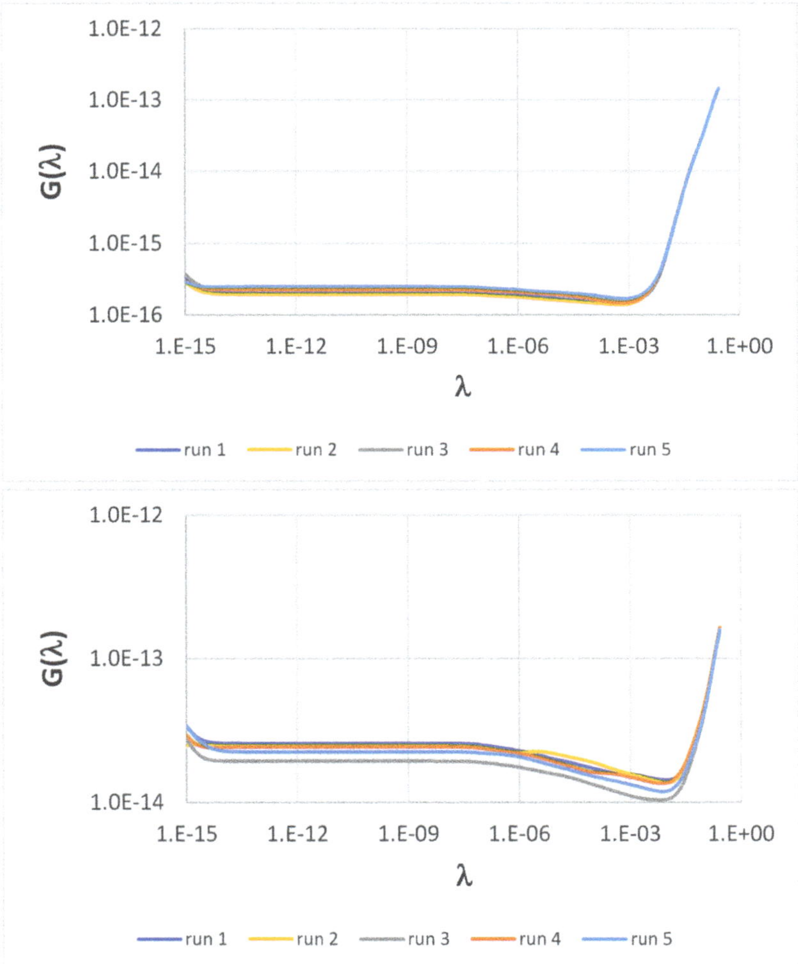

Figure G.9. G(λ) as a function of λ with noise at a level of (top) $N = 1 \times 10^{-7}$ and (bottom) $N = 1 \times 10^{-6}$.

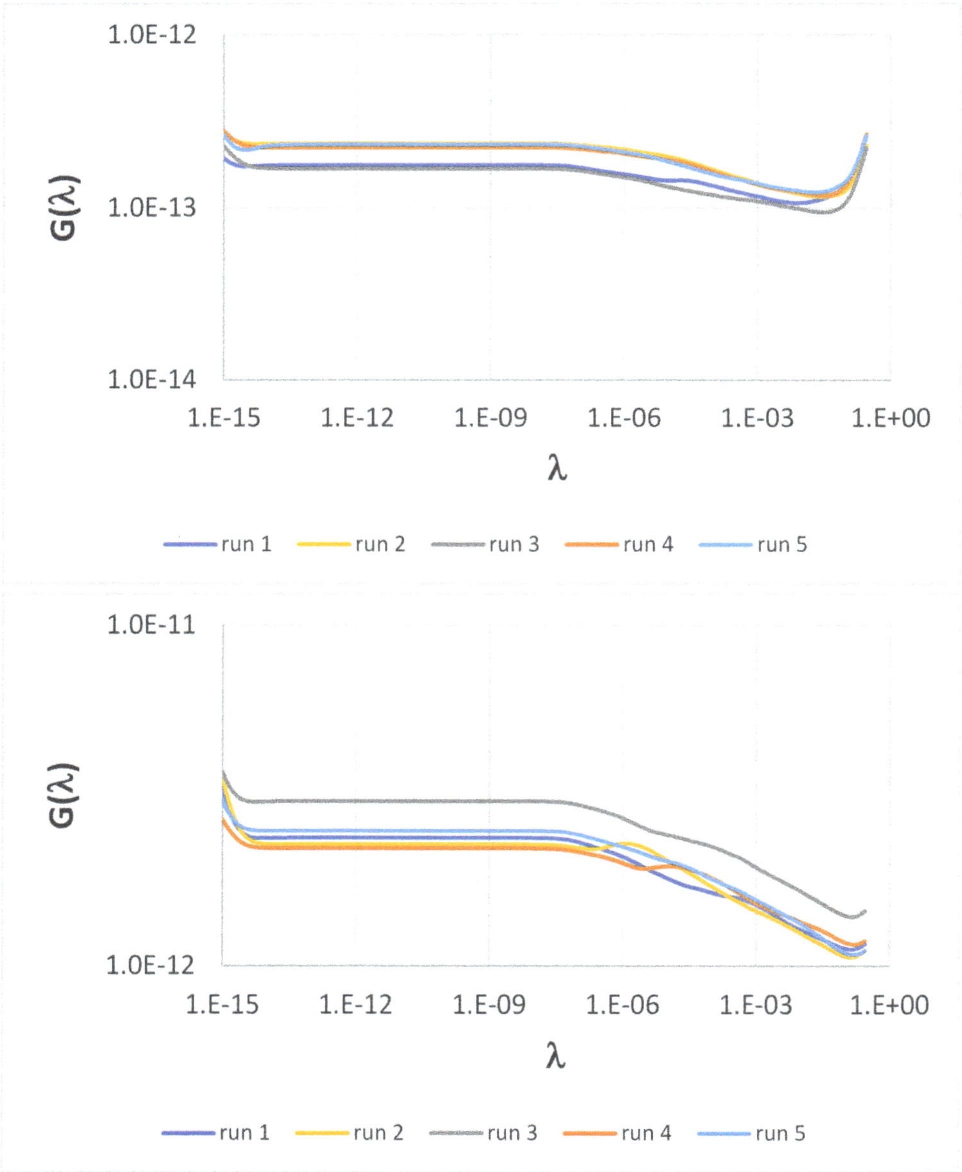

Figure G.10. G(λ) as a function of λ with noise at a level of (top) $N = 3 \times 10^{-6}$ and (bottom) $N = 1 \times 10^{-5}$.

G.10 EIT Images for N_{th}, L-Curve, and GCV methods of finding λ (related to section 7.1)

EIT and threshold images for the same four levels of noise as in section G.9 are shown in figure G.11–G.14 for five replicates. The images were created from the same underlying **Δ** using the three methods.

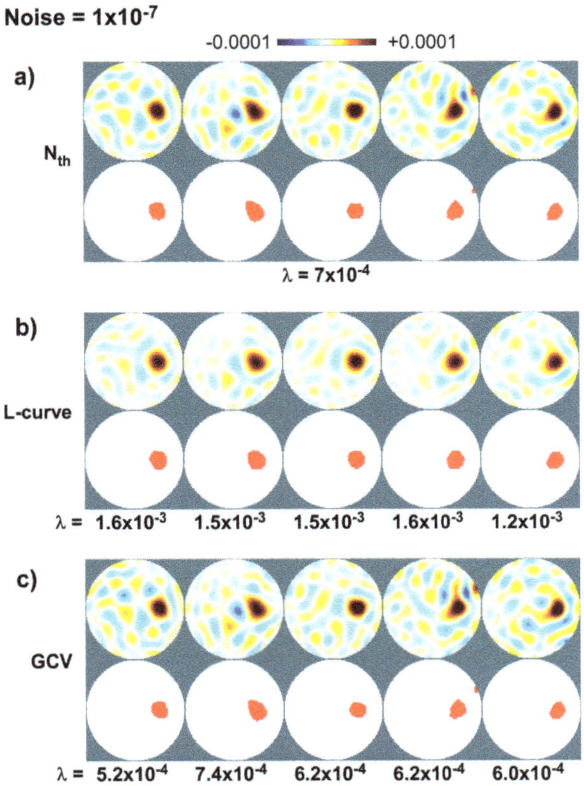

Figure G.11. EIT and half-max threshold images produced with noise $N = 1 \times 10^{-7}$ in five trials using (a) the fixed N_{th} hyperparameter and (b) the optimal L-curve, as well as (c) the GCV hyperparameters found in each trial.

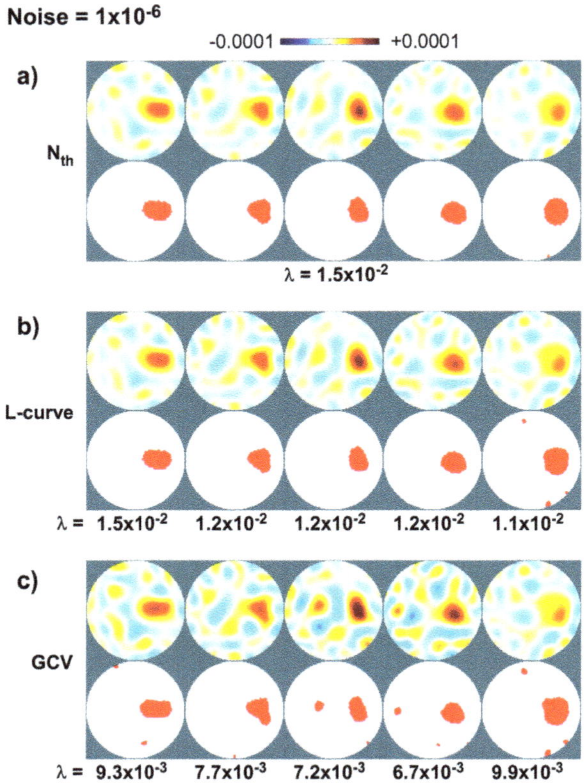

Figure G.12. EIT and half-max threshold images produced with noise $N = 1 \times 10^{-6}$ in five trials using (a) the fixed N_{th} hyperparameter and (b) the optimal L-curve as well as (c) the GCV hyperparameters found in each trial.

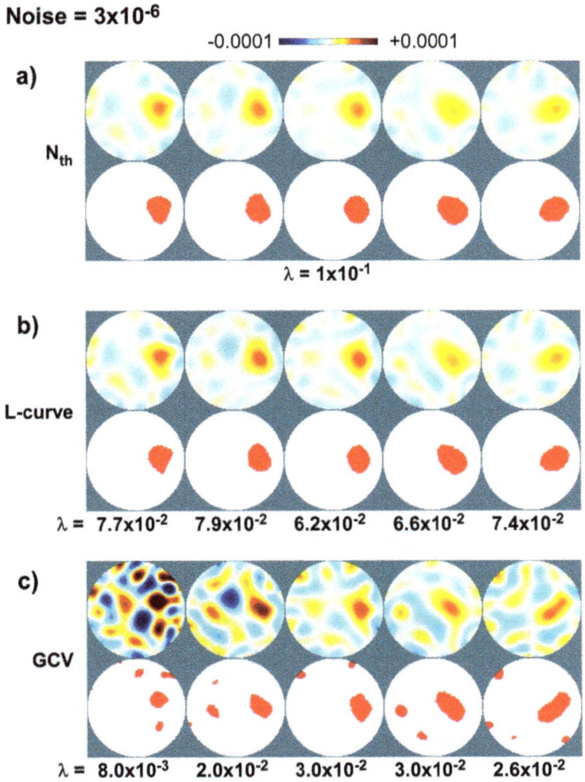

Figure G.13. EIT and half-max threshold images produced with noise $N = 3 \times 10^{-6}$ in five trials using the (a) fixed N_{th} hyperparameter and (b) the optimal L-curveas as well as the (c) GCV hyperparameters found in each trial.

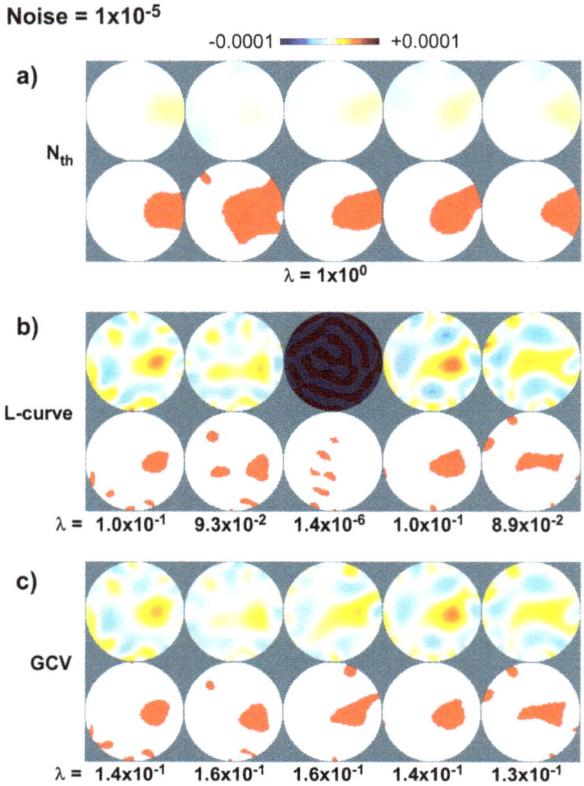

Figure G.14. EIT and half-max threshold images produced with noise $N = 1 \times 10^{-5}$ in five trials using (a) the fixed N_{th} hyperparameter, (b) and the optimal L-curve, and (c) the GCV hyperparameters found in each trial.

G.11 Resolution as a function of noise, fixed λ (related to section 7.1)

The average total area A_R (region of interest, ROI) above $\Delta\sigma_R/2$ in all the features in five trials and the resolution, which is the square root of that (section 7.1, equation (7.4)), are shown in figure G.15 for two targets, along with the standard deviations. The procedure was the same as that used for finding N_{th}: at a fixed λ the noise was increased and the metrics were obtained. The points in (b) are from the same data set as those in figure 7.3(a).

With only five trials, the standard deviations are so large that it is difficult to determine the point at which the area is a minimum. A large number of trials would be needed to reduce the error bars to reasonable levels.

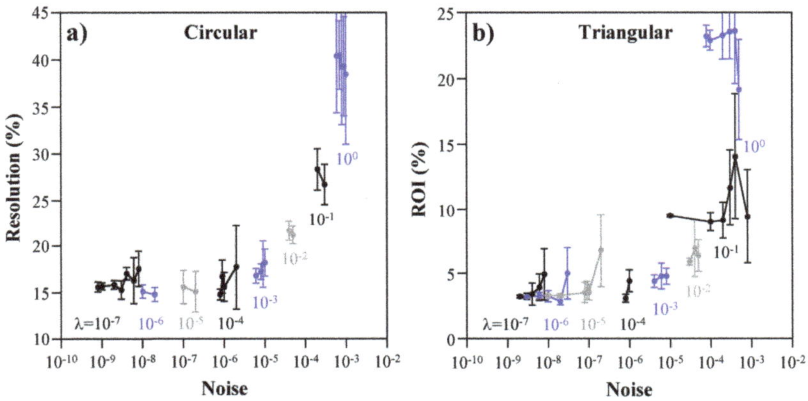

Figure G.15. (a) Resolution as a function of noise at seven hyperparameters for a circular target at $x = 0.5$. (b) Half-max area A_R (or ROI) versus noise for a triangular target at $x = 0.5$. (16 electrodes, I–M = 7–1, $\sigma_0 = 10^{-2}$, $\sigma_T = 0.6\sigma_0$, $I = 10^{-3}$, $r_T = 0.2$)

G.12 Additional threshold images at various values of N, λ (related to section 7.1)

The first three sets of images in figure G.16 used a target of $r_T = 0.05$ and correspond to the data in figure 7.5. The fourth set of images used a target of larger radius,

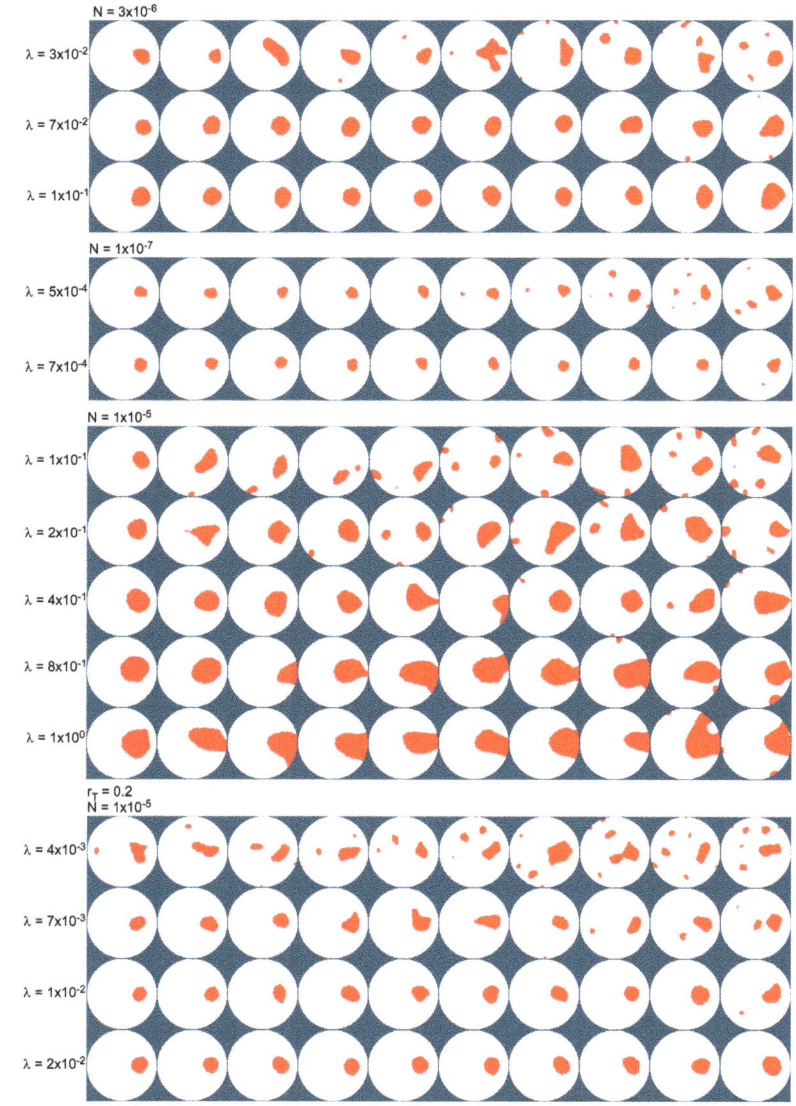

Figure G.16. EIT images corresponding to the data in figure 7.5 (first three groupings) (r_T = 0.05), plus additional images for a larger target (fourth grouping) (r_T = 0.2).

$r_T = 0.2$. At the hyperparameters used, the blur radii of the two targets were similar, but the actual hyperparameter for the larger target was smaller because of its higher SNR.

G.13 N_{th} for the three-circle target (related to section 7.1)

The noise threshold for the three-circle target of figure 6.17 is comparable to that of a one-circle target with $r_T = 0.1$ as shown in figure G.17.

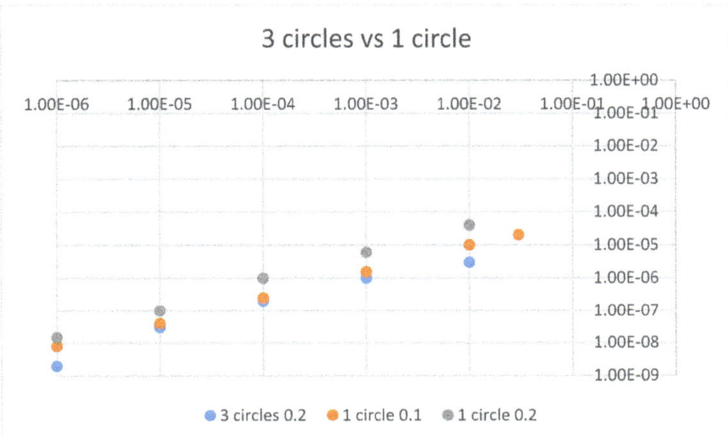

Figure G.17. Noise thresholds as a function of hyperparameter for three-circle target $r_T = 0.2$ of figure 6.17 and one-circle target of $r_T = 0.1$. (16 electrodes, I–M = 7–1, $\sigma_0 = 10^{-2}$, $\sigma_T = 0.9\sigma_0$, $I = 10^{-3}$)

G.14 N_{th} for contrasts 0.1 versus 0.4 for a 32-electrode system (related to section 7.1)

Figure G.18 shows noise thresholds at two contrasts, 0.1 and 0.4, for a triangular target at $x = 0.5$ with $r_T = 0.2$, using I–M = 15–1 (equivalent to 7–1 in a 16-electrode system).

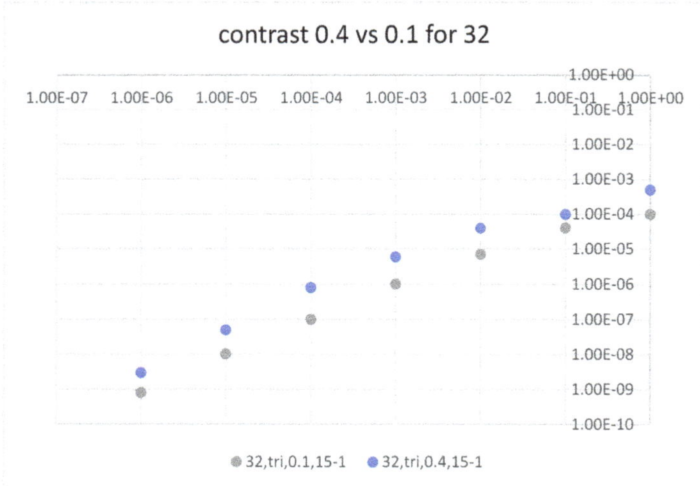

Figure G.18. Noise thresholds at two contrasts, 0.1 and 0.4, for a triangular target at $x = 0.5$. (16 electrodes, I–M = 15–1, $\sigma_0 = 10^{-2}$, $\sigma_T = 0.9\sigma_0$, $I = 10^{-3}$, $r_T = 0.2$)

G.15 Resolution and N_{th} for 7–1 and 1–1 (related to section 7.1)

The comparison of the I–M patterns at the same λ in figure 7.4(a) is not entirely 'apples to apples'. Raising λ has a greater effect on 1–1 than on 7–1. One would hence need to employ a smaller λ with 1–1 to obtain a resolution similar to that of 7–1. Cross-sections are shown in figure G.19 to demonstrate this difference in resolution. At $\lambda = 10^{-1}$ the peak for 7–1 (black) is more focused than the peak for 1–1 (red), and this is true in the absence and in the presence of the same amount of noise. Thus, while the performance of 1–1 and 7–1 are similar at small λ, at large λ 7–1 is both less susceptible to noise and less affected by the deleterious effects of regularization.

G.16 N_{th} for circular versus triangular targets (related to section 7.1)

Noise thresholds are shown in figure G.20 for triangular and circular targets at $x = 0.5$ with $r_T = 0.2$, using I–M = 7–1, $I = 1 \times 10^{-3}$, and contrast 0.4.

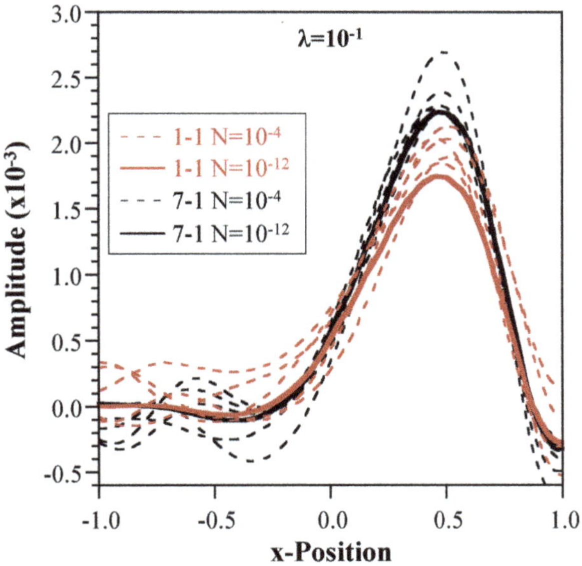

Figure G.19. Cross-sections ($y = 0$) for $\lambda = 10^{-1}$ with noise (dashed lines) and with negligible noise (solid lines) for a triangular target at $x = 0.5$. (16 electrodes, $\sigma_0 = 10^{-2}$, $\sigma_T = 0.6\sigma_0$, $I = 1 \times 10^{-3}$, $r_T = 0.2$)

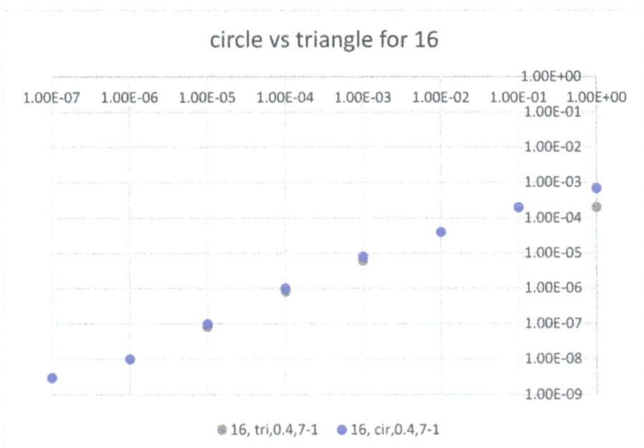

Figure G.20. Noise thresholds for triangular and circular targets at $x = 0.5$. (16 electrodes, I–M = 15–1, $\sigma_0 = 10^{-2}$, $\sigma_T = 0.6\sigma_0$, $I = 10^{-3}$, $r_T = 0.2$)

G.17 Additional targets at negligible noise, small hyperparameter (related to section 7.2)

Images with little noise and a small hyperparameter will have the finest resolution and greatest amplitude uniformity. Figure G.21 shows reconstructions of triangle and three-circle targets using $\lambda = 10^{-5}$ and noise $N = 10^{-12}$. The images are shown with the current injection pair on the horizontal axis and the measurement pair on the vertical axis, going in opposite directions for the two targets.

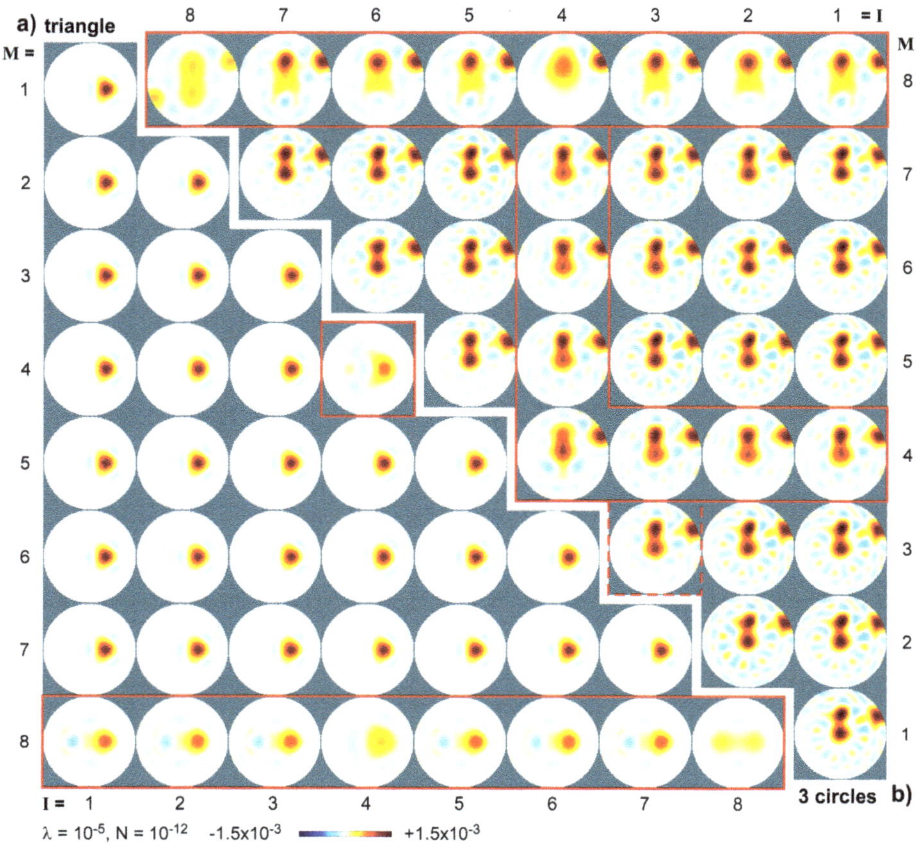

Figure G.21. EIT images obtained using different I–M patterns with targets (a) II-0.4 and (b) III-0.0. Red outlines indicate visibly poor reconstructions. (16 electrodes, $N = 10^{-12}$, $\lambda = 10^{-5}$, $r_T = 0.2$, $\sigma_0 = 10^{-2}$, $\Delta\sigma = 0.9\sigma_0$ (−10% target contrast), $I = 10^{-3}$)

The highest symmetry patterns are 4–4 and those with at least one opposite pair (8–#), as shown by the ranks in figure 7.10. In figure G.21 these patterns resulted in obviously poor reconstructions, as indicated by the red outlines. I–M = 8–8 had positive mirror image peaks, while other 8–# patterns had a negative-mirror peak, as is well known. The three-circle target shows that the 4–# patterns had a small amplitude for the circle at (0,0). A smaller number of terms used in the reconstructions results in lower quality, or even incorrect, representations of the target.

Figure G.22 shows reconstructions with five patterns for a circular target at different positions between the center and the perimeter, also using a small λ and little noise. Reconstructions from the high symmetry configurations were reasonably accurate only near the perimeter, except for 8–8, which was inaccurate everywhere. The energy going into the mirror feature is siphoned from the main feature, and the mirror feature's amplitude decreases with distance from the center, except for 8–8.

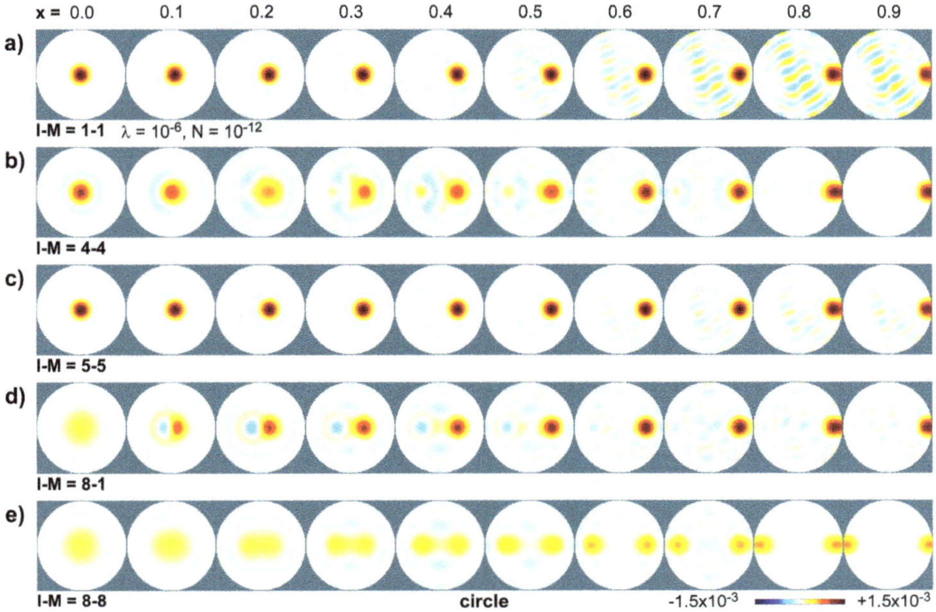

Figure G.22. EIT images of a circular target (I) at different x-positions for five I–M patterns: (a) 1–1, (b) 4–4, (c) 5–5, (d) 8–1, and (e) 8–8. (16 electrodes, $N = 10^{-12}$, $\lambda = 10^{-6}$, $r_T = 0.2$, $\sigma_0 = 10^{-2}$, $\Delta\sigma = 0.9\sigma_0$, $I = 10^{-3}$)

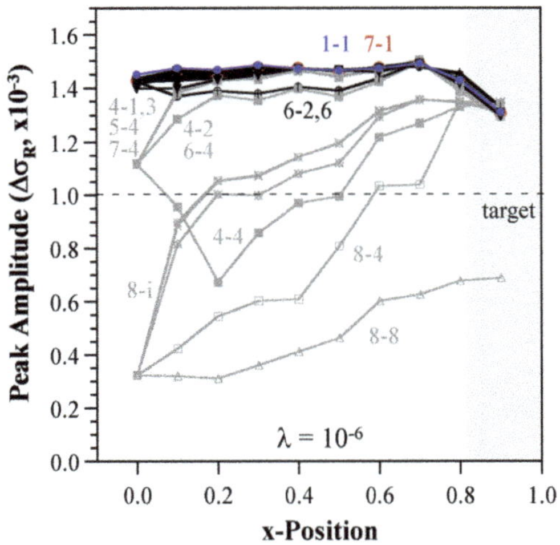

Figure G.23. Peak amplitude for a circular target (I) as a function of x-position for the 36 I–M patterns using $\lambda = 10^{-6}$. Pattern 1–1 is shown in blue, 7–1 in red, the highest symmetry configurations in gray, and the rest in black. (16 electrodes, $r_T = 0.2$, $\sigma_0 = 10^{-2}$, $\Delta\sigma = 0.9\sigma_0$, $I = 10^{-3}$, $N = 10^{-12}$)

The peak amplitudes of the circular target reconstructions are shown for all of the I–M as a function of x-position in figure G.23 for $\lambda = 10^{-6}$. The most closely studied patterns in the book are shown in blue (1–1) and red (7–1). At this small λ, every pattern with a spacing of 4 or 8 showed a diminution of the peak near the center. The other patterns were similar to each other except for 6–2 and 6–6, which had slightly lower amplitudes. In summary, since the total volume of the feature is relatively constant, the area of the feature followed as expected from the peak value. The position and shape errors were small and similar for all except the 4–4 and 8–# patterns. As indicated in figure G.22, ringing generally grew in size as the target moved beyond $x = 0.3$, increasing with distance from the center and varying considerably between I–M patterns. The greatest ringing was experienced by 1–1, 2–1, 6–1, 3–1, and 5–1, in decreasing order, and the lowest ringing was seen in 2–2, 4–2, 6–2, 6–4, and 6–6.

Based on the results of this section, it is clear that with a small hyperparameter, no configurations involving a spacing of 4 or 8 should be used in a circular 16-electrode system. By analogy, 180° and 90° orientations should also be avoided for 8- and 32-electrode systems. (By using 17 electrodes, these symmetries are broken.)

G.18 16-electrode system—resolution and volume versus I–M at $x = 0.1$ (related to section 7.2)

Figures G.24 and G.25 show the resolution and volume of a circular target at $x = 0.1$ as a function of I–M pattern number at different hyperparameters.

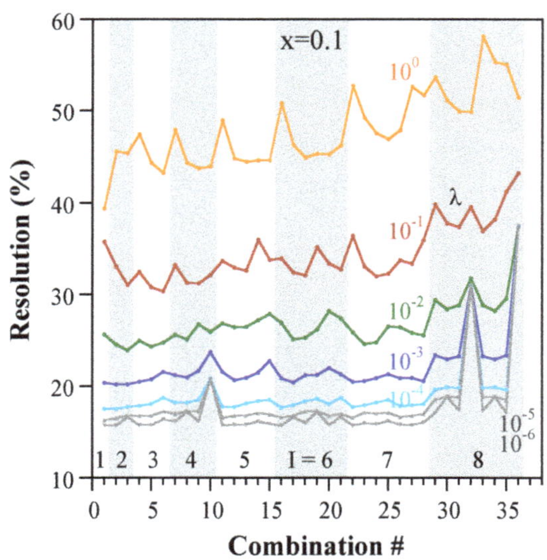

Figure G.24. Resolution for a circular target for the 36 I–M patterns at different hyperparameters. (16 electrodes, $I = 10^{-3}$, $\sigma_0 = 10^{-2}$, $\Delta\sigma = 0.9\sigma_0$, $r_T = 0.2$, $N = 10^{-12}$)

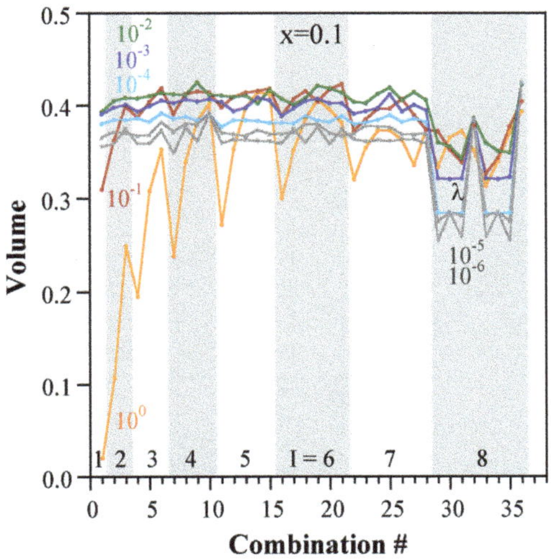

Figure G.25. Volume of circular target at $x = 0.1$ for the 36 I–M patterns at different hyperparameters. (16 electrodes, $I = 10^{-3}$, $\sigma_0 = 10^{-2}$, $\Delta\sigma = 0.9\sigma_0$, $r_T = 0.2$, $N = 10^{-12}$)

G.19 16-electrode system—amplitude and resolution at $x = 0.5$ (related to section 7.2)

Figure G.26 begins at $\lambda = 10^{-4}$, at which the metrics began to be significantly affected. The onset of the -$a$log(λ) dependence was delayed for $x = 0.5$ relative to $x = 0.1$ because a higher λ is needed to have effect at the perimeter.

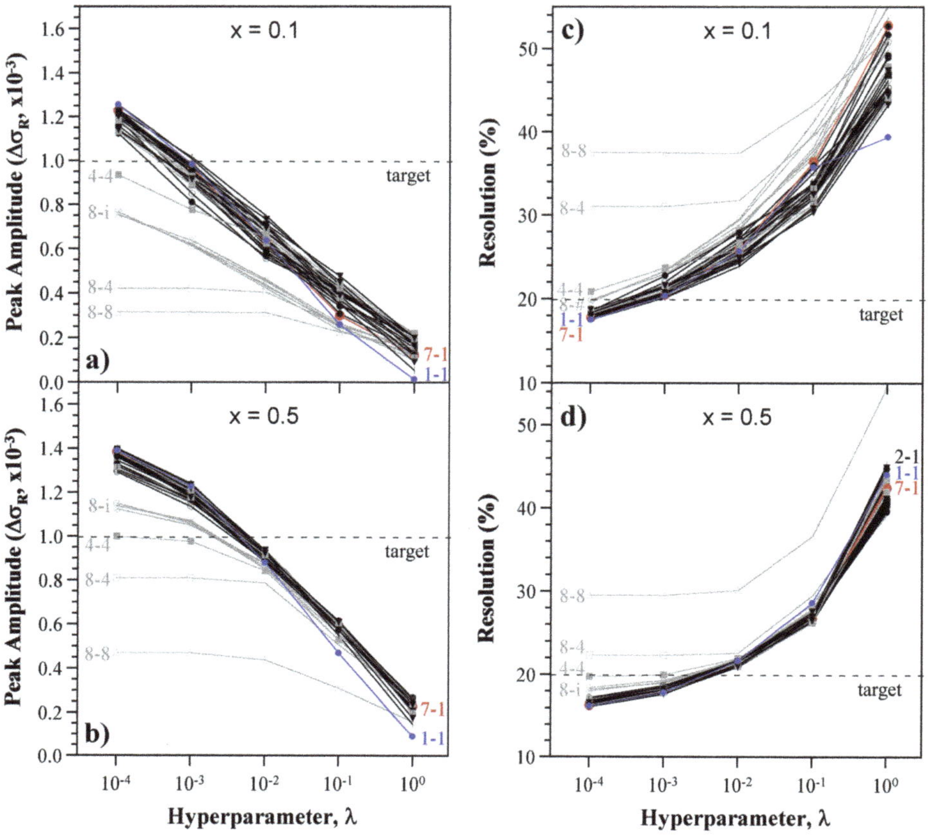

Figure G.26. (a),(b) Peak amplitude and (c), (d) resolution for a circular target for the 36 I–M patterns as a function of hyperparameter at (a), (c) $x = 0.1$ and (b), (d) $x = 0.5$. Pattern 1–1 is shown in blue, 7–1 in red, the 4–4 and 8–# configurations in gray, and the rest in black. (16 electrodes, $I = 10^{-3}$, $N = 10^{-12}$, $\sigma_0 = 10^{-2}$, $\Delta\sigma = 0.9\sigma_0$, $r_T = 0.2$)

G.20 16-electrode system—peak amplitude versus I–M, small and large targets (related to section 7.2)

Figures G.27 and G.28 show, for all the I–M patterns, the peak amplitudes of a feature at $x = 0.1$ with radii of $r_T = 0.02$ or 0.4, respectively.

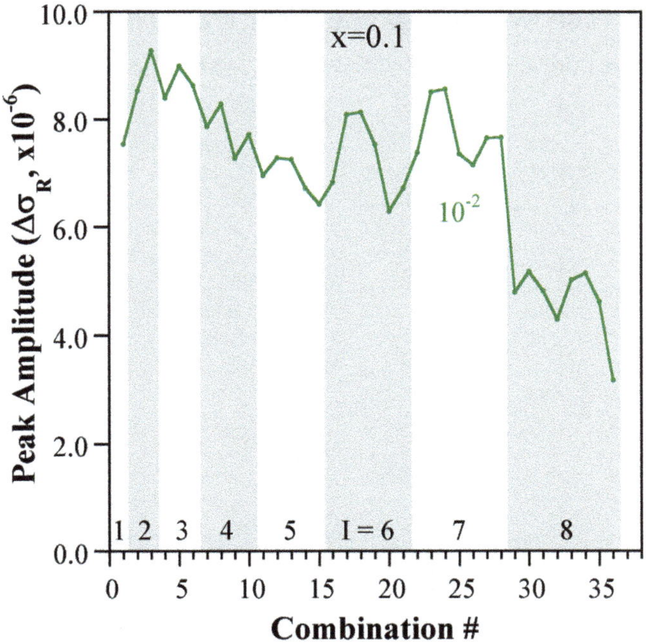

Figure G.27. Peak amplitude for a circular point target of $r_T = 0.02$ for the 36 I–M patterns at $\lambda = 10^{-2}$. (Compare figure 7.16 in the main text). (16 electrodes, $I = 10^{-3}$, $\sigma_0 = 10^{-2}$, $\Delta\sigma = 0.9\sigma_0$, $r_T = 0.02$, $N = 10^{-12}$)

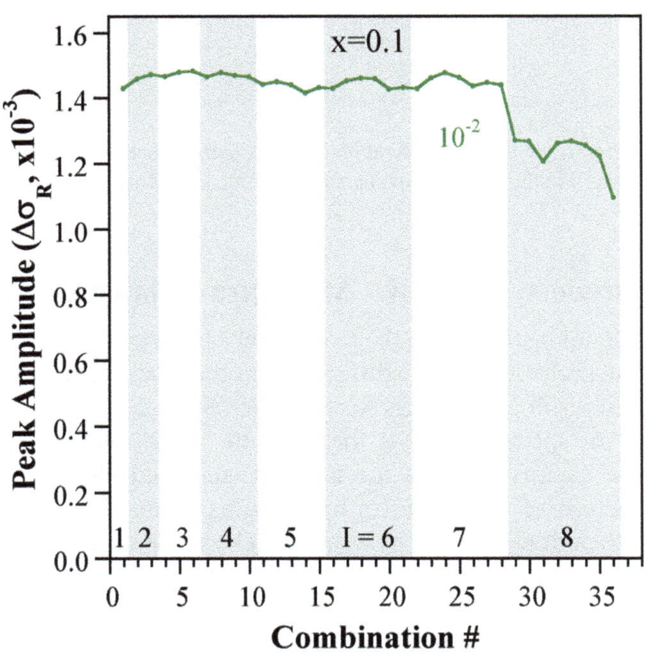

Figure G.28. Peak amplitude for a circular point target of $r_T = 0.4$ for the 36 I–M patterns at $\lambda = 10^{-2}$. (Compare figure 7.16 in the main text). (16 electrodes, $I = 10^{-3}$, $\sigma_0 = 10^{-2}$, $\Delta\sigma = 0.9\sigma_0$, $r_T = 0.02$, $N = 10^{-12}$)

G.21 16-electrode system—shape error (related to section 7.2)

Figure G.29 shows the shape errors for various I–M patterns and hyperparameters.

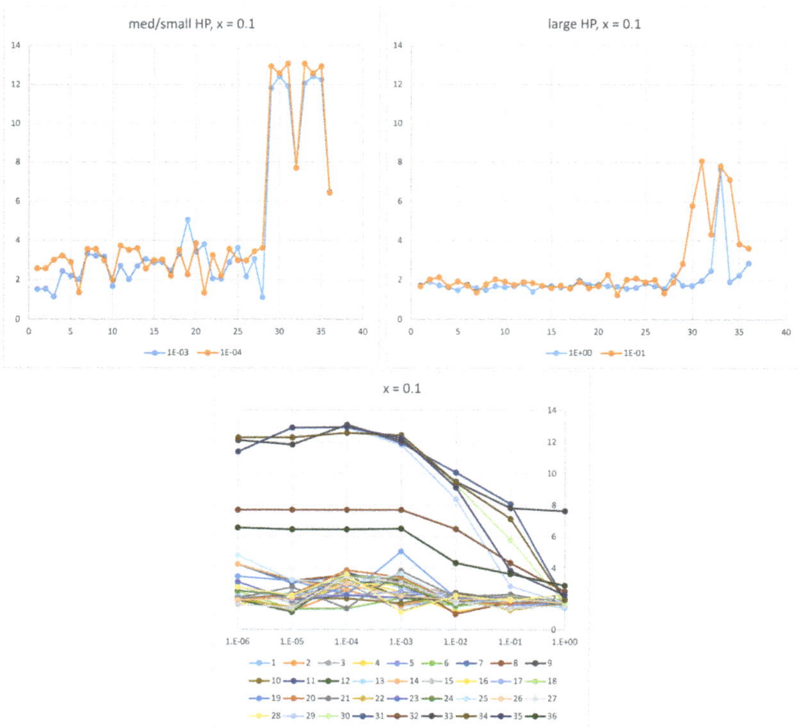

Figure G.29. Shape error at $x = 0.1$ as a function of (top) I–M pattern number for different hyperparameters and (bottom) shape error as a function of hyperparameter for all 36 I–M patterns.

G.22 16-electrode system—$|\mathbf{U}^{\mathrm{T}}\boldsymbol{\Delta}|$ spectra (related to section 7.2)

As discussed in detail in chapter 6, the noise level can be compared to $|\mathbf{U}^{\mathrm{T}}\boldsymbol{\Delta}|$ spectra [4], where $\boldsymbol{\Delta}$ is the vector of voltage differences in the measurement frame and the $\mathbf{u}_i$ in $\mathbf{U}$ are a set of orthogonal basis vectors, or 'eigen-Δs', with which $\boldsymbol{\Delta}$ can be expressed. A $|\mathbf{U}^{\mathrm{T}}\boldsymbol{\Delta}|$ spectrum shows the absolute values of the amplitudes of the coefficients in the 'expansion' of $\boldsymbol{\Delta}$ into $\mathbf{u}_i$. These so-called Picard coefficients P_i are plotted as a function of their size (rather than as a function of their index i) in figure G.30 for the circular target at $x = 0.1$. The noise amplitude can be directly compared to these coefficients: a P_i that is smaller than the noise is corrupted, necessitating the use of a larger λ to remove the corresponding corrupted eigen-image $\mathbf{v}_i$ from the final EIT image. If λ is too small, as noise increases the image first develops artefacts, or extra peaks that do not correspond to the target, and then the image breaks up completely. The largest P_i (see the inset), at the lowest sort

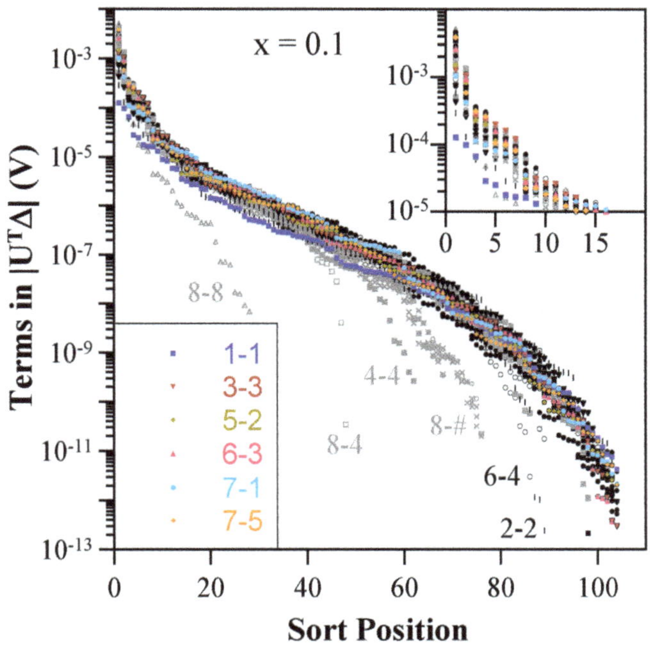

Figure G.30. The size-sorted, absolute values of the terms in $\mathbf{U}^{\mathrm{T}}\mathbf{\Delta}$ for the 36 I–M patterns for a one-circle target at $x = 0.1$. (16 electrodes, $I = 10^{-3}$, $\sigma_0 = 10^{-2}$, $\Delta\sigma = 0.9\sigma_0$, $r_{\mathrm{T}} = 0.2$, $N = 10^{-12}$)

numbers, are unaffected until noise is very high. At large λ, only the $\mathbf{v}_i$ associated with the large P_i contribute to the image, the others having been filtered out.

The number of terms shown in figure G.30 is equal to the rank of the I–M pattern; thus 4–4 and 8–# patterns are clearly identified from the small number of terms. From these curves, no candidates emerged among the I–M_{80+} that would be expected to have a markedly better performance over all noise levels. The largest several P_i for 1–1, 2–1, and 3–1 were exceptionally small, and for 7–6 the second-largest P_i was exceptionally small. Thus, they would be expected to be most susceptible to high noise, when a large λ is employed.

The small N_{th} for 1–1, 2–1, 3–1, and 7–6 at $\lambda \geqslant 10^{-1}$ in figure 7.20 were as predicted from figure G.30.

As shown in chapter 6, the best way to view these coefficients is ordered by index, since the index is related to the hyperparameter. The Picard coefficients for six of the spectra are shown in figure G.31.

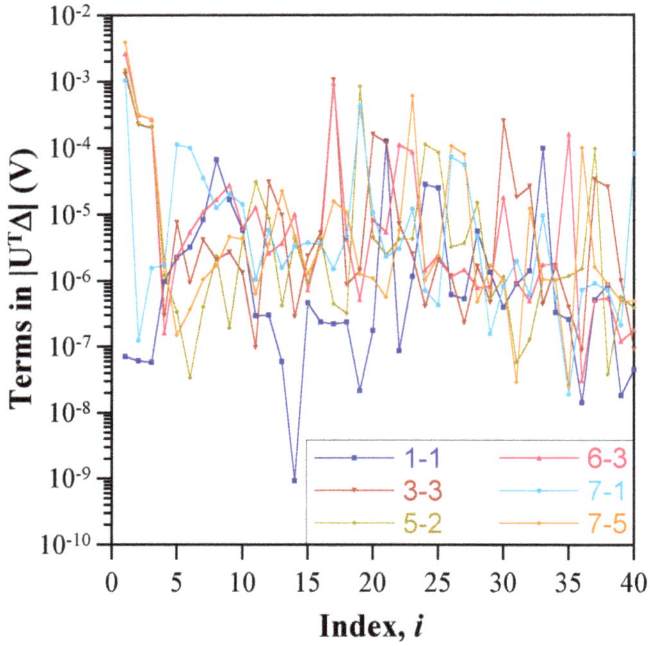

Figure G.31. The Picard coefficients P_i, or absolute values of the terms in $\mathbf{U}^T\mathbf{\Delta}$ sorted by index i, for six of the I–M patterns for a one-circle target at $x = 0.1$. (16 electrodes, $I = 10^{-3}$, $\sigma_0 = 10^{-2}$, $\Delta\sigma = 0.9\sigma_0$, $r_T = 0.2$, $N = 10^{-12}$)

G.23 13-electrode system—metrics and $|\mathbf{U}^T\mathbf{\Delta}|$, $x = 0.1$, circular target (related to section 7.2)

Additional metrics for the 13-electrode system are shown in figures G.32–G.34, along with the Picard coefficients in figure G.35. The best patterns overall were 4–2, 4–3, 5–2, 5–3, and 6–2. Figure G.32 shows that the worst patterns for conservation of feature volume ('energy') were: #–1, 2–2, 6–5. Figure G.33 shows that the worst patterns for position error were: 4–4 and 6–#, especially 6–5. Figure G.34 shows that there were no worst patterns for shape error.

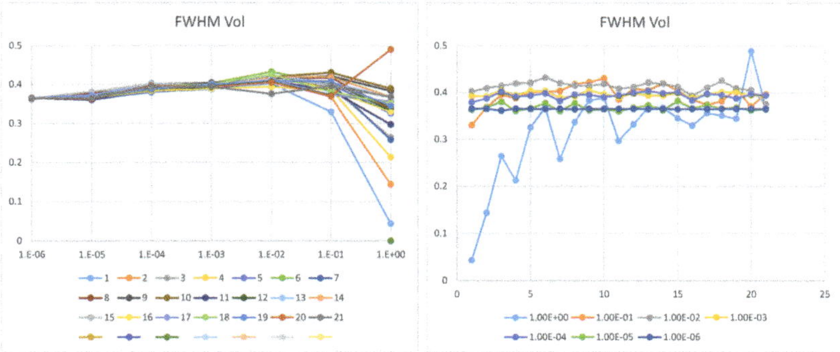

Figure G.32. Full width at half maximum volume (feature 'energy') as a function of hyperparameter for the 21 I–M patterns, and as a function of I–M pattern number at different hyperparameters.

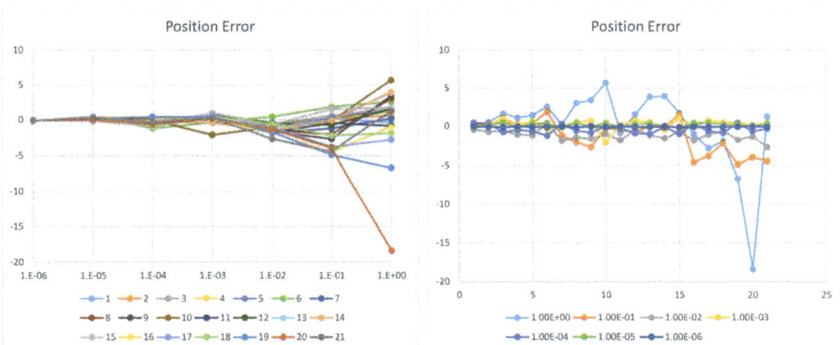

Figure G.33. Position error as a function of hyperparameter for the 21 I–M patterns, and as a function of I–M pattern number at different hyperparameters.

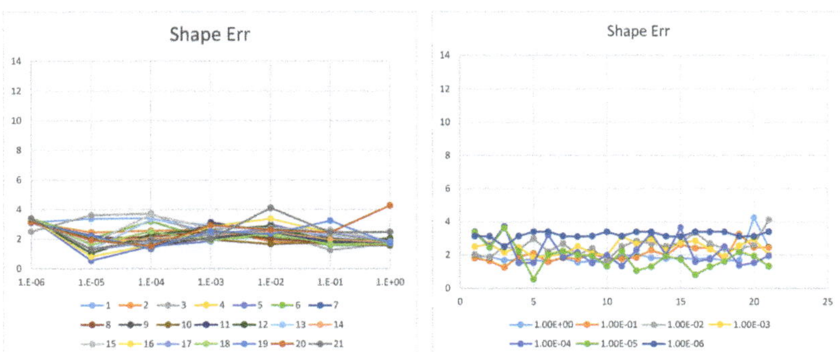

Figure G.34. Shape error as a function of hyperparameter for the 21 I–M patterns, and as a function of I–M pattern number at different hyperparameters.

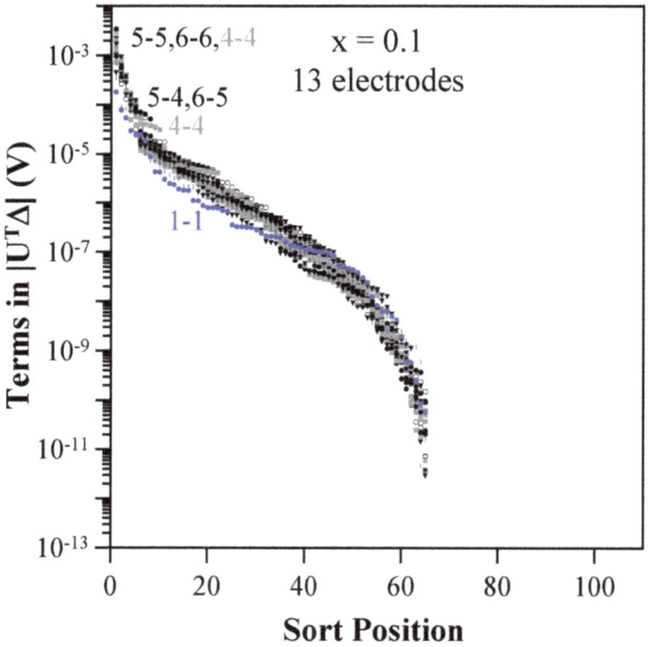

Figure G.35. The Picard coefficients P_i, or absolute values of the terms in $\mathbf{U}^T\boldsymbol{\Delta}$ as a function of sort position for six of the I–M patterns for a one-circle target at $x = 0.1$. (13 electrodes, $I = 10^{-3}$, $\sigma_0 = 10^{-2}$, $\Delta\sigma = 0.9\sigma_0$, $r_T = 0.2$, $N = 10^{-12}$.)

G.24 15-electrode system—metrics at different λ, $x = 0.1$, circular target (related to section 7.2)

The patterns with the best performance in the 15-electrode configuration were 2–2, 3–2, 4–2, 4–3, 4–4, 6–2, and 6–4.

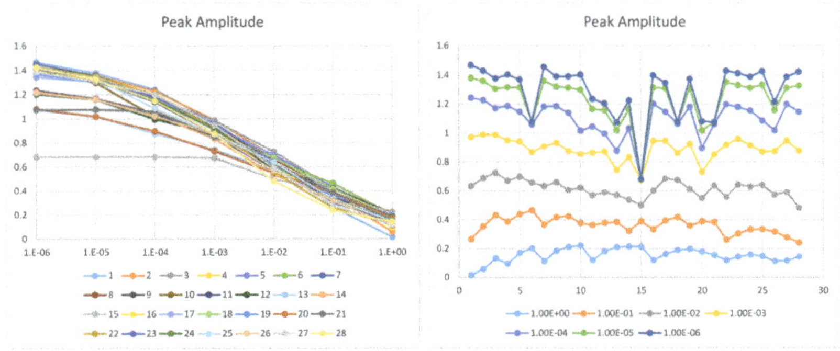

Figure G.36. Peak amplitude as a function of hyperparameter for the 28 I–M patterns, and as a function of I–M pattern number at different hyperparameters.

Figure G.36 shows that the worst patterns for peak amplitude were: 5–5, #–1, 3–3, 5–#, #–5, 6–1, 6–6, 7–#.

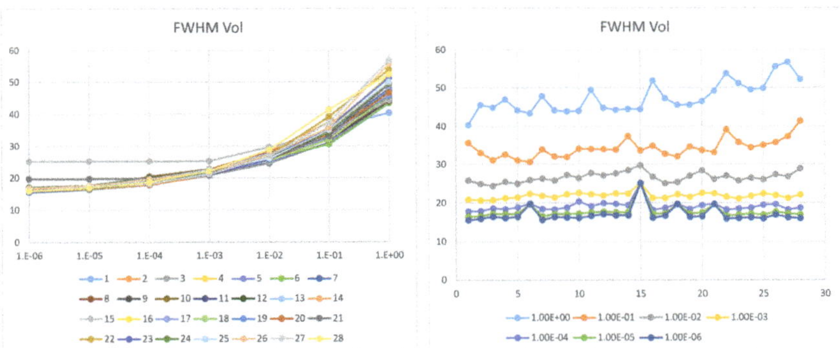

Figure G.37. Resolution as a function of hyperparameter for the 28 I–M patterns, and as a function of I–M pattern number at different hyperparameters.

Figure G.37 shows that the worst patterns for high resolution were: 5–5, #–1, 6–6, 7–5, 7–6, 7–7.

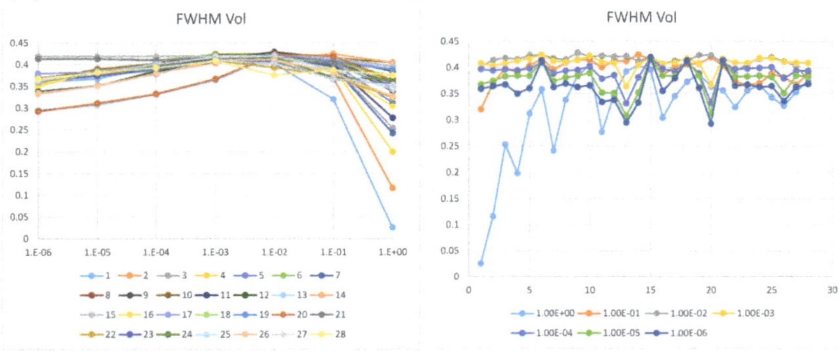

Figure G.38. Full width at half maximum volume (feature 'energy') as a function of hyperparameter for the 28 I–M patterns, and as a function of I–M pattern number at different hyperparameters.

Figure G.38 shows that the worst patterns for conservation of feature volume ('energy') were #–1, 5–3, 5–4, 6–5, 7–5 and that the best patterns for conservation of feature volume were 3–3, 5–5, 6–3, 6–6.

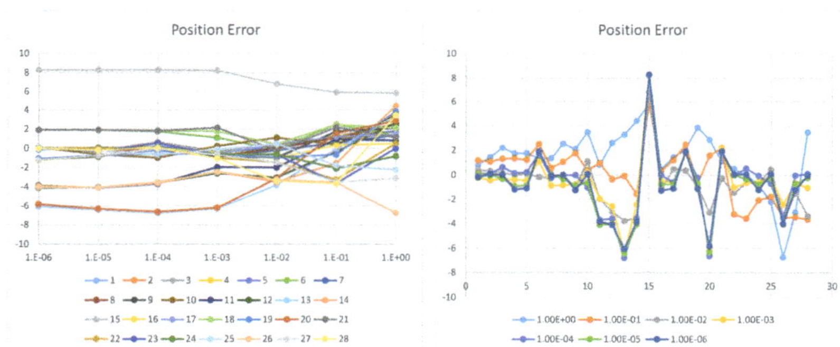

Figure G.39. Position error as a function of hyperparameter for the 28 I–M patterns, and as a function of I–M pattern number at different hyperparameters.

Figure G.39 shows that the worst patterns for position error were 5–#, 6–3, #–5, 6–6.

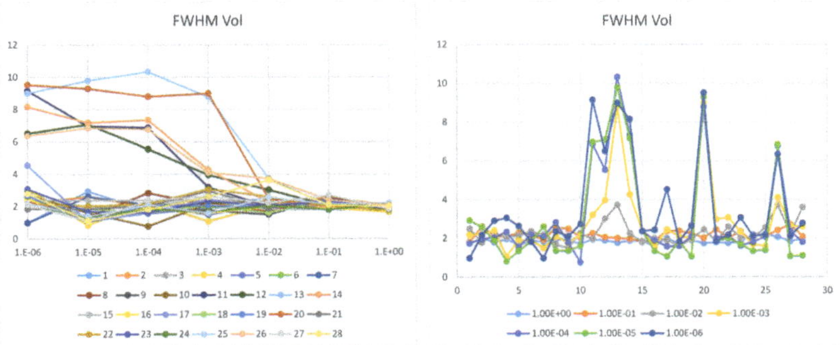

Figure G.40. Shape error as a function of hyperparameter for the 28 I–M patterns, and as a function of I–M pattern number at different hyperparameters.

Figure G.40 shows that the worst patterns for shape error were 5–# and #–5.

G.25 16-electrode system—noise susceptibility N_{th} at $x = 0.5$ (related to section 7.2)

The noise threshold N_{th} is shown at $x = 0.5$ in figure G.41 as a function of hyperparameter λ and in figure G.42 as a function of I–M pattern number. Note that both N_{th} and noise are specified in units of V.

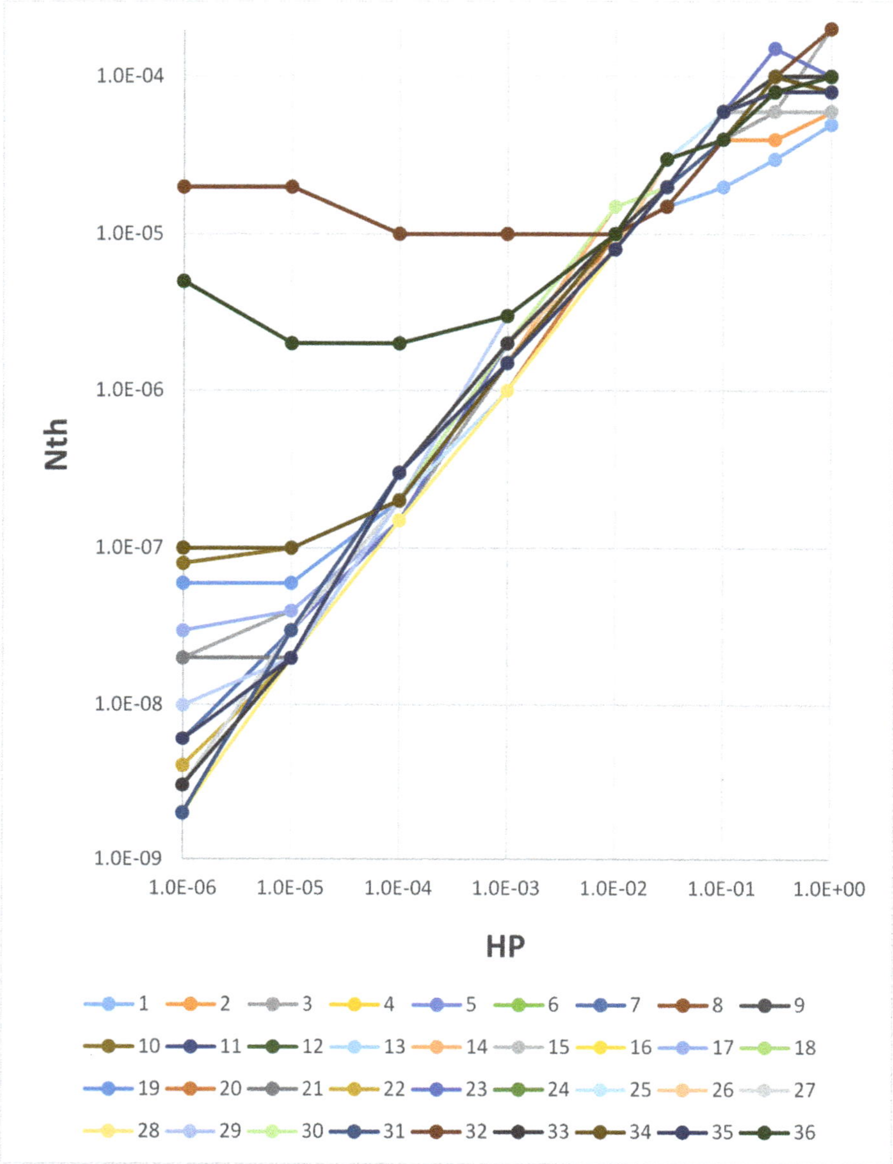

Figure G.41. Noise threshold as a function of hyperparameter for the 36 I–M patterns.

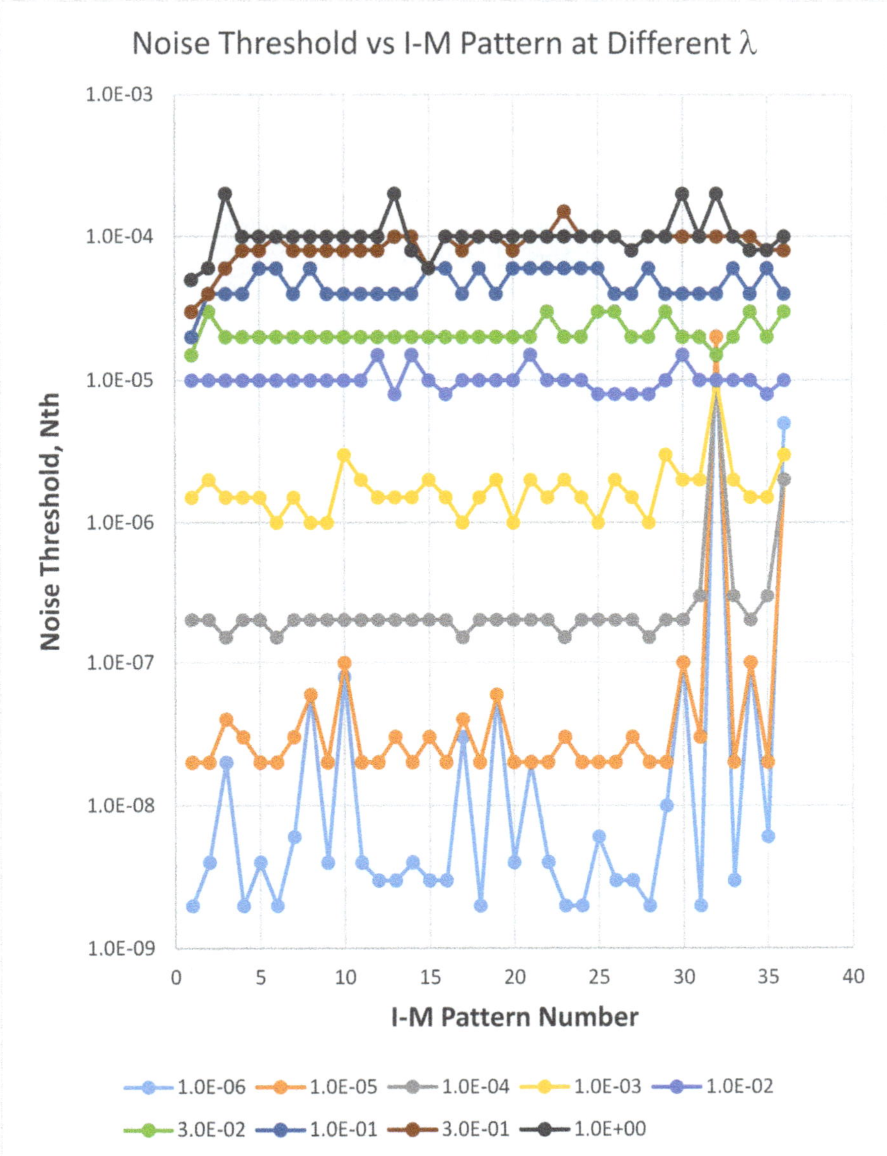

Figure G.42. Noise threshold as a function of I–M pattern number for different hyperparameters.

References

[1] Smela E 2022 EIT for tactile sensing: considering artefacts in hyperparameter selection *Eng. Res. Expr.* **4** 035057

[2] Polydorides N and McCann H 2002 Electrode configurations for improved spatial resolution in electrical impedance tomography *Meas. Sci. Technol.* **13** 1862–70

[3] Hansen P C 2010 *DIAS 006—Discrete Inverse Problems—Day 1, Slides Based on Discrete Inverse Problems: Insight and Algorithms vol 2020, Fundamentals of Algorithms* (Philadelphia, PA: Society for Industrial and Applied Mathematics (SIAM)

[4] Lionheart W, Polydorides N and Borsic A 2005 The reconstruction problem *Electrical Impedance Tomography: Methods, History and Applications, Series in Medical Physics and Biomedical Engineering* ed C G Orton, J H Nagel and J G Webster (Bristol: IOP Publishing) ch 1

www.ingramcontent.com/pod-product-compliance
Ingram Content Group UK Ltd.
Pitfield, Milton Keynes, MK11 3LW, UK
UKHW051906100926
8556IPUK00005B/787

9 780750 354004